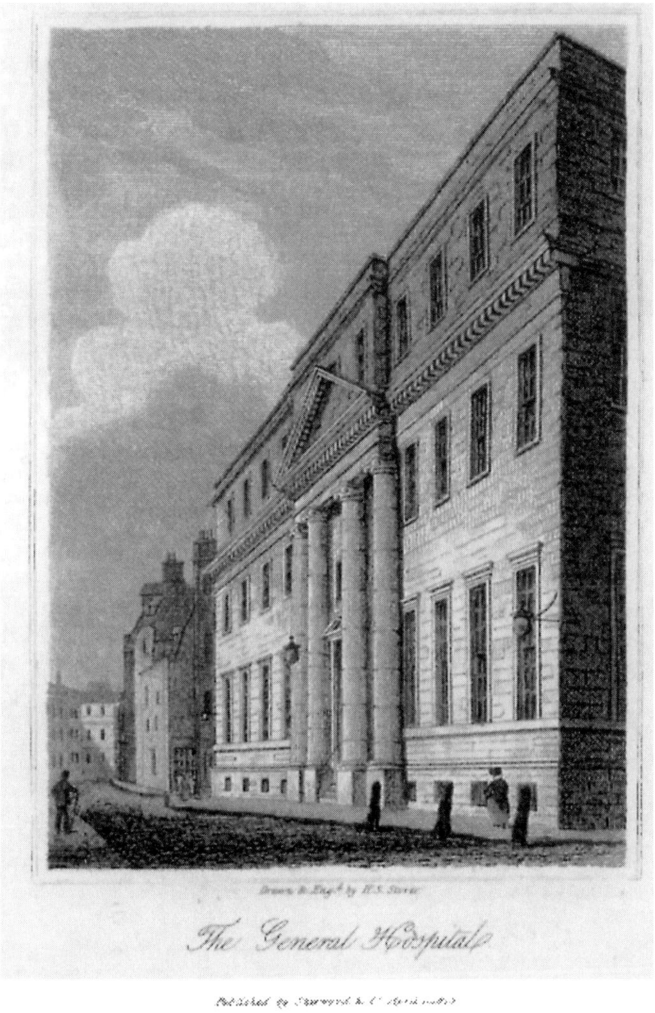

Frontispiece Bath General Hospital, 1819: engraving by H.S. Storer

Medicine and Charity in Georgian Bath

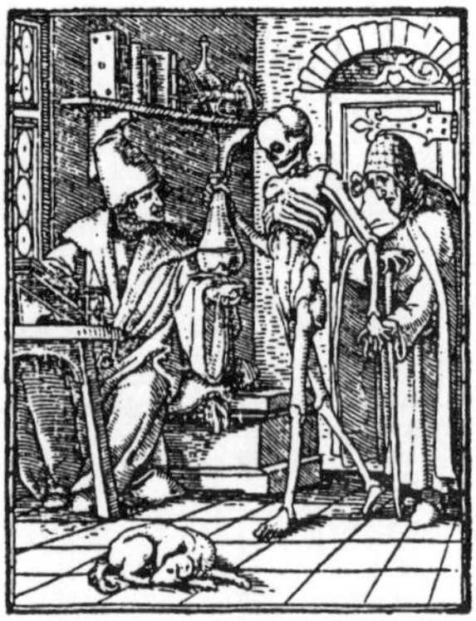

The History of Medicine in Context

Series Editors: Andrew Cunningham and Ole Peter Grell,
Department of History and Philosophy of Science,
University of Cambridge

Titles in this series include:

Medicine from the Black Death to the French Disease
edited by Roger French, Jon Arrizabalaga,
Andrew Cunningham and Luis García-Ballester

Faith, Medical Alchemy and Natural Philosophy:
Johann Moriaen, Reformed Intelligencer, and the Hartlib Circle
J. T. Young

The Making of the Dentiste, c. *1650–1760*
Roger King

'The Battle for Health': A Political History of the
Socialist Medical Association, 1930–51
John Stewart

Medicine and Charity in Georgian Bath

A Social History of the General Infirmary, *c.* 1739–1830

ANNE BORSAY

Ashgate

Aldershot • Brookfield USA • Singapore • Sydney

Published by
Ashgate Publishing Limited
Gower House
Croft Road
Aldershot
Hants GU11 3HR
England

Ashgate Publishing Company
Old Post Road
Brookfield
Vermont 05036–9704
USA

British Library Cataloguing in Publication Data

Borsay, Anne
Medicine and Charity in Georgian Bath: A Social History of the General Infirmary, *c.* 1739–1830.
(The History of Medicine in Context)
1. General Hospital, Bath—History. 2. Public health—England—Bath—History. 3. Bath (England)—Social conditions.
I. Title.
362.1'1'0942398

Library of Congress Catalog Card Number: 99–63692

ISBN 0 7546 0060 2

This book is printed on acid free paper

Typeset in Sabon by Manton Typesetters, Louth, Lincolnshire
Printed and bound in Great Britain by
MPG Books Ltd, Bodmin, Cornwall

Contents

List of Figures

List of Tables

List of Appendices

Acknowledgements

During the preparation of this book, I have been given assistance from many quarters. The University of Wales, Lampeter (formerly St David's University College) has allowed me three periods of study leave to pursue the project. I have been awarded two Small Personal Research Grants from the British Academy, one which financed my first and most substantial period of archival work in Bath and one which enabled the computerization of patient records. Subsequently, I received a Grant for Research Expenses (M/91/3759) from the Wellcome Trust which met the cost of additional research visits, and a sum from my Department's Research Fund which facilitated setting up a database.

The Royal National Hospital for Rheumatic Diseases NHS Trust (known initially as the General Hospital or Infirmary and later as the Mineral Water Hospital) has kindly granted permission to reproduce the 'Plan and Elevation' of 1738 and William Hoare's portrait of Dr Oliver and Mr Pearce examining patients. These two illustrations were included in Roger Rolls, *Hospital of the Nation: The Story of Spa Medicine and the Mineral Water Hospital at Bath* (Bath: Bird, 1988), and the author and publisher have obligingly agreed to their use here. Moreover, Clive Quinnell not only consented to the reproduction of his photographs from this volume, but has also generously supplied new prints from the negatives. In addition, I am grateful to the copyright holders for permission to reproduce extracts from my articles previously published in *Archives*, 21 (1994), pp. 172–82; *Disability and Society*, 13 (1998), pp. 645–63; *Medical History*, 35 (1991), pp. 281–94; *Social History*, 24 (1999), pp. 269–86; and *Social History of Medicine*, 4 (1991), pp. 207–29.

A study of this sort is heavily dependent upon the efforts of others. Therefore, I am indebted to the authors whose work I have used, to Trevor Fawcett for making available his encyclopaedic knowledge of eighteenth-century Bath, to the audiences at conferences and seminars who have commented on papers derived from aspects of this book, and to those who have commented on earlier versions of the full text, notably Dorothy Porter, Tim Hitchcock, William Price and the publisher's anonymous referees. Thanks are also due to Colin Johnston at Bath City Record Office, to the staff of the Bath Central Library, the Somerset County Record Office and the British Library in London, and to the personnel of the Royal National Hospital for Rheumatic Diseases for the hospitality that I was shown whilst consulting the archive. At Lampeter, I have enjoyed excellent library and computing services.

Kathy Miles willingly fielded numerous requests for Inter-Library Loans, and Alan Rogers demonstrated skill and patience in developing a computer program for my more awkward data. Ceinwen Jones, Gromette Walker, Mark Merrony and Neil Caddick helped with data processing, and Joan Williams word-processed sections of the text with admirable accuracy. I am also grateful to my colleagues in the Department of History for providing a congenial working environment, and to the Series Editors, Andrew Cunningham and Ole Peter Grell, and Caroline Cornish and the editorial staff at Ashgate, for their efficient but careful handling of the final manuscript. However, my biggest debt is to Peter Borsay. Without his intellectual and emotional support and his willingness to shoulder equal responsibility for the care of two young children, it is doubtful whether this book would have ever been completed.

PART ONE
Introduction

In memory of my grandparents

Albert Grimes (1902–85)
Hilda Grimes (1901–82)

Sidney Howard (1891–1955)
Alice Howard (1896–1992)

CHAPTER ONE

Britain in the Long Eighteenth Century

In January 1740, the governors of the newly founded General Hospital or Infirmary at Bath commissioned Vincent Mattyssens to carve a sculpture of the Good Samaritan for the tympanum of the building then under construction. Despite being paid fees of 30 guineas, Mr Mattyssens produced no more than drawings and a model;[1] and the Hospital had to wait for more than a century before a nineteenth-century artist, 'obviously influenced by Mattyssen's studies', completed his version of the parable for the west wing added in the early 1860s.[2] Yet though lacking a visual emblem of good works, the Georgian Bath Infirmary exuded the virtues of altruism. Even without any improvement in 'the knowledge and the use of the Bath waters' ran a 'Plan and Elevation', published to raise funds in 1738, 'the relief of our miserable fellow creatures ... [was] sufficient to induce all good-natured persons to promote this Charity'.[3] A letter for insertion in the press was still more effusive. The trustees 'judged proper to advertise [their scheme to] the public, that persons of a benevolent disposition and easy fortunes may be acquainted with the glorious opportunity they now have of assisting, and relieving their distressed fellow-creatures, by becoming liberal benefactors to this good work'.[4] Disinterested giving was similarly exhorted by clerics like Robert Leyborne, preaching on behalf of the Infirmary in 1754:

> Do those in high stations not always mind high things, but condescend sometimes ... to men of low estate, to be strength to the weak, and feet to the lame, and for the stript, and wounded, and half-dead, to provide both medicines and an house, saying, like the Good Samaritan to the host, Take care of him; and what thou spendest, when I come I will repay?[5]

This celebration of altruism was not confined to publicity strategies sponsored by the Hospital itself. The *London Evening Post*, describing the ceremony for laying the foundation-stone in July 1738, also reported how 'all demonstrations of joy possible [were] shewn on this occasion, every one appearing pleased with a design so excellently well calculated for the good of mankind in general, and the welfare and the happiness of the poor, wretched, and miserable in particular'.[6]

The historiography of the Georgian voluntary hospital

Throughout the long eighteenth century, the commitment of the General Infirmary to the ideal of the Good Samaritan was shared by other voluntary hospitals.[7] Bath was the fifth provincial foundation in a movement which between 1720 and 1800 acquired over 30 members in England and a further five north of the border.[8] The historiography of these institutions can be traced back to the empiricism of the Victorian age. One strand was demographic. Infirmaries – accused of calamitous mortality rates by Florence Nightingale and other nineteenth-century critics – were during the 1920s accredited with aiding population growth, only to be castigated 30 years on for being dens of death.[9] The second strand in hospital historiography was administrative. Less controversial than the demographic debate, this viewpoint concentrated on the collection of facts and figures, telling tales of endeavour which often lauded doctors, governors and the humanitarian values that their institutions represented.[10] This genre of medical history continues.[11] Yet though 'the public good' undoubtedly prompted donations which repaid their donors with the warm glow of giving,[12] voluntary infirmaries were also arenas for the acting out of ulterior motives. This was appreciated by more cynical contemporaries when they penetrated beneath the charitable veneer. 'Pride and vanity', quipped Bernard Mandeville, 'have built more hospitals than all the virtues together.'[13]

The explosion of the social sciences from the 1960s, together with persistent deficiences in the health care of the welfare state, encouraged a sceptical disposition towards medicine which affected historical as well as contemporary research. Therefore, the past 30 years have witnessed the development of a *social* history of medicine, free of the shackles of hagiography and wedded to 'social constructionist' perspectives which place medical 'ideas and practices' within their societal contexts.[14] There were prodromal signs in *The Hospitals* by Brian Abel-Smith: a piece of administrative history, published in 1964, which nevertheless noted the necessity of 'a fairly wide social and economic background'.[15] A decade later, John Woodward prefaced his assessment of health, mortality and the voluntary hospital with a substantial review of the economic and social benefits of philanthropy, while in the mid-1980s Guenter Risse's exposition of medical care and teaching at the Edinburgh Infirmary during the Scottish Enlightenment began with a comment on medical charity and the sick poor.[16] More recently, the historiography of the Georgian voluntary hospital has been advanced by two excellent monographs on the theme of medical authority: Susan Lawrence's study of how the growth of clinical training in London fragmented the traditional division of labour between physicians, surgeons and apothecaries, and Mary Fissell's account of how institutional routines marginalized popular remedies by linking them to superstition and political agitation.[17] Whereas the principal focus of these works was medical practice, Roy Porter – in a seminal essay on 'The Gift Relation' – used a wider aperture to include the 'reciprocity of giving and receiving' enacted through the voluntary hospital.[18] This interface was put under detailed empirical scrutiny in Amanda Berry's thesis on 'Patronage, Funding and the Hospital Patient, c.1750–1815': a comparison of the Bristol, Northampton, and Devon and Exeter Infirmaries. As the author says in her introduction, 'An attempt is made ... to broaden the scope of the discussion away from the narrow focus on hospital history to incorporate details of contemporary demographic, social and economic change and to place the hospitals in the broader context of late-eighteenth and early-nineteenth-century society'.[19] In this investigation of medical charity at the Bath Infirmary, the Georgian context is the starting-point, the hospital being envisaged as 'an organ of society', only comprehensible if related to 'political and economic conditions, social structure, value systems, [and] cultural organization'.[20]

National society: commerce and the Enlightenment

The commitment to contextualize the General Infirmary calls for a historiographical interpretation of both national society and local Bath society. For the revisionist historian, J.C.D. Clark, Georgian Britain was an *ancien régime* much akin to the absolutist states of continental Europe.[21] Rejecting the progressive orthodoxies propagated by the Whig and Marxist schools, Clark has argued that 'English society between the Restoration and the Reform Bill may be best understood as a mutually reinforcing system of three main components: monarchy, patrician élite [and] clerical intelligensia'.[22] Such a static, paternalist model has room for neither a commercial economy nor a secular Enlightenment, yet both are vital to our comprehension of Georgian society. The origins of the commercial economy lay in the unprecedented prosperity generated by agricultural improvement, industrialization and foreign trade in the second half of the seventeenth century. The international dimension was most telling. Not only did the volume of trade increase by more than a third in the 40 years after 1660, but its direction also changed so that by 1700 the profitable re-export of goods from the Plantations had dislodged Dutch imports to Europe.[23] After 1689, this mercantile expansion became spliced to a Financial Revolution which saw the ascent of the joint-stock company and the development of a system of public credit based on the Bank of England, and the South Sea and East India

Companies.[24] As Paul Langford has observed, attempts by economic historians to measure the growth unleashed by this trade and commerce 'necessarily employ crude and unreliable estimates to arrive at disarmingly precise conclusions'. Nevertheless, they do indicate an increase in real national output of just under 2 per cent per annum by the first three decades of the nineteenth century.[25] This prosperity was moreover redistributed. Though rental incomes, largely stationary since the mid-seventeenth century, were undermined by the agricultural depression of the 1730s and 1740s, they took off from mid-century. Members of the aristocracy and gentry also seized opportunities to profit from mineral exploitation and urban growth. Above all, the new wealth began to filter down beyond this traditional élite to the middling ranks of society. Price rises from the 1760s, and the imposition of additional taxes, provoked howls of protest from both the landed and the middle orders. In practice, however, they were affordable burdens.[26]

The surplus income produced and allocated by the commercial economy was directed towards projects inspired by the Enlightenment, among them medical philanthropy. Even those who view the Georgian period as an 'aristocratic century' concede that the ideas of the Enlightenment had a 'slow but relentless impact'.[27] That they are missing from Clark's *ancien régime* is unsurprising since the unifying thread of Enlightenment – multi-faceted and regionally diverse – was a commitment to critique the old order. Confidence in the prospects for a better future abounded. Man was to be released from ignorance, superstition and clerical control. And wealth was to be created, law and government reformed, religious toleration and intellectual freedom permitted, and individuality nurtured. The means to this more liberal and humane world were knowledge and education. The Enlightenment privileged experience and experiment over the *a priori* reasoning which had underpinned the classical Renaissance and the Protestant Reformation; and with humanity no longer condemned by original sin, a science of man ripened to inform strategies for personal and social improvement.[28] This intellectual mind-set was differential in its impact. A preoccupation with the early eighteenth-century philosophers has led historians to neglect such thinking outside France.[29] But England in the later seventeenth century was home to the Scientific Revolution, to religious pluralism and to a constitutional monarchy. Therefore, Enlightenment came early. With the *ancien régime* after 1688 in retreat if not defeated, the mission was not to denounce the old ways but to construct a cohesive modern society in which disruptive economic and social, political and religious changes were mediated.[30] From the 1760s, the precepts of the 'Age of Reason' were themselves increasingly refined by political radicalism and the French Revolution, Romanticism and the

Evangelical Revival; and as the process of industrialization gained momentum, the values of the Enlightenment were transmuted into the *laissez-faire* and utilitarian ideologies which became the leitmotiv of early Victorian Britain.[31] It follows that Clark's ferocious anti-modernism is unconvincing. For though the Georgian élite may have avoided parliamentary reform until 1832, the commercial economy set in motion fundamental social, political and moral transitions which were negotiated with the help of an Enlightenment agenda.

Local society: Georgian Bath in transition

Urbanization supplied important locations for the transaction of these changes, trends in national society interacting with the local context. Bath was a premier site.[32] In 1700 under 3 000 people occupied the town. By 1760, the population had climbed to 10 000. It more than trebled again to reach 33 000 in 1801 and during the next 30 years there was a further increase of 50 per cent.[33] In his trenchant study of the city as *A Valley of Pleasure, yet a Sink of Iniquity*, R.S. Neale was adamant that 'while Bath was invented as a pre-industrial leisure city its growth was also bound up with the industrial transformation of England from the second half of the eighteenth century'.[34] Commentators have conveniently forgotten the manufacturing on the geographical periphery and spuriously claimed that Bath was not a place of commerce.[35] None the less, the phenomenal demographic expansion was triggered by the spa and its associated service industries rather than by the industrialization which drove urban centres of comparable size. Bathing in the hot springs – which had drawn visitors since Roman times – was of little economic significance to medieval Bath: a small West Country ecclesiastical, market and textile town. However, the regional woollen cloth industry went into decline from the late sixteenth century and the spa began to play a modest compensatory role. By the 1680s, Celia Fiennes was observing that 'the town and all its accommodations is adapted to the bathing and drinking of the waters, and to nothing else'.[36] Consequently, Bath did not take advantage of the revival of the textile industry from which its hinterland benefited after the Restoration. Already, it had become a dedicated watering-place.[37]

Although the spa purveyed a combination of medicine and amusement, the real pull was exerted by visitors from fashionable society, known as the Company. Bath, wrote Daniel Defoe in the 1720s, 'is the resort of the sound, rather than the sick; the bathing is made more a sport and diversion, than a physical prescription for health; and the town is taken up in raffling, gaming, visiting, and in a word, all sorts of gallantry and levity.'[38] The patronage of the future Queen Anne had helped the city to consolidate its exclusive reputation but, from the beginning of the eighteenth century, a programme of enhancement commenced. Social intercourse was regulated through the introduction of rules and routines.[39] There was also substantial investment in visitor amenities. The Corporation, which on medical advice built a Pump Room in 1706, continued to maintain and upgrade roads, streets and public walks, and when the growing town yielded higher rental incomes, more ambitious civic schemes were embarked upon, notably the Guildhall complex completed in 1777 and the grandiose new Pump Room opened in 1795. However, private enterprise was responsible for the majority of initiatives from the first assembly rooms of 1708 to lodgings, hotels and houses, proprietary chapels, coffee shops, bookshops, circulating libraries, theatres, pleasure gardens and horse-racing.[40] This splendid array of facilities enabled Bath to flourish in the face of stiffening competition.[41] So too did its cultivation of the non-summer business, with a spring season running from late February to early June and an autumn season running from late September to mid-December.[42] The estimated number of visitors rose accordingly, from an annual figure of 8 000 in the early eighteenth century to 10 000 in 1766 and no fewer than 25 000 in 1791.[43] Yet, paradoxically, this success was also Bath's downfall. With so many arrivals, the city was no longer a select enclave for the aristocracy, gentry and wealthy bourgeoisie who up to mid-century had been the keynote patrons. Instead, it became a destination for the middling sort who not only holidayed but increasingly settled as permanent residents. The Napoleonic Wars granted a temporary reprieve. But with the continental spas once more open to British travellers after 1815, Bath gradually sank into sedate and respectable repose, religiosity replacing the fame for fun and elegance.[44]

The General Hospital or Infirmary

The aim of *Medicine and Charity in Georgian Bath* is to write the social history of a medical charity which is firmly rooted in both the national context and the local community. In some respects, the General Hospital is a curious choice for this exercise because it has unique characteristics which distinguish it from other voluntary hospitals. These institutions were typically managed by governors picked from among the annual subscribers and casual benefactors who were also granted patient nomination rights in return for their donations.[45] At Bath, on the other hand, only contributors of at least £40 automatically joined the governing body, access to which was by election for subscribers and donors who had not fulfilled the financial requirement.[46] The General Infirmary was also distinctive in being established to give 'poor cripples and other indigent strangers' access to the spa waters:[47] a brief which led to the exclusion of town residents and the admission of patients by medical recommendation instead of lay patronage.[48] Reflective of the Hospital's intersection with the spa, however, these departures from the norm make it an ideal case study.

There are two reasons. First, balneology pointed up broader changes in medicine. Though water was integral to the Hippocratic tradition, bathing during the Middle Ages was recreational rather than therapeutic. The 'moral rigorism' of the Reformation and the Counter Reformation encouraged more serious, medical usage, and from the 1750s inland spas were joined by seaside resorts as venues for the consumption of water cures.[49] Balneology was invested with scientific credibility through the chemical analysis of mineral content. Furthermore, the treatment programme embraced pharmacology and minor surgical techniques as well as drinking, pumping and bathing. Nineteenth-century hydrotherapy abandoned the peripherals on the grounds that they impeded the natural expulsion of body pollutants, and prescribed only a grim regime of pure cold water baths and bandages allied to an austere diet.[50] Even by 1800, however, the holism which this theory shared with gentler eighteenth-century balneology was moving to the margins of mainstream medicine as doctors increasingly viewed the human frame in terms of its constituent parts. The second justification for using the General Infirmary is Bath's position as a stylish resort. Each year a large proportion of the nation's élites took part in the Season, making the city a microcosm of their world. Consequently, the attitudes and activities of residents and visitors throw into sharp relief major themes in the historiography of the long eighteenth century and the dynamics of fashionable philanthropy: the adaptation of classical notions of civic virtue to the organization of charity and the ethics of giving; the interplay between paternalism, *laissez-faire* and the Evangelical Revival; the defusion of political and religious conflict through sociability, symbolism and the ordering of the poor; the professionalization of medicine and the rise of the middling sort.

The Bath General Infirmary is blessed with a rich archive with which to trawl this Georgian past, comprising printed Acts of Parliament and *Annual Reports*, and Minute Books and financial records, rules and correspondence, an Admissions Register and a Casebook in manuscript. Additional primary material of relevance includes medical texts, charity sermons and reports, local newspapers, Poor Law records, and the Minute Books of the Bath Corporation and the Bath United Hospital. These sources have been consulted to varying degrees by previous historians of the General Infirmary. In his contemporary *Description of Bath*, first published in 1742, the locally born architect, John Wood, included a substantial but idiosyncratic section on the initial development of the institution which contained the only account of its protracted origins before the archive starts in 1738.[51] Later guides often repeated this material.[52] Dr Randle Wilbraham Falconer also relied on Wood when preparing the first 'proper' history of the Hospital in 1860, but he went on to quote heavily from a range of sources in a chronicle which italicized personalities: the instigators of the scheme, physicians and surgeons, benefactors and governors.[53] P.V. Turner's *Brief History* of 1921[54] was in a different vein. Prompted by a shortage of money brought about by the 'new surgical science' and experienced across the voluntary hospital movement during and after the First World War,[55] it adopted a thematic layout. There were sections on the early days, the buildings and arrangements for bathing, management structures, special events and the treatment of soldiers. This last patriotic subject then provided the pretext for two muffled pleas for research funds from the medical staff.

The professional reputation of the Hospital was likewise paramount for George Kersley and John Cosh. Published in 1965 and reprinted in 1980, their pamphlet was in the progressive mould. Having made a ritual bow to the eighteenth-century legacy, discussion moved to 'Improvements and Extensions' between 1742 when the wards opened and 1862 when a new wing was completed. The century to 1962 was described as 'A Period of Increasing Work' which culminated in the successful rebuilding programme which the history marked, and the concluding catalogue of clinical achievements reaffirmed the ethos of betterment. Old and new were compatible, even in an era renowned for its technology. Therefore, despite 'the beautiful Georgian exterior', the Hospital housed 'modern equipment for the treatment of all types of rheumatic disease, for postgraduate teaching and for postgraduate research'.[56] The most recent history of the Bath Infirmary is *The Hospital of the Nation* by Roger Rolls, with fine illustrations from Clive Quinnell. Covering the first 250 years to 1988, this volume is sub-titled *The Story of Spa Medicine* and five of its nine chapters deal with medical matters: the nosology of eighteenth-century ailments, developments in rheumatology, physiotherapy and pharmacology, and the evolution of the spa doctor. The first four chapters do examine the origins of the institution, its architecture and construction, finance and administration, and life on the wards for nurses and patients. Given the chronological span, however, the picture is inevitably painted with bold but broad brush strokes.[57]

Structure of the book

Medicine and Charity in Georgian Bath offers a close and systematic analysis of the General Infirmary to 1830 which applies recent developments in the social history of medicine to the philanthropic as well as the clinical aspects of the voluntary hospital. The organizing principle is not a particular problem in the history of medicine or charity. Nor is a biography constructed, narrating the twists and turns of institutional life. Rather, the book arises from the conviction that the Georgian medical institution – like other health and welfare services past and present – evolved as an integral part of its host society, national and local. Central to the environment of eighteenth-century Britain was economic prosperity and the endorsement of an Enlightenment agenda. Therefore, the General Hospital is analysed thematically in terms of the commercial, professional, moral, social and political relationships which grew out of this new context. Each chapter presents a historiographical setting for its construction of the primary sources. The Infirmary's records document copiously the minutiae of finance and administration, and its medical and ethical dimensions are accessible via printed tracts and sermons. The evidence relating to social and political roles is more piecemeal, but the *Annual Reports* normally list governors and the Minute Books normally indicate those who attended hospital meetings. Therefore, biographical tools are used to recover occupation and political background, and profiles are compiled for cohorts of governors throughout the long eighteenth century in order to explore their socio-economic status and their affiliation to faction or party. Particular attention is paid to the employment categories of the men who administered the Hospital, on the grounds that time was a more stringent test of charitable commitment than money and its donors more pivotal to the operation of the institution.

The aspiration to view the Bath Infirmary in societal context shapes the content and structure of the book. Chapters 2 and 3 address the commercial economy and tease out how the concept of civic virtue was used in the management of the Hospital, both to alleviate fears of corruption and to achieve financial solvency in an era when gifts were erratic and inflation rampant. Chapters 4 and 5 are concerned with medical practitioners. Balancing the limitations imposed upon the autonomy of physicians and surgeons against the economic, socio-cultural and clinical rewards for honorary service, it is suggested that the institutional endorsement of spa therapy furthered the professionalization of medicine in Bath and hence the position of local doctors. In Chapters 6 and 7, attention turns to the moral economy of medicine. The diminishing currency of the paternalist ideal espoused by the landed classes, and the substitution of this tributary relationship between rich and poor with a proprietary bond based on market relations, is linked to the Evangelical belief in the retrievability of sinful man and the rationalist belief in the improving qualities of *laissez-faire* economics and Benthamite utilitarianism.

All these ideas, maturing within the middling sort from the late eighteenth century, had their genesis in the Enlightenment search for order and control. Integration is also the preoccupation of the next three chapters on the social and political ramifications of the Hospital. Chapter 8 tackles social status: the public statement of benevolence that was moral tender for all supporters; the financial and administrative contributions made by different economic and social groups; and the opportunities afforded by an Enlightenment project for middling men to encounter the patrician presence, satisfy their social ambitions and join a broader social élite. The resolution of religious and party conflict was no less pressing. Chapter 9 deduces from their biographical profiles that governors were recruited from Whigs and Tories, Anglicans and Dissenters. But if the Infirmary signified that the enlarged social élite was capable of unity, the restricted entry to its governing body led to an exclusive oligarchy rather than an open democracy which seriously challenged the existing structures of power. The consolidation of traditional authority extended to the education of the lower orders discussed in Chapter 10. Committed to the Enlightenment programme of physical and moral rehabilitation, the governors strove for a disciplined environment. Its patients were in the main willing collaborators. Irrespective of the gaps in supervision, therefore, the Hospital stood as an icon of order, symbolizing the enduring subservience of the poor in a changing society.

Running throughout this synopsis of *Medicine and Charity in Georgian Bath* have been the dual influences of the economy and the Enlightenment, and their roles in shaping a prosperous and civilized middling sort whose values were increasingly grafted on to the political agenda despite the unreformed parliamentary system. The book concludes by asking whether these middle men had become a 'middle class' by 1830? Whatever the answer to this question, the social history of the Georgian Bath Infirmary demonstrates that Britons during the long eighteenth century were 'a polite and commercial people',[58] not inhabitants of an *ancien régime*.

Notes

1. Minute Book, 3 January 1740; 3 April 1740.

2. Walter Ison, *The Georgian Buildings of Bath from 1700 to 1830* (Bath: Kingsmead Reprints, 1969), p. 91. See also Mowbray A. Green, *The Eighteenth Century Architecture of Bath* (Bath: George Gregory, 1904), p. 104.
3. Minute Book, 16 February 1738, 'Plan and Elevation'.
4. Minute Book, January 1738, 'A Copy of a Letter to be Inserted in the Public Papers'.
5. Robert Leyborne, *Charity Conducive to God's Glory: A Sermon for the Benefit of the General Hospital, in Bath* (Bath: Thomas Boddely, 1754), p. 13. See also Edward Bayly, *A Sermon Preached at the Abbey-Church at Bath* (Bath: Thomas Boddely, 1749), 'Dedication'; Joseph Hunter, *The Ameliorated Condition of the Poor, One Benefit Derived to the World from Christianity* (Bath: Richard Cruttwell, 1811), pp. 21–2.
6. *London Evening Post*, 8 July 1738.
7. See, for example, J.G. Humble and Peter Hansell, *Westminster Hospital 1716–1974* 2nd edn (London: Pitman Medical, 1974), pp. 12, 21; Claire Daunton, *The London Hospital Illustrated: 250 Years* (London: B.T. Batsford, 1990), pp. 42, 44; *Gentleman's Magazine*, **13** (20 September 1743), p. 496; George McLoughlin, *A Short History of the First Liverpool Infirmary 1749–1824* (London and Chichester: Phillimore, 1978), pp. 16–17; William Brockbank, *Portrait of a Hospital 1752–1948 to Commemorate the Bi-Centenary of the Royal Infirmary, Manchester* (London: William Heinemann, 1952), p. 6; A.W. Langford, 'The History of Hereford General Hospital', *Transactions of the Woolhope Naturalists' Field Club*, 37 (1959), pp. 153–4; F. Marcus Hall, Richard S. Stevens and John Whyman, *The Kent and Canterbury Hospital 1790–1987* (Canterbury: Kent Postgraduate Medical Centre, 1987), p. 42.
8. John Woodward, *To Do the Sick No Harm: A Study of the British Voluntary Hospital to 1875* (London: Routledge and Kegan Paul, 1974), pp. 147–8.
9. F.B. Smith, *The People's Health 1830–1910* (London: Weidenfeld and Nicolson, 1979), p. 249; Woodward, *To Do the Sick No Harm*, pp. 114–16, 124–5.
10. See, for example, Frank H. Jacob, *A History of the General Hospital near Nottingham* (Bristol: John Wright and Sons, and London: Simpkin Marshall, 1951), 'Preface'; John Daniel Leader, *Sheffield General Infirmary: A Brief Sketch of a Century's Work* (Sheffield: Published on behalf of the Infirmary Board by Mr G.H. Day, Secretary, 1897), p. 6; William Henry McMenemey, *A History of the Worcester Royal Infirmary* (London: Press Alliances, 1947), p. ix.
11. See, for example, F.F. Cartwright, *A Social History of Medicine* (London: Longman, 1977), p. 36; Anthony Batty Shaw, *Norfolk and Norwich Medicine: A Retrospect* (Norwich: Norwich Medico-Chirurgical Society, 1992), p. 53.
12. Donna Andrew, *Philanthropy and Police: London Charity in the Eighteenth Century* (Princeton: Princeton University Press, 1989), pp. 21, 36; Roy Porter, 'The Gift Relation', in Lindsay Granshaw and Roy Porter (eds), *The Hospital in History* (London: Routledge, 1989), p. 162.
13. Bernard Mandeville, 'An Essay on Charity and Charity-Schools', in *The Fable of the Bees*, ed. Phillip Harth (Harmondsworth: Penguin Books, 1970), p. 269.

14. Ludmilla Jordanova, 'The Social Construction of Medical Knowledge', *Social History of Medicine*, 8 (1995), pp. 361–3.
15. Brian Abel-Smith, *The Hospitals 1800–1948: A Study in Social Administration in England and Wales* (London: Heinemann, 1964), pp. x–xi.
16. Woodward, *To Do the Sick No Harm*; Guenter B. Risse, *Hospital Life in Enlightenment Scotland: Care and Teaching at the Royal Infirmary of Edinburgh* (Cambridge: Cambridge University Press, 1986).
17. Susan Lawrence, *Charitable Knowledge: Hospital Pupils and Practitioners in Eighteenth-Century London* (Cambridge: Cambridge University Press, 1996); Mary Fissell, *Patients, Power and the Poor in Eighteenth-Century Bristol* (Cambridge: Cambridge University Press, 1991).
18. Porter, 'Gift Relation', p. 151. The term, 'gift relationship', was coined in an important study of altruism and blood donation. See Richard M. Titmuss, *The Gift Relationship: From Human Blood to Social Policy* (London: George Allen and Unwin, 1970).
19. Amanda Berry, 'Patronage, Funding and the Hospital Patient, c.1750–1815: Three English Regional Case Studies' (unpublished doctoral thesis, University of Oxford, 1995).
20. George Rosen, *From Medical Police to Social Medicine: Essays on the History of Health Care* (New York: Science History Publications, 1974), p. 274. See also Henry E. Sigerist, 'The History of Medicine and the History of Science', *Bulletin of the Institute of the History of Medicine*, 4 (1936), pp. 5–6; Peregrine Horden, 'A Discipline of Relevance: The Historiography of the Later Medieval Hospital', *Social History of Medicine*, 1 (1988), p. 359; John V. Pickstone, 'Medicine in Industrial Britain: The Uses of Local Studies', *Social History of Medicine*, 2 (1989), p. 203; David Cantor, 'Contracting Cancer?: The Politics of Commissioned Histories', *Social History of Medicine*, 5 (1992), p. 141.
21. See J.C.D. Clark, *English Society 1688–1832* (Cambridge: Cambridge University Press, 1985); J.C.D. Clark, *Revolution and Rebellion: State and Society in England in the Seventeenth and Eighteenth Centuries* (Cambridge: Cambridge University Press, 1986). For assessment of Clark's thesis, see Joanna Innes, 'Jonathan Clark, Social History and England's "ancien regime"', *Past and Present*, **115** (1987), pp. 165–200; Roy Porter, 'English Society in the Eighteenth Century Revisited', in Jeremy Black (ed.), *British Politics and Society from Walpole to Pitt 1742–1789* (London: Macmillan, 1990), ch. 1; G.S. Rousseau, *Perilous Enlightenment: Pre- and Post-Modern Discourses: Sexual, Historical* (Manchester: Manchester University Press, 1991), ch. 10.
22. J.C.D. Clark, 'On Hitting the Buffers: The Historiography of England's *ancien régime* – a response', *Past and Present*, **117** (1987), p. 199.
23. Michael Hunter, *Science and Society in Restoration England* (Cambridge: Cambridge University Press, 1981), p. 4; Charles Wilson, *England's Apprenticeship 1603–1763,* 2nd edn (London: Longman, 1984), pp. 160–61.
24. J.G.A. Pocock, *Virtue, Commerce and History: Essays on Political Thought and History, Chiefly in the Eighteenth Century* (Cambridge: Cambridge University Press, 1985), p. 108; W.A. Speck, 'Conflict in Society', in Geoffrey Holmes (ed.), *Britain after the Glorious Revolution 1689–1714* (London: Macmillan, 1969), pp. 135–6; Wilson, *England's Apprenticeship,* p. 172.
25. Paul Langford, *A Polite and Commercial People: England 1727–1783*

(Oxford: Clarendon Press, 1989), p. 162; N.F.R. Crafts, 'British Economic Growth, 1700–1831: A Review of the Evidence', *Economic History Review*, **36** (1983), p. 187, table 5. See also Pat Hudson, *The Industrial Revolution* (London: Edward Arnold, 1992), ch. 2; John Rule, *The Vital Century: England's Developing Economy 1714–1815* (London: Longman, 1992), pp. 28–31.

26. J.V. Beckett, *The Aristocracy in England 1660–1914* (Oxford: Basil Blackwell, 1986), pp. 195–7, 231–2, 280–82; Peter Borsay, *The English Urban Renaissance: Culture and Society in the Provincial Town 1660–1760* (Oxford: Clarendon Press, 1989), pp. 199–200; Asa Briggs, *The Age of Improvement 1783–1867* (London: Longmans, 1959), pp. 169–70; M.C. Buer, *Health, Wealth and Population in the Early Days of the Industrial Revolution* (London: George Routledge, 1926), p. 43; Langford, *Polite and Commercial People*, pp. 68, 447–52, 644–6; Porter, 'English Society', p. 41; John Rule, *Albion's People: English Society 1714–1815* (London: Longman, 1992), ch. 3.
27. John Cannon, *Aristocratic Century: The Peerage of Eighteenth-Century England* (Cambridge: Cambridge University Press, 1984), p. 179.
28. Hugh Dunthorne, *The Enlightenment* (London: Historical Association, 1991), pp. 5–13; Norman Hampson, *The Enlightenment: An Evaluation of its Assumptions, Attitudes and Values* (Harmondsworth: Penguin Books, 1968), pp. 16, 23; Thomas L. Hankins, *Science and the Enlightenment* (Cambridge: Cambridge University Press, 1985), chs 1 and 6; Geoffrey Hawthorn, *Enlightenment and Despair: A History of Social Theory*, 2nd edn (Cambridge: Cambridge University Press, 1987), pp. 8–10; Roy Porter, *The Enlightenment* (London: Macmillan, 1990), pp. 1–11, 18–20, 68–9, 71–3.
29. See, for example, Peter Gay, *The Enlightenment: An Interpretation – the Rise of Modern Paganism* (London: Weidenfeld and Nicolson, 1967), pp. 3–19; David Spadafora, *The Idea of Progress in Eighteenth-Century Britain* (New Haven: Yale University Press, 1990), p. 10.
30. Roy Porter, 'The Enlightenment in England', in Roy Porter and Mikulas Teich (eds), *The Enlightenment in National Context* (Cambridge: Cambridge University Press, 1981), ch. 1; Arthur M. Wilson, 'The Enlightenment Came First to England', in Stephen B. Baxter (ed.), *England's Rise to Greatness 1660–1763* (Berkeley: University of California Press, 1983), ch. 1.
31. H.T. Dickinson, *Liberty and Property: Political Ideology in Eighteenth-Century Britain* (London: Methuen, 1977), pp. 197–205; Ludmilla Jordanova, 'The Authoritarian Response', in Peter Hulme and Ludmilla Jordanova (eds), *The Enlightenment and its Shadows* (London: Routledge, 1990), pp. 202–3, 210; Porter, 'Enlightenment', pp. 16–17.
32. Borsay, *English Urban Renaissance*, pp. 257–63.
33. Trevor Fawcett and Stephen Bird, *Bath: History and Guide* (Stroud: Alan Sutton, 1994), pp. 44, 57, 72; Sylvia McIntyre, 'Bath: The Rise of a Resort Town, 1660–1800', in Peter Clark (ed.), *Country Towns in Pre-Industrial England* (Leicester: Leicester University Press, 1981), p. 214.
34. R.S. Neale, *Bath: A Social History 1680–1850 or a Valley of Pleasure, yet a Sink of Iniquity* (London: Routledge and Kegan Paul, 1981), p. 45. This argument is also pursued in Graham Davis and Penny Bonsall, *Bath: A New History* (Keele: Keele University Press, 1996).

35. *The Improved Bath Guide* (Bath: Wood and Co., 1812), p. 18. See also John Collinson, *The History and Antiquities of the County of Somerset*, introduced by Robert Dunning, 3 vols, first pub. 1791, repr. (Gloucester: Alan Sutton, 1983), vol. 1, p. 28.
36. *The Journeys of Celia Fiennes*, ed. Christopher Morris (London: Cresset Press, 1949), p. 21.
37. McIntyre, 'Bath', pp. 199–201. See also John Barrett, 'Spas and Seaside Resorts, 1660–1780', in *The Rise of the New Urban Society*, Open University Third Level Course, English Urban History 1500–1780, Units 13, 14, 15 and 16 (Milton Keynes: Open University Press, 1977), pp. 43, 64.
38. Daniel Defoe, *A Tour through the Whole Island of Great Britain*, eds G.D.H. Cole and D.C. Browning, 2 vols, first pub. 1724–26, repr. (London: Dent, 1962), vol. 2, p. 34.
39. Phyllis Hembry, *The English Spa 1560–1815: A Social History* (London: Athlone Press, 1990), pp. 92–3, 135–6.
40. Fawcett and Bird, *Bath*, pp. 45, 50–51, 54–7, 60–67, 73, 76; Sylvia McIntyre, 'Towns as Health and Pleasure Resorts' (unpublished doctoral thesis, University of Oxford, 1973), pp. 129–30.
41. Brigitte Mitchell, 'English Spas', *Bath History*, **1** (1986), pp. 196–8. See also Peter Borsay, 'Health and Leisure Resorts, 1700–1840', in Peter Clark (ed.) *The Cambridge Urban History of Britain*, 3 vols (Cambridge: Cambridge University Press, forthcoming), vol. 2; Trevor Fawcett, 'Selling the Bath Waters: Medical Propaganda at an Eighteenth-Century Spa', *Somerset Archaeology and Natural History*, **134** (1991), p. 194.
42. Barrett, 'Spas', p. 51; Hembry, *English Spa*, p. 114.
43. Fawcett and Bird, *Bath*, p. 68; Hembry, *English Spa*, p. 155; McIntyre, 'Towns', pp. 41–2.
44. Barrett, 'Spas', p. 69; McIntyre, 'Towns', pp. 58–9; McIntyre, 'Bath', pp. 212, 214, 222, 243. See also A. Barbeau, *Life and Letters at Bath in the Eighteenth Century* (London: William Heinemann, 1904), pp. 298–9, 302–6; Davis and Bonsall, *Bath*, pp. 61, 63–5; Fawcett and Bird, *Bath*, pp. 60, 71–2; A.B. Granville, *Spas of England and Principal Sea-Bathing Places*, 2 vols, first pub. 1841, repr. (Bath: Adams and Dart, 1971), vol. 2: *The Midlands and South*, pp. 432–3; Austin J. King, 'Bath – its General History from the Norman Conquest to the Nineteenth Century', in J.W. Morris (ed.), *Handbook to Bath Prepared on the Occasion of the Visit of the British Association 1888* (Bath: Isaac Pitman and Sons, 1888), pp. 90–91.
45. Porter, 'Gift Relation', pp. 156–7; Woodward, *To Do the Sick No Harm*, pp. 18, 21.
46. 12 Geo. II, *An Act for Establishing and Well Governing an Hospital or Infirmary in the City of Bath* (London, 1739), pp. 572–3, 582.
47. John Wood, *A Description of Bath 1765* (Bath: Kingsmead Reprints, 1969), p. 279.
48. 12 Geo. II, pp. 571, 575.
49. Roy Porter, 'Introduction', in Roy Porter (ed.), *The Medical History of Waters and Spas*, *Medical History* Supplement No. 10 (London: Wellcome Institute for the History of Medicine, 1990), pp. viii, x; Roy Porter, 'The Eighteenth Century', in Lawrence I. Conrad, Michael Neve, Vivian Nutton, Roy Porter and Andrew Wear, *The Western Medical Tradition 800 BC to AD 1800* (Cambridge: Cambridge University Press, 1995), p. 420.

50. Roy Porter, *The Greatest Benefit to Mankind: A Medical History of Humanity from Antiquity to the Present* (London: HarperCollins, 1997), p. 392.
51. Wood, *Bath*, pp. 275–301.
52. See, for example, *The Bath and Bristol Guide; Or, The Tradesman's and Traveller's Pocket-Companion*, 3rd edn (Bath: T. Boddely, 1755), p. 17; *Improved Bath Guide*, p. 46.
53. Randle Wilbraham Falconer, *History of the Royal Mineral Water Hospital, Bath*, rev. by Anthony Beaufort Brabazon, first pub. 1860 (Bath: Charles Hallett, 1888).
54. P.V. Turner, *The Royal Mineral Water Hospital, Bath: A Brief History, 1742–1921* (Bath: William Lewis and Son, 1921).
55. Steven Cherry, *Medical Services and the Hospitals in Britain, 1860–1939* (Cambridge: Cambridge University Press, 1996), pp. 60–63, 72–4.
56. George D. Kersley and John A. Cosh, *The History of the Royal National Hospital for Rheumatic Diseases, Bath 1742–1965* (Bath: Royal National Hospital, 1965); George D. Kersley and John A. Cosh, *The History of the Royal National Hospital for Rheumatic Diseases, Bath 1742–1979* (Bath: Royal National Hospital, 1980).
57. Roger Rolls, *The Hospital of the Nation: The Story of Spa Medicine and the Mineral Water Hospital at Bath* (Bath: Bird, 1988).
58. Paul Langford borrowed this phrase for the title of his masterful New Oxford History of England covering the years 1727 to 1783. The source was William Blackstone's *Commentaries on the Laws of England*, 4 vols (Oxford: Clarendon Press, 1765–69). See Langford, *Polite and Commercial People*, pp. 1–2.

PART TWO
The Commercial Economy

CHAPTER TWO

The Promotion of Civic Virtue

Charity thrived in early modern Britain. During the century to 1760, it is estimated that the number of trusts alone grew twofold, while a parliamentary enquiry in 1788 judged their yearly income to be over £250 000.[1] By the late eighteenth century, however, these traditional forms of giving had been significantly undermined and though benefactors continued to leave bequests, they did so at a declining rate. Changing attitudes to property were partly responsible; in 1736, for example, the Mortmain Act had introduced controls on the charitable disposition of land to prevent men at the end of their lives from discarding wealth that properly belonged to their descendants. But in addition to this anxiety about inheritance rights, the inflexibility and mismanagement of posthumous benevolence became a matter of increasing concern.[2] Therefore, rather than relying on trustees to implement their wishes, donors chose associated philanthropy in accelerating numbers and subscribed to collective projects whose relevance and organization they were able to approve during their lifetimes. This subscription system not only matched the modest surplus incomes of the prospering middle orders, but also resonated with corporate civic traditions and the organization of both religious sects, and the clubs and societies upon which post-Restoration urban sociability rested.[3] However, its greatest debt was to the joint-stock company, thrown up by the Financial Revolution to meet the need for large quantities of capital, for benefactors – like small investors – became 'shareholders' in the charity they helped to finance. Thus, from the 1690s, associated schemes became a common feature of cultural life, permeating hunts and balls, libraries and music no less than good works.[4] The initial philanthropic applications were charity schools, workhouses and Societies for the Reformation of Manners. By the 1730s, these enthusiasms were waning; but the principle of associated charity had been taken on board by the nascent voluntary hospital movement,[5] whose history was to prove more enduring. This part explores the adaptation of the joint-stock company to the charitable purposes of the Bath Infirmary. Chapter 2 considers the extent to which its administrative structures and practices offset the allegations of corruption sown by commerce and politics. Chapter 3 then charts the Hospital's income and expenditure, and asks how effectively the associational method of financing tapped the resources of the volatile Georgian economy.

The concept of civic virtue

As an early member of the hospital movement, the Bath Infirmary was founded while joint ventures of all kinds were at a low ebb. In 1720, the South Sea Bubble had traumatized the commercial sector, after the conversion of high-interest annuities into stock, without an agreed ratio of exchange, precipitated the inevitable crash. Yet though this affair brought financial ruin to many, it was the outcome of an 'infatuation' with profit-making rather than fraud on the part of the Company's directors.[6] More destructive for associated philanthropy was the departure to France in 1732 of the cashier and banker of the Charitable Corporation, having embezzled 'more than half a million of money' meant to provide employment and relief for the poor.[7] As Ruth McClure has observed: 'Not one of the charitable institutions still operating in London in 1810 had been founded between 1720 ... and 1739 ... although prior to 1720 associational charity in non-corporate form had flourished in the heyday of the charity school movement'.[8] Institutional fraud was reinforced by the misdemeanours of politicians: in 1725, for instance, the Lord Chancellor was fined no less than £30 000 for corruption offences; and the integrity of the government was further undermined by Walpole's willingness to shield those of his supporters implicated in illegal or irregular activities.[9] The frequency with which corruption erupted into Hanoverian politics is indicative of how the *ancien régime* was adjusting to the commercial conditions of a modern society. Landed critics of the increasingly powerful 'monied interest' bolstered their attack by resuscitating the paternalist model of civic humanism, which had originally revived with the classical Renaissance. According to this paradigm, civic virtue depended upon the 'good' man who used his property to acquire the independence and the leisure to engage in public affairs and pursue the public interest with impunity.[10] Commercial exchanges, on the other hand, were treated with considerable suspicion, especially if they involved the stock market rather than solid commodities; as a disenchanted MP complained in 1702, 'a merchant finds a better return between the Exchequer and the Exchange than he makes by running a hazard to the Indies'.[11]

The case against the new commercial élite rested on the dependence of its members. Without an income derived from property, they were said to possess neither the time nor the autonomy to work for the public good. During the wars against France, financiers had been accused of a vested interest in the continuation of hostilities, as they reaped huge profits from loans to the government while property owners sank under the burden of a heavy land tax. The indictment lived on. The 'monied interest' was accused of being caught in a web of symbiotic economic and political relationships, whose servicing took priority over the public interest. Therefore, corruption was always lurking and civic virtue unavoidably compromised.[12] By mid-century, commercial institutions were losing their pejorative image as tax reductions for the landed classes and their gradual investment in government loans eased conflict with the men of commerce.[13] However, when political radicalism emerged in the late 1760s and 1770s, the ethic of civic virtue was again used to expose government waste and the perverse effects of patronage, and the American War of Independence similarly rekindled hostility towards profiteering suppliers, not least among the landed élite aggrieved by high taxes and the spiralling yields from government stock. The economical reform campaign of the early 1780s gained modest successes, notably with the departure of government contractors from the House of Commons. But that exclusion, together with a reduction in offices and sinecures, had little effect on the 'Old Corruption', which drew the government into a series of commercial and professional relationships within the unreformed political system.[14] Criticisms of foul play, moreover, were not confined to the state. In 1811, the *Gentleman's Magazine* published a hard-hitting account of philanthropic corruption, which drew attention to longstanding evidence of 'the fraudulent or negligent abuses of public charities' and called for new legislation, 'that justice may be done to the poor ... and punishment inflicted on those who have been guilty of wilful frauds and known peculations'.[15] Therefore, concern about public morality, which found cultural expression in the art of Hogarth and the literature of writers from Defoe to Wordsworth,[16] was ongoing throughout the Georgian period.

If corruption was perceived as endemic, however, a new moral code was evolving from the early eighteenth century, imbued with the optimism of the Enlightenment. As Pocock has argued: 'the rise of commerce and culture ... vastly enhanced the human capacity for production and consumption, exchange, inter-dependence, and sympathy, and on this foundation there might be erected new ethical systems which displayed how man's love of himself might be converted into love of his fellow social beings'.[17] The direction of wealth into associated philanthropy was an excellent way of achieving this end because it used the commercial idea of a joint-stock company to fulfil moral goals. In the first place, the objective was charitable rather than profit-making. But to ensure that this version of corporate collaboration was free of corruption, strenuous efforts were also made to encourage open management and to challenge 'the customary operation of clientage'.[18] The utility of such associated philanthropy, modelled on the principles of civic virtue, outlived the birth pangs of the commercial economy and continued to be a valuable antidote to Georgian corruption, helping to retrieve the moral standing of civil society by demonstrating a capacity to put aside self-interest for the public good. Essential to this exemplification of propriety were the administrative arrangements. Although based on the joint-stock company, associated charities were not necessarily its legal equivalent; for unless incorporated, they were unable to sue in a court of law and faced restrictions when acquiring leases. In the case of voluntary hospitals, not all immediately sought or achieved corporate status: a request from St George's Infirmary in the capital was turned down in 1735, and upon learning that this lack of a charter caused 'no inconvenience', the London Hospital deferred an application for more than 15 years until in 1756 legal action was required.[19] At the Bath Infirmary, as elsewhere, the leasehold restriction was overcome by naming trustees 'to receive the lands on which the said Hospital is intended to be built', but 'When the building was advanced almost to the second story', an application was submitted to Parliament for a charter.[20] Correspondence from the Somerset MP, Thomas Carew, to one of the leading trustees indicates that a bid for exemption from the Mortmain Act was rejected; in his words, 'the purchase of land ... I fear will not be admitted to extend to above one thousand pounds'.[21] That aside, the Bill passed and the charter came into effect on 1 May 1739.[22] Therefore, the Foundling Hospital was not the first 'eleemosynary' or charitable corporation in Britain because its charter received Royal Assent on 14 August 1739,[23] more than two months after the Bath Hospital became a corporate body.

The most valuable documents for quarrying the administrative history of this early incorporated charity are the minutes relating to the general court and the weekly committee which co-ordinated hospital affairs. Their paleography suggests that routine business – in particular, financial transactions, the appointment of the duty physician and surgeon, and the admission and discharge of patients – was normally compiled in advance by the register or secretary, whilst incidental decisions, together with a list of the governors present, were added during or after the meeting in a different hand. Needless to say, neither these Minute Books nor the other remaining 'traces' of the Bath Infirmary offer direct access to its Georgian past.[24] Not only were errors and inadvertent omissions almost inevitable; but the material was also deliberately constructed to meet both the internal requirements of the institution and the external requirements of the outside world. Moreover, priorities altered over time, and so though changes in content or format are unlikely to be without meaning, they cannot be read as simple variations in practice. Critical as these qualifications are, however, they oblige not the historical abandonment of medical records but a healthy scepticism towards their use.

Administrative structures and participation

Although important for legal reasons, a charter no more assured civic virtue for voluntary hospitals than for the South Sea Company or the Charitable Corporation. Corruption had to be banished by the adoption of credible managerial structures and procedures. The available sources indicate that propriety was a prime concern for the Georgian Bath Hospital. Following the first subscription in 1723, a general meeting of all contributors was convened at which a treasurer was nominated 'to keep the money' and 13 representatives chosen 'to manage the charity'.[25] By 1731, however, the link between financial sponsorship and administrative participation had been forged. It was initially determined that 'every person contributing 20 pounds, or upwards, shall be admitted a governor of this Hospital'.[26] The 'Plan and Elevation', prepared in 1738, retained the same amount, but when corporate status was conferred a year later the position of governor was reserved for contributors of at least £40.[27] Compared with other institutions, this was substantial.[28] As we have seen, the Bath Infirmary was also unusual in not tying governorship to annual subscriptions. The effect of these two attributes was to preserve an element of clientage alien to the concept of civic virtue. For smaller contributors, the only route to participation in the affairs of the institution was through the patronage of existing members of the corporation, who were permitted to elect governors who had not fulfilled the financial criterion.[29]

Whether elected or appointed on account of their donations, governors of the Bath Hospital became members of its corporation, by law numbering at least 50.[30] Managerial responsibilities were then executed via an organizational framework that bore strong resemblance to the administrative structures found throughout the voluntary infirmary sector.[31] Brian Abel-Smith relegated to a footnote the fact that 'Some "house committees" were started in the eighteenth century'; only during the early nineteenth century, did governors begin to appoint 'small sub-committees to supervise day-to-day management'.[32] The sophisticated administrative structure of Georgian infirmaries belies this chronology. At Bath, all governors were entitled to attend the general court, legally required to meet annually at the beginning of May to select a president, three treasurers and the weekly committee of 32 assistants from among members of the corporation to serve for the forthcoming Hospital year. Day-to-day control was vested in this group, which was expected to convene on a weekly basis. As well as overseeing the Hospital's financial and material assets, the assistants had three further functions: 'to appoint ... and at their pleasure remove' officers, servants and other staff; to fix 'salaries, perquisites, or other rewards, for their labour or service'; and to admit those patients for whom the charity was intended, making 'such provision for their maintenance and cure, as they shall think necessary and convenient'. This work was 'subject to the inspection of the corporation', but unless summoned by the weekly committee due to special circumstances,[33] the general court was at first obliged to assemble only once a year to fulfil its electoral functions. In 1744, however, the governors decided to hold three additional general meetings each year at quarterly intervals, an order confirmed in the 1790s.[34]

The creation of a closed weekly committee, manned by a panel of governors, was augmented by a series of subcommittees, to which specific tasks were given. In the early 1750s, committees of all the governors were formed, one to consider the most appropriate bye laws for the Hospital and a second to examine the best method of controlling infestations.[35] The same decade saw the delegation of duties to the honorary physicians and surgeons: revising the Infirmary's rules, for example; overseeing the conversion of a store room into a ward; and negotiating with the Corporation of the city over the use of the King's and Queen's Baths by patients.[36] Much more common, however, was the establishment of subcommittees of lay governors, occasionally joined by representatives of the medical staff. Some of these subcommittees were a regular feature of the administrative landscape. The ball began rolling as early as 1744, when not only was a monthly 'committee of the governors' set up 'to review the patients', but a benefaction of £100 was made conditional upon the appointment of a tradesmen's bills committee 'to examine the prices of all goods and provisions bought in the preceeding month and to audit the bill for the treasurer's payment thereof'.[37] By 1758, management of the Charmy Down Estate, purchased in 1750, had been hived off to a subcommittee,[38] and after 1760 a small group of governors was commissioned to enlist preachers prior to charity services on behalf of the Hospital.[39] Finally, in 1783, 'a committee of accounts' was inaugurated to inspect the register's record of the caution money[40] which patients deposited on arrival to pay for their return journey or burial in the event of death.[41] Over and above these ongoing arrangements, no fewer than 53 *ad hoc* subcommittees were set up between 1742/43 and 1830/31, in response to particular situations (Table 2.1). Though used most widely in the decade of the 1820s, this mechanism had taken root by the mid-eighteenth century. By far the most common application was to the management of premises and amenities: almost 40 per cent of subcommittees up to 1830 addressed themselves to furniture, repairs and sanitation,[42] enlargement of the building[43] and the piping of spa water from the city's baths.[44] None the less, legal matters (usually associated with the Infirmary's Acts of

Table 2.1 Bath General Hospital: the establishment of subcommittees, 1742–1830

Decade	*Premises and Amenities*	*Legal*	*Financial*	*Staff and Patients*	*Other*	*Total*
1742/43–1750/51	—	1	—	—	—	1
1751/52–1760/61	6	—	1	1	—	8
1761/62–1770/71	1	—	—	—	1	2
1771/72–1780/81	2	1	—	2	2	7
1781/82–1790/91	—	—	2	1	1	4
1791/92–1800/01	6	2	1	—	—	9
1801/02–1810/11	1	—	1	—	—	2
1811/12–1820/21	1	2	3	—	1	7
1821/22–1830/31	5	4	2	3	1	15
Total	22	10	10	7	6	55

Source: Minute Books.

Parliament or its lease from a local almshouse) generated ten subcommittees,[45] as did money raising, legacies, insurance and other financial affairs.[46] Staff and patient issues, including the rules which prescribed their behaviour, were responsible for seven subcommittees,[47] while publicity, food and provisions, and the establishment of a chaplain's fund fell into the miscellaneous category.[48]

Complementing this array of general courts, weekly committees and subcommittees was the supervision of house visitors, two of whom were chosen from among the assistants every week. The 'Scheme of Rules', approved in 1742 and printed in John Wood's *Description of Bath*, designated three principal duties for house visitors, typical of the responsibilities imposed at other voluntary infirmaries.[49] First, visitors were to 'enquire into the management of the whole House, receive the complaints of patients, and servants, each of whom they shall examine apart, and enter an account thereof into a book kept for that purpose ... [to] be read at the next Committee'. Secondly, house visitors were to 'examine the meat, malt liquor, and other provisions brought into the House, to see if they be wholesome, and proper for the family'. And, thirdly, in the last week of April, they were to prepare an annual inventory of household goods and furniture, compare it with the previous year and, after allowing for wear and tear, decide whether any embezzlement had taken place. Additionally, 'for the time being', house visitors were expected to ensure that the admission conditions laid down by Act of Parliament were complied with and to transfer the patients' caution money to the treasurers.[50] When the rules were reviewed during the 1770s, and later 'fairly transcribed in a book',[51] the temporary duties were dropped, but the house visitors' brief had been extended to include directing 'the beadles, who are to be appointed from among the porters and chairman, to take up vagrants'. This job appears to date from at least 1750.[52]

Although the structure of general courts and weekly committees, subcommittees and house visitors created a basis for effective supervision, its ability to deliver an institution managed in the public interest depended upon the participation of governors and the practices which they adopted. Restricted access to governorships meant that the huge attendances stirred up at other institutions by a controversial agenda were not matched.[53] However, the Minute Books for the general court and weekly committee, which are extant for the entire long eighteenth century, suggest that governors were less than conscientious in exercising their rights of attendance. The collapse of two general courts is documented, one in 1768 and the other in 1791 when a mere seven governors appeared to consider enlarging the Hospital.[54] Furthermore, a count of listed participants, taken at five-yearly intervals after 1745/46, indicates that the proportional turnout was never high and deteriorated noticeably in the late eighteenth and early nineteenth centuries (Table 2.2). Throughout the Georgian period, contention or crisis had pulling power – the number of honorary physicians in 1757, paying for a chaplain in 1775, financial problems ten years later.[55] The first meeting in May was usually quorate, but from the 1760s general courts later in the administrative year did not always hit the legal minimum of nine.[56] With a governor population of 106 in 1750, rising to 147 by 1830,[57] dedication to duty was in short supply.

Weekly committees were likewise sparse gatherings. Activists were not largely confined to the physicians, as at Worcester where in 1748 the governors were urged to 'take the general management more entirely into their own hands ... [to give] an acceptable relief to the worthy and learned gentlemen'.[58] However, absentee assistants resident near Bath, who were chosen because they were more likely to attend,[59] did receive reminders of meetings or requests to help with particular jobs.[60] Decisions were also postponed due to poor attendance: in May 1759, the purchase of sheets and table-cloths, proposed by the house visitors, was deferred until the next week 'there not being a committee'; in February 1781, the discharge of 'Nurse Vezey for insolent behaviour to the matron' was recommended to the next full committee because the meeting was inquorate; and in August 1801, the election of a chairman to convey patients to the baths was thwarted altogether, again 'for want

Table 2.2 Bath General Hospital: attendance at general courts, 1739–1830

Year	*No. of Meetings*	*Average Attendance*	*1 or 2 May Attendance*	*No. of Inquorate Meetings*
1739/40	1	—	—	—
1740/41	1	15.00	15	0
1741/42	1	11.00	11	0
1742/43	1	16.00	16	0
1743/44	8	13.50	21	0
1744/45	4	18.75	—	0
1745/46	5	12.80	—	0
1750/51	8	15.63	21	0
1755/56	4	16.50	17	0
1760/61	5	13.00	22	2
1765/66	4	11.50	16	2
1770/71	4	15.25	23	0
1775/76	5	13.80	14	3
1780/81	5	14.60	14	0
1785/86	4	17.00	28	0
1790/91	4	15.50	22	1
1795/96	4	10.00	14	2
1800/01	4	8.75	18	3
1805/06	4	8.25	17	3
1810/11	4	9.00	16	2
1815/16	4	8.75	19	3
1820/21	5	13.60	24	2
1825/26	5	15.00	13	2
1830/31	5	14.80	18	0

Notes:
1. The Hospital year ran from 1 May to 30 April.
2. Only meetings with a list of attenders are included. There was no list for one meeting in 1739/40, 1740/41, 1744/45 and 1745/46.
3. The quorum for a general court was nine governors.
4. The average figure for 1825/26 includes an exceptional attendance of 39 on 15 February 1826 when a new Hospital register was elected.

Source: Minute Books.

of a committee'.[61] Table 2.3 demonstrates that in the years sampled quinquennially after 1745/46, half-hearted participation by assistants was a regular trait of the Hospital's administration. Interest peaked in

Table 2.3 Bath General Hospital: average attendance at weekly committees, 1739–1830

Year	*Total attendance*	*No. of meetings*	*Average attendance per meeting*
1739/40	120	19	6.31
1740/41	46	5	9.20
1741/42	165	16	10.31
1742/43	577	52	11.09
1743/44	520	50	10.40
1744/45	432	48	9.00
1745/46	386	48	8.04
1750/51	452	47	9.62
1755/56	316	49	6.45
1760/61	289	48	6.02
1765/66	315	49	6.43
1770/71	277	49	5.65
1775/76	339	49	6.92
1780/81	356	48	7.42
1785/86	307	49	6.27
1790/91	311	49	6.35
1795/96	235	49	4.80
1800/01	173	48	3.60
1805/06	105	48	2.19
1810/11	226	49	4.61
1815/16	188	49	3.84
1820/21	191	48	3.98
1825/26	193	48	4.02
1830/31	291	50	5.82

Notes:
1. The Hospital year ran from 1 May to 30 April.
2. Only meetings with a list of attenders are included. In 1739/40 there was no list for four meetings, and in 1740/41, 1741/42 and 1744/45 no list for one meeting.
3. The average figure for 1795/96 includes three meetings where more than a dozen assistants were present.

Source: Minute Books.

1742/43, when patients were first admitted, but even then only 11 of the 32 assistants were on average present at meetings. Thereafter, numbers fell away, dropping to a nadir in the early nineteenth century. The predicament of the Bath Infirmary was not unique. In 1792 concern that attendance was 'far less than the efficient supervision of the charity rendered necessary' prompted the Salop Hospital to reform its 'ordinary government', replacing the 'open' format for weekly meetings with a 'closed' structure of 12 directors elected from among the trustees.[62] At Bath, where weekly committees had always been 'closed', a modest recovery in participation had occurred by 1830/31. However, from the 1750s average attendance was below the quorum of seven prescribed by law and when a new Act – designed primarily to permit the supply of spa water to the Infirmary – was passed in 1830, the quorum for weekly committees was reduced to three.[63] Pragmatism prevailed.

If general courts and weekly committees were thinly populated, house visiting and the subcommittee structure were more diligently staffed. Though some institutions had difficulty in establishing routine house visiting or abandoned the practice,[64] experience at Bath was consistent with Howie's conclusion that the system generally worked well.[65] Throughout the long eighteenth century, house visitors were routinely nominated by the weekly committee rather than appointed on an impersonal rota basis.[66] There were instances of default as in 1744 when Mr Bush was reappointed on the grounds that he had 'neglected last week'.[67] But, equally, house visitors stood in for colleagues[68] and reasons for absence are reported: on 21 December 1758, for example, 'Mr Scott was prevented from further attending the Hospital this week, by being confined with a very bad cold'; and in April of the following year, it was recorded that 'Mr Leake set out for London this morning'.[69] The survival of two House Visitors Books, one covering 1742 to 1743 and the other 1754 to 1759, enables a systematic analysis of day-to-day supervision (Table 2.4). Though daily calls were not an explicit requirement, the attendance rate for two house visitors was 85 per cent when managing the Hospital was a novelty. That degree of commitment quickly evaporated, and the governors became very reliant upon the paid apothecary, John Morris, who was a member of the governing body. Even after his retirement in 1757, however, at least one visitor arrived on almost seven days out of ten and the lapses that did occur were typically brief and interspersed rather than long and concentrated. Therefore, the mid-century Hospital was able to sustain an acceptable level of house visiting.

The servicing of subcommittees was likewise satisfactory. With the Charmy Down Estate, there were occasional breakdowns. In April 1767, four governors had to be reminded of a request to inspect the farmhouse, which had been made by a general court in March. Problems arose again in 1786, after the weekly committee decided to reject recommendations from the subcommittee, which had been signed only by two and not the minimum of three members. A professional survey was

Table 2.4 Bath General Hospital: the attendance of house visitors, 1742–43 and 1754–59

No. of house visitors	*1742 (26 June– 31 December)*		*1743 (1 January– 16 November*		*1754 (28 March– 31 December)*		*1755 (1 January– 31 December)*		*1756 (1 January– 31 December)*		*1757 (1 January– 31 December)*		*1758 (1 January– 31 December)*		*1759 (1 January– 27 September)*		*Total*	
	No. of days	*%*	*No. of days*	*%*	*No. of days*	*%*	*No. of days*	*%*	*No. of days*	*%*	*No. of days*	*%*	*No. of days*	*%*	*No. of days*	*%*	*No. of days*	*%*
2	163	85.79	210	65.63	88	31.77	81	22.31	79	21.70	75	20.60	105	28.77	58	21.48	859	34.18
1	27	14.21	109	34.06	157	56.68	217	59.78	173	47.53	212	58.24	152	41.64	128	47.41	1 175	46.76
0	—	—	1	0.31	32	11.55	65	17.91	112	30.77	77	21.15	108	29.59	84	31.11	479	19.06
Total	190	100.00	320	100.00	277	100.00	363	100.00	364	100.00	364	100.00	365	100.00	270	100.00	2 513	100.00

Notes:

1. Between March and December 1754, and January and December 1755, there were two days where no names of house visitors were recorded.
2. Between January and December 1756, and January and December 1757, there was one day where no names of house visitors were recorded.

Sources: House Visitors Book, 1; House Visitors Book, 2.

commissioned instead but when, almost 12 months later, the report was submitted and referred to the subcommittee, a general court had to be adjourned because no response had been received.[70] New blood was introduced, and from the 1790s the subcommittee was periodically reappointed.[71] In 1827, however, following an examination of the estate by the Hospital's register, the weekly committee was once more forced to urge those governors responsible for Charmy Down 'to meet upon some early day' and take the necessary measures.[72] Yet despite these intermittent problems, the Subcommittee Book which survives for the years 1778 to 1823 indicates that in the early nineteenth century between a half and four-fifths of the governors appointed to oversee the estate attended Charmy Down meetings. This degree of participation was typical of the subcommittee system as a whole, only the chaplaincy generating lower attendance during the 1780s (Table 2.5). Taken together with the performance of house visitors, such levels of engagement imply that throughout the long eighteenth century a hard core within the governing body was prepared to invest time and energy in managing the Hospital.

Keeping accounts and records

In many respects, the procedures followed by these active governors were of more significance for civic virtue than crude rates of participation in the administrative structure. To mediate successfully between economics and ethics, charitable institutions had to exemplify administrative good practice; they had to be free of corruption and visibly managed in the public interest, not for personal or sectional advantage. At the Bath Hospital, maintaining accurate records and accounts, and closely supervising expenditure were pivotal to the achievement of this propriety. When the first subscription opened in 1723, each collector kept separate records of the donations he received, which were 'transcribed into the book, wherein all the proceedings, touching the charity, were directed to be entered'.[73] After the proposal for a Hospital was resuscitated in the late 1730s, the trustees ordered the purchase of 'proper books for keeping the accounts'.[74] The surviving archival material indicates that the main Committee Minute Book was at the heart of this accounting system. Thus, contributions and the monthly payment of tradesmen's bills and servants' wages were cross-referenced to entries in a Journal, Ledger, House Incidents Book and Cash Book.[75] Annual details of investment income from the Hospital's London banker were also included after 1767.[76] Care was apparently taken to ensure reliability. First, contributions made at the end of the financial year were

Table 2.5 Bath General Hospital: attendance at subcommittees, 1778–1823

Subcommittee	*Date*	*No. of meetings*	*No. of members*	*Average attendance*	*Standardized attendance rate*
Mortmain	1778–89	15	5	3.93	0.79
Chaplain	1780–87	4	9	3.50	0.39
Caution Money	1783	1	5	5.00	1.00
Additional Male Patients	1789	1	11	11.00	1.00
Hospital Enlargement	1791	1	7	7.00	1.00
Hospital Finances	1792	1	18	14.00	0.78
Purchasing a House	1792	9	12	5.89	0.49
By-Laws	1793	4	7	3.75	0.54
Attic Storey	1793	4	15	8.00	0.53
Offensive Sewers	1796	12	5	3.50	0.70
Financial Statement	1797	1	8	6.00	0.75
Charmy Down Estate (1)	1800–06	5	5	4.20	0.84
Charmy Down Estate (2)	1810–14	8	9	5.00	0.56
Charmy Down Estate (3)	1822	2	6	4.50	0.75
Subscriptions in Arrears	1802	1	6	4.00	0.67
Removing the Hospital	1806	2	9	5.50	0.61
Financial State	1812	1	9	6.00	0.67
Additional Ward	1818	2	11	6.50	0.59
St John's Hospital (1)	1818–19	5	7	5.20	0.74
St John's Hospital (2)	1819–23	29	9	6.20	0.69
Mr Parish	1819	5	5	4.60	0.92

Notes:
1. The standardized attendance rate has been calculated by dividing average attendance by the number of members appointed to the subcommittee.
2. The following subcommittees included the six honorary medical staff: Hospital Finances (1792); Purchasing a House (1792); and the Attic Storey (1793).
3. The composition of a 1792 by-laws subcommittee is not minuted.
4. The Attic Storey Subcommittee was reappointed later in 1793, but the entry in the Subcommittee Book contains neither minutes nor the names of those present.

Source: Subcommittee Book.

carried forward: 'The above £5.5 being too late to receive them in the balance of this year's account, they are only entered in this place by way of memorandum.'[77] Secondly, overlooked income and expenditure were subsequently added: 'The treasurer, Charles Phillott Esq., reported that he had paid two shillings for a stamp for Mr Geo. Toghill's rent, in April last, and omitted to report it at that time.'[78] And, finally, mistakes were rectified. In May 1769, for example, the weekly committee 'surmised ... that some entries in the receipts and payments for the [last] year and also one entry in the book kept at the coffee house are erroneous'. A small subcommittee was duly set up to investigate and when the inaccuracies were confirmed, a general court ordered the necessary corrections.[79] Similarly, after a subscription of five guineas was wrongly recorded in 1801, the Minute Book noted not only the error but the folio number in the treasurer's Ledger.[80]

The statements compiled from these records were audited at the end of the financial year. Before the first *Annual Report* was prepared for January 1739, the treasurers were instructed to 'draw out an account of the receipts and disbursements that have been already made', to be reviewed by the rest of the trustees; and every member of the trust residing in Bath was invited to take part in the auditing exercise.[81] From 1745 the procedure was formalized, with a group of three or four governors examining and signing the accounts prior to their approval by the general court.[82] A sample of the resulting accounts, taken at five-yearly intervals after 1745/46, offers little ammunition with which to attack their accuracy. In a few instances, the ageing process has rendered the figures illegible.[83] A number of internal inconsistencies have also arisen from transcription or small calculating errors. In the 1744/45 *Annual Report,* for instance, the income and expenditure columns balanced only because the former embodied a mistake of £4, while in 1749/50, receipts for the year were five shillings adrift because a 'three' was transcribed as an 'eight'. In 1830/31, there was a more serious discrepancy: the subtotal for sums received was quoted as £2 131 instead of £4 227, though the total balance for receipts was correct and tallied with total disbursements. However, on just two occasions during the sample years was there a major error in the financial statement: in 1740/41, £60 was omitted from the credit side; and in 1765/66, receipts and payments were reconciled only by over-calculating the former by £148.[84]

These generally reliable annual accounts were joined in 1829 by an annual statement, prepared by the 'court of committees' to enable the 'general board' to decide 'how far the members of the court are deserving of their continued confidence'. The procedure was repeated in 1830.[85] From a much earlier stage, the minutes of past proceedings had been submitted for acceptance. On 16 June 1762, the Minute Book noted that 'the meetings of the committee since the 1st of May, were ... read, and are approved, confirmed and ratified'. The recording of this delay, explained by the constitutional failure of the president to appoint a deputy, implies that ratification was the norm. A similar entry appeared in 1763; and from the later 1760s, confirmation of the minutes was logged as a matter of routine, albeit with varying regularity.[86] In 1829, however, the Minute Book became the focal point of controversy, after an angry governor used it to express a personal grievance without approval, protesting that only the general court had the 'power of ratifying and confirming the acts of the court of committees'. The dispute about this critical relationship rumbled on: motions to defer decisions on structural alterations and the installation of gas lighting fell because no seconder came forward; while the report from a sub-committee charged with repairing the Hospital was received by the weekly committee only after a motion to call a special general court had collapsed.[87] At the next routine meeting of the court, the chairman received a unanimous vote of thanks 'for the very able, polite and *conciliating* [my italics] manner of conducting the business'.[88] After a temporary truce, however, conflict broke out again in 1830, when two assistants tried unsuccessfully to delay permission for the apothecary to take an apprentice. Moreover, dissident members of the general court also attempted, without success, to refer back to the weekly committee an instruction leaflet on the admission of patients.[89] The Minute Book documented this more contested approach to the management of the Hospital, but from the official perspective. After the incident in 1829, the register was directed to disallow future entries which had not been 'sanctioned by the committee'.[90]

The supervision of expenditure

The production of confirmed minutes and audited accounts may have assumed more significance in the pursuit of civic virtue as the government of the Bath Hospital became more discordant. From the outset, however, the detailed supervision of expenditure played a crucial role in the quest for financial propriety. The governors developed complex procedures to control building and maintenance, purchasing and the quality of goods supplied. In common with other institutions,[91] a tight rein was kept on the construction programme. To acquire additional property adjacent to the site, the trustees drove a hard bargain. In March 1738, Francis Fauquier – a financial expert who later became governor of Virginia[92] – reported that after negotiation, he and Dr

Oliver had concluded that it was in the Hospital's interest to buy the White House for £100, 'that being the lowest sum for which the said proprietors would part with it'.[93] Other property valuations were subjected to independent assessment, so that when Mr Boyce was asked to have his stables in Vicarage Lane valued 'by some skilful person whom he shall approve', the architect governor, John Wood, was requested to undertake the same exercise on behalf of the trustees.[94] Moreover, when Mr Fauquier was delegated 'to treat with Mr Boyce for his stable' after the valuation had taken place, a cash ceiling of £140 was imposed.[95] Craftsmen were recruited with equal care using competitive tendering. Before construction began, advertisements were placed in the *Bristol Journal* inviting proposals from masons and carpenters; and Mr Emes and Mr Bushell were chosen, their tenders 'being adjudged the lowest'. Articles were duly drawn up 'for the due performance of their contract', which included phased payments linked to the advance of the work.[96] Painters and plasterers were later signed up in the same way.[97] Finally, with their workforce *in situ*, the trustees gave detailed specifications for materials like wood and glass,[98] and kept a keen watch on progress, instructing Mr Rolph to finish immediately 'the painting of the Committee Room and Secretary's Office and then to desist till further orders'.[99]

Despite the presence of John Wood within their midst, the governors were not induced to extricate themselves from supervising the building process. Once completed, the Infirmary underwent no substantial alterations until the 1790s when a top storey, consisting of two extra wards, was added. The management of this project was very different. True, an independent opinion was sought on the plan and estimate, and phased payments were negotiated.[100] But whereas between 1739 and 1742 weekly committees and general courts co-ordinated construction, now a special subcommittee was set up, which drafted a contract with the architect and left him to handle day-to-day management.[101] A major refurbishment 30 years later was also overseen by a specialist subcommittee. Convened in the autumn of 1828,[102] this group brought detailed costings to a weekly committee covering repairs, improvements, furniture, painting, alterations to the laundry, and the heightening of passage ceilings on the second floor.[103] These were approved, but the assistants continued to influence the programme of work by acting as a conduit for proposals which ranged from the installation of gas lighting and a new heating and ventilation system to the relocation of the Committee Room and the Register's Office and the composition of bedding and bedsteads.[104] Professional opinion was not spurned where appropriate; indeed, an analogous subcommittee, investigating the more technical problem of constructing baths within the Hospital, did co-opt expert advisers and Mr Charles Capper of Birmingham was subsequently employed as a consulting engineer.[105] The high profile of the governors, however, contrasts sharply with the architect's supervision of the attic storey and reflects the revival of interest in the administration of the Hospital from the early nineteenth century. Such close involvement did not stop the total cost exceeding the estimate by over £1 000. But this was a genuine overspend due to extra commitments and 'dilapidations ... much more extensive than was at first supposed'.[106] There is no suggestion of runaway expenditure caused by extravagance or poor management.

The control of basic maintenance – redecoration,[107] repairs[108] and minor alterations[109] – also evolved during the course of the long eighteenth century. Specialist arrangements were not always made. In 1754, for example, the Hospital apothecary was asked to oversee the modification of the nurses' rooms, 'in such manner as may best prevent bugs from harbouring'. At other times, responsibility was devolved to the relevant craftsman as when, in 1792, Edward Mullins was commissioned to stop 'the offensive smells arising from the privies' by taking those measures 'he thinks will answer the purpose'.[110] The governors themselves were also enlisted. In 1753, Mr Emes and Mr Jelly were employed to alter the wash-house and the servants' bedchamber for 'such sums ... as shall be approved of by the committee appointed to examine the tradesmen's bills'.[111] More often the house visiting system was harnessed, with visitors either flagging repairs which were later sanctioned by the weekly committee[112] or taking executive action: 'There was a hole in the floor of the Princess Ward, which I ordered to be mended' read one entry in the House Visitors Book for November 1757.[113] After mid-century, however, the premises and their amenities became the most common rationale for subcommittees (Table 2.1); and from the later Georgian period a more professional style of maintenance management emerged. Estimates were sought for smaller jobs,[114] if not without complaint: in 1826, one of the honorary physicians deplored the expense and delay caused by putting out to tender the restoration of decayed timbers in the Queen's Ward when the integrity of the Infirmary's carpenter had 'never been questioned'.[115] Greater reliance was also placed on expert advice. In 1796, for instance, a subcommittee – set up 'to examine into the nuisance arising from the offensive sewers of this Hospital' – was recommended 'to consult with Mr Palmer or some experienced workman on the best means of remedying the same'. Similarly, the weekly committee in 1819 'Ordered that the pitching and paving be done according to the notice delivered by the surveyor'.[116] Maintenance no less than construction was being subjected to more formalized and professional scrutiny.

Whereas managerial procedures for building, decoration and repair matured over the long eighteenth century, the controls for purchasing furniture, equipment and provisions were relatively static, and showed a continuing reliance on competitive tendering and the delegation of authority to paid officers, individual governors and house visitors. Though competitive tendering was used for bedsteads when the Infirmary was first fitted out,[117] its most common application was to the supply of food and provisions. Just before the wards opened in 1742, the governors 'publicly advertised' their readiness 'to receive proposals from persons willing to supply ... meat, cheese, butter, sugar, malt, salt, milk, rice, candles, soap, faggots, coal, flour and oat meal'.[118] A small group was put together to determine the best way of organizing provisions and the first contracts were awarded on 27 May 1742.[119] A repeat of this procedure is recorded for 1743 and 1744,[120] whereupon the weekly committee as a whole apparently assumed responsibility. Competitive tendering remained in use for the purchase of food and provisions throughout the Georgian period. Thus, in October 1819, the weekly committee instructed that 'the *usual* [my italics] advertisements for proposals to serve the Hospital with flour, cheese and malt be inserted in the several Bath papers'.[121] Comparable notices had been ordered from the 1770s, covering soap and candles, malt, butchers' meat, butter, milk and cheese.[122] Their intermittent occurrence suggests that annual tendering may not have been rigidly enforced. In 1747, for instance, Mr Paul Bertrand met the person who supplied the Hospital with butter to negotiate the best future terms; and in 1803, an increase in the agreed price of milk was conceded following a report from 'J. Churchill ... that he cannot serve the same any longer, under two pence farthing a quart'.[123] When existing contracts broke down, moreover, the Infirmary on occasions turned to the open market. Obtaining the large quantities of cheese consumed by patients and servants proved most troublesome; and at one time or another, the steward, the apothecary and a representative of the governors were all charged with buying this product on behalf of the Hospital.[124] However, meat,[125] raisins,[126] salt butter,[127] hops[128] and coal[129] were likewise temporarily withdrawn from tendering, especially in the 1740s and 1750s. During this period at least, rival proposals for food and provisions may have been sought selectively with a view to value for money. Competitive bidding was durable but flexible.

Recourse to governors and paid officers was the dominant strategy where medical supplies, furniture, cooking and eating utensils, and linen for bathing and domestic purposes were concerned. Six months before the Infirmary opened, the 'gentlemen of the faculty' were invited to consider the equipment necessary for the apothecary's shop.[130] Whilst the institution was expanding to its full complement of patients, the extra household goods required were normally purchased by the matron, who was given varying amounts of discretion: at one extreme, she was ordered in March 1742 to 'provide 4 dozen of bowls at 4s a dozen (9 inches diameter)'; at the other, she was permitted in 1748 to 'provide such bathing linen as are wanted'.[131] The matron was also involved in buying furniture,[132] but this task was more typically the province of the steward, the honorary medical staff, or governors. Though the straightforward purchase of items like rugs, lamps and chairs was devolved to the steward, he was also given the more complex job of acquiring 'a mashing tub large enough to mash 12 bushells of malt' and disposing of 'the old mash tub to the best bidder'.[133] Physicians and surgeons purchased non-medical as well as medical items;[134] and the governors in general were commissioned to act in a personal capacity in a number of situations. In 1747, Mr Bertrand was 'desired to provide four chairs for the use of the wards'.[135] Five years previously, the treasurers collectively had been asked by the weekly committee 'to provide desks for the House' and their co-operation was later sought in purchasing 'such a number of Bibles and Prayer Books for the use of the patients as they shall think convenient'.[136] Governors were also entrusted as house visitors with procuring 'frocks' for the chairmen and a supply of wood and candles for the winter, as well as locating 'a proper person to supply the House with water'.[137] Discretion was apparently conferred in the same way that the approval of repairs was permitted. Entries in the House Visitors Books report not merely the 'want' of items, but the purchase (or making) of lamp oil, household equipment, clothing, furniture and religious literature.[138] In some instances, the power to buy was quite explicit: 'an ironing cloth for the laundry being entirely worn out a new one was ordered to be got'.[139] What is more, the visitors designated who was to undertake the acquisition: the matron in the case of 'two table cloths for the Princess Ward and some cloth to cover a quilt';[140] the apothecary when 'lump sugar for the wards' was sought.[141] Therefore, it seems likely that the house-visiting system was an integral part of the procurement process.

The supervision of expenditure was not confined to purchasing; nor did it end with the monthly auditing of invoices by the tradesmen's bills committee. In addition, effective financial control required mechanisms to ensure that demands were justified and that the goods supplied were of a satisfactory quality. When the new extension opened in 1794, the weekly committee commissioned 'the house visitors for the ensuing week ... to examine and report ... on Wednesday next what furniture will be necessary for the new wards'.[142] The presence of house visitors in the Infirmary on a regular basis was vital to both the legitimation of demand and the monitoring of supply because, if conscientious, they were able to keep an ear to the ground and identify any difficulties. The

House Visitors Books catalogue a string of requests for medical supplies,[143] linen and clothing,[144] utensils and cutlery,[145] foodstuffs and provisions,[146] furniture and equipment[147] which the visitors authorized. However, they also took seriously their duty to 'enquire in to the management of the whole House' and themselves initiated projects. As well as recommending repairs and redecoration, the visitors anticipated a need for wood in the winter,[148] suggested leather jacks instead of jugs for fetching bath water,[149] and put forward a number of structural alterations. In March 1743, for instance, they speculated that: 'It may be convenient to make another door way into the cook's pantry, to keep the bake house more private which is at present liable to some abuses.' An eye to savings also prompted them to query in January of the same year: 'Is it worth while to keep constant fire in the pantry below for the rice and sugar?' There are signs that the advice of house visitors was heeded. Not only did the Minute Books order 'that the necessaries mentioned in the Visiting Book of the foregoing week' be provided;[150] but in October 1757, one of the visitors commented that the committee had allowed 'all the articles ... in this week's visitation'. Equally, the implementation of instructions was recorded in February 1743, when the visitors noted that they had 'sent in two great chairs at 2s 6d each as was desired at the last meeting'.[151]

Just as important as the approval of demand was the quality of goods supplied. In monitoring the apothecary's shop, the Hospital followed the common practice of vesting responsibility in the physicians, surgeons and apothecaries who were governors;[152] and when they reported in September 1742 that certain drugs did not 'answer their expectations', the paid apothecary, Mr John Morris, was asked to apply to his druggist in London 'for what shall be wanting'.[153] The shop was included in the overall tours of the Hospital conducted by the house visitors.[154] In general, they 'found all in good order and the provisions very good'.[155] In the words of the meticulous Mr Scott, visiting on 16 November 1757: 'As I have been very exact in looking into the several parts of the House, and seeing what provisions were used in it ... I cannot but declare in favour of all persons concerned, that I am well pleased with everything I have seen.' After a subsequent visit, he was to find 'all in good order ... as seldom is to be seen in any other of our hospitals'.[156] None the less, mid-century house visiting at Bath did throw up shortcomings across a range of areas. In 1742/43, the medical governors were accused of failing to inspect the apothecary's shop;[157] there were also grumbles about bathing linen;[158] and after bedsteads had failed to comply with the original proposal, a house visitor confirmed that a later delivery was 'as good as the pattern from London and better than the first sent in'. 'The man', he concluded, 'should have his money.'[159] By far the most frequent cause of complaint, however, were foodstuffs.[160] Though isolated criticism of bread and cheese surfaced,[161] small beer, meat and malt provoked most negative comment. Sour small beer in June 1743 led the house visitors to order 'a new cooler and tub' to improve its storage, but in July of the same year the beer was again described as 'bad'.[162] The poor quality of meat, which attracted the attention of house visitors in the 1740s and 1750s, re-emerged as an issue in May 1784, when Mr William Sheppard, butcher to the Hospital, was summoned before the weekly committee 'to answer a complaint made by the house visitors of his sending in bad provisions'. Later in the same month, the visitors were asked in future to call at the Hospital on Wednesdays and Saturdays between 9 o'clock and 11 o'clock in the morning, so that if the meat was 'improper' it could be returned. In January 1785, however, terms were struck with a new butcher 'provided that the quality of the meat be such as shall be approved by the house visitors'.[163] In the case of malt, quantity as well as quality was at stake. During 1743, the visitors received a complaint from the Hospital brewer that 'the malt was not good'. Short weight can be inferred from a resolution of 1766 in which a proposal, linked to the price of barley at Warminster or Devizes market, was accepted with the proviso that the visitors 'see the measurement of the malt'. Neither problem was easily rectified. In 1811, the Hospital terminated a contract for malt on the grounds that the product was 'deficient in quantity and quality', and entered into an agreement with a new supplier who had 'sent a sample approved by ... [the general] court'.[164]

Advertising good practice

Such prudent monitoring of how resources were expended, even when allied to careful accounting and recording procedures, was not enough to secure the institutional embodiment of civic virtue; the propriety of the Hospital's behaviour also had to be advertised vociferously if it was to serve as a model of good practice. The publication of *Annual Reports*, and their circulation to all governors and subscribers,[165] provided a basic publicity tool and offered a safeguard against errors and misappropriation; benefactors could see that their gifts were accurately reported. Charity sermons too tackled accountability, assuring congregations that all donations were soundly deployed. As the Reverend Mr Bayly, Rector of Kilkeel in Ireland, told Bath Abbey worshippers in 1749: 'The proper application of what you give, can admit of no doubt, since the management of it is in the hands of persons of distinguished rank, fortune and character.'[166] The accounts of the Infirmary attached to published sermons reiterated its trustworthy management of expenditure: 'least anything should be charged too high, and overlooked by the treasurer', advised a statement appended to a sermon preached in 1759 by the Reverend Mr Olive of Burnham, 'every bill is inspected by gentlemen appointed for that purpose ... and the provisions are bought in by the house steward at the market, for ready money; by which means the Hospital is served with as good provisions and cheaper than any family in Bath, which any person who visits the Hospital may be convinced of'.[167] The sermons also tried to anticipate allegations of misconduct by drawing attention to special circumstances, in particular the diseconomies of scale when it was wise to keep the Infirmary only partially full and the cost, peculiar to Bath, of arranging for bathing in the spa waters.[168] During the late 1740s and the 1750s, the *Annual Reports* likewise explained that wages amounted 'to more than in other hospitals, for the same number of patients, on account of the extraordinary expenses for bathing patients, and servants for that purpose'.[169]

The financial and administrative practices of the Bath Hospital were presented to a wider audience through the pages of the press. In January 1738, a letter designed for the public papers pledged that all contributions would be 'faithfully applied to the purposes intended by the donors' and publicly acknowledged.[170] This promise of publicity, repeated in the slightly later printed 'Plan and Elevation',[171] was honoured. Large benefactions attracted their own newspaper coverage, local and national. 'We hear His Royal Highness the Prince of Wales has given one hundred pounds, to the General Hospital in this city' noted the *Bath Journal* for 30 May 1748;[172] while in February 1749, the *Gentleman's Magazine* divulged that Mr Robert Dingley, a wealthy London merchant and philanthropist, had included the Bath Infirmary among a clutch of charities to receive benefactions of £50 each.[173] Some years previously, both periodicals almost simultaneously disclosed that £500 had been received 'out of the money left by the late Lord Thanet',[174] and legacies and donations were still being reported in the local press during the 1820s.[175] More modest gifts were also broadcast. In March 1743, the weekly committee 'Ordered that a list of all the casual benefactions from 1 May last be fixed in a frame and hung in the Pump Room'.[176] Furthermore, writing to their London banker, Mr Benjamin Hoare, in February 1738, the governors requested him 'once a month [to] insert in the *Gazette* a list of what money may from time to time be paid to you for the carrying out of this charity': every contributor was to be named, and each issue containing the advertisement transmitted to the Hospital register 'for public view'. Mr Hoare was not left to his own devices, for in December 1739, the weekly committee 'Ordered that Mr Benjamin Hoare be desired to make a publication of the subscriptions received by him since his last'.[177] Presumably, there had been a lapse. Summaries of the Hospital's account with its London banker appeared in the *Gentleman's Magazine* in 1739, and in early issues of the *Bath Journal*.[178] This local paper also carried incidental reports of the sums removed from collection boxes placed at the Hospital, pump rooms and libraries[179] and regular announcements of the money raised by charity sermons.[180] Such publicity for benefactions, and for the propitious way in which affairs were managed, was not peripheral to the operation of the Infirmary. On the contrary, it was essential to its moral purpose. Alone, exemplary administrative structures and procedures were not enough. Civic virtue had to be seen to be done.

Although financial complaints about Georgian charities were not uncommon, and loomed in the press on several occasions at the neighbouring Bristol Infirmary,[181] the General Infirmary was largely successful in preserving a reputation for propriety; even the satirical critic of Bath society, Philip Thicknesse, pronounced 'the General Hospital, and another called the Pauper scheme[182] ... excellent, and well regulated charities ... highly worthy of the support of those who have the power and means, to contribute towards maintaining them'.[183] In 1819, therefore, the governors were swift to act when accusations of extravagance appeared in a paper circulated privately to the committee of the Bath Penitentiary. The author was John Parish, a former Hamburg merchant and 'eccentric philanthropist'[184] who had been president of the General Hospital in 1817. Parish alleged that when 'foreign invalids' arrived in Bath to drink the waters:

> they will be not only comfortably lodged, but that when the weather is cold, warmed rooms will be kept for them; that they will be well fed; and that the best of medical and surgical aid will be administered to their complaints: and to make their comforts complete, that the house is provided with careful *nurses* to attend them; a stud of *twelve chairmen*, to carry them to and from the baths: and to their knowing that nothing can be wanting to administer to their wants, and to their cure, they will find this spacious Hospital provided with servants, to the number of 40, to attend on 106 patients, the number limited by the Governors – FORTY SERVANTS *to attend on* ONE HUNDRED AND SIX *poor invalids*!!!

There followed a calculation which put the annual cost of such a luxurious existence at over £35 per patient, far greater than the level for other Bath charities.[185] After Mr Parish refused to retract his remarks in a counter-statement, the governors went into print, publishing the original allegations and taking them apart step by step: eight, not a dozen, chairmen were employed; their duties were broader than simply transporting patients to the bath; and the overall size of the servant community was 'immaterial' because the only relevant question was 'whether the service of any one individual could, with justice to the sick, be dispensed with'. Moreover, Mr Parish had got his sums wrong; due to under-counting the patient population and misrepresenting the Hospital's financial circumstances, he had overestimated per capita costs by more than £25.[186] In a published reply, Mr Parish denied that he had meant harm and claimed that his light treatment of the subject – the 'careless and even jocose form of expression' – was 'sufficient proof' that 'no serious and injurious attack' was intended.[187] For the Hospital governors, however, even observations thrown 'very unreservedly upon paper' for the private consumption of another philanthropic organization were sufficiently in the public domain to threaten the reputation of the institution; there was no option but to defend its 'good name' against 'fallacious and unfounded assertions'.[188]

Countering corruption

Though profligacy was a serious charge, embezzlement posed a graver threat to the respectable image of voluntary hospitals. The everyday control of financial matters was, of course, capable of picking up irregularities and proposing remedial action. At Bath, for example, the apothecary, John Morris, was unable to produce receipts for goods delivered in 1747 by Richard Walker of London and Samuel Smith of Bristol. A general court resolved that Morris himself should be answerable for all demands in respect of these items, unless he found the missing documentation. Furthermore, new procedures were introduced to prevent a recurrence, stipulating that the duty physician or surgeon should sign orders for medical supplies, and that vendors from outside Bath should appear in person to collect payment or appoint a proxy in writing.[189] To strengthen their anti-corruption brief, however, voluntary hospitals also adopted specific measures to root out abuse. In particular, the emptying of charity boxes was regulated;[190] the acceptance of gratuities forbidden;[191] inventories of furniture, linen and equipment collated;[192] bonds demanded as security from governors and paid officers with access to substantial funds or resources;[193] and steps taken to minimize conflicts of interest within the governing body.

The Bath Infirmary deployed some but not all of these mechanisms. From the point at which the Pump Room Box was installed in February 1738, the trustees agreed that at least two of the treasurers should empty it every Thursday morning and report to the next meeting. Moreover, from 1746–47 until 1778–79, *Annual Reports* named the governors responsible for opening both the Pump Room and the Hospital Boxes, after which they were simply described as 'gentlemen of the committee'.[194] The banning of gratuities was enshrined in the formal rules, which forbade fees, rewards and gratifications for services 'done on account of the Hospital'. The directive was enforced in 1743 when Mr Hyatt was 'forthwith discharged ... for having taken prerequisites contrary to the rules of this House'. But the proscription was obeyed too. In 1749, £1 from the parish of Rowde in Wiltshire was transmitted to a treasurer by the steward, who had been offered it 'as a gratuity ... for his care and trouble of a patient which sum he refused as being against the rules of the Hospital'.[195] Over and above the annual exercise that was a duty of house visitors throughout the Georgian period, inventories were carried out additionally in the late 1770s when matrons resigned or were sacked following criticism from a subcommittee investigating malpractice by a former steward.[196] There is little evidence that any of these listings uncovered embezzlement, but in April 1749 the weekly committee did order 'that the following kitchen furniture be purchased ... to make good the deficiency of the inventory taken the 25 instant, viz. 2 dozen wooden bowls, ten trenchards, 2 wooden dishes, six knives, six forks and six pewter spoons'. It was also decided to enter the linen and bathing linen in the inventory 'as they now stand',[197] perhaps insinuating that items were missing.

Bonds from governors were eschewed at the Bath Infirmary throughout the Georgian period. This was due in part to the high status of its treasurers who, unlike the local tradesmen handling the accounts at, say, Shrewsbury, were men of substance or national standing for whom such down payments might have been judged demeaning. But the governing body as a whole was also socially exclusive and hence predisposed towards the traditional notion of civic virtue based on personal integrity rather than impersonal procedure.[198] None the less, the potential for corruption was appreciated and addressed. At a meeting in 1739, the trustees endorsed 'an unlimited number of governors' for their proposed corporation on the grounds that they would not only 'render the management of this Hospital less liable to abuse but ... more especially clear it from all suspicion of monopoly or private interest'. The same gathering recommended three treasurers rather than just one, 'so that they were proper checks on each other'. A year previously the Hospital's banker had been advised to make no payments without the authorization of at least two named trustees.[199] Bonds were not originally expected of paid officers either, but upon election in 1755 Mr Noah Elliot was required 'to give £100 security for the faithful discharge of his stewardship'. This bond did not ensure his integrity and in 1773 he was dismissed for sharp practice. When a subcommittee, set up to investigate his behaviour, compared 'the list of patients kept in the Committee Room with the account of caution money' stating their date of arrival and departure, the number on the steward's list exceeded 'the real number of patients in the House upon an average above ten a week'. Discovery had been thwarted because 'he most artfully omitted the entry of one whole week's expenses, beginning his account on the 9 May instead of 2 May'. As well as perpetrating false patient records, Mr Elliot was accused in the two weeks ending 23 January 1773 of charging 'upwards of ninety pounds a week ... more [meat] than could possibly be consumed ... according to the usual allowances'; the duration of this deceit was uncertain, but there was 'reason to believe it began long before the year 1769 to which time ... the imposition' was tracked. Finally, the disgraced steward was said to have sent 'faggots and cheese from the Hospital to his own house, putting, as he pretended, the value into the box'.

Several proposals for reform resulted from this episode. First, the subcommittee suggested that in future the register and not the steward should 'keep up a full complement of patients'. Secondly, the practice of staff buying provisions from the Infirmary was disallowed, not only because it made 'an opening ... for fraud' but also because 'the article of House expenses [was] swollen beyond reality'. Thirdly, the opportunity presented by an example of abuse was seized to highlight the scope for savings if the steward paid 'due attention ... to the internal management' of the Hospital: in particular, the heavy consumption of flour and malt was noted; the purchase of raisin wine rather than its in-house distillation advocated; and the presence of a Hospital servant urged to 'see the coal weighted ... keep with the wagon till it is loaded' and so stall foul play by carriers. But it seems that the steward's role remained unsatisfactory, for in 1774 the post was abolished and his duties divided between the matron, apothecary and register.[200] Reforms of a long-term nature also flowed from a misappropriation of patients' caution money a decade later. In the autumn of 1783, following the death of a Hospital register called John Jarman, the general court resolved that future incumbents of this post should 'give security for two hundred pounds'. Simultaneously, two subcommittees were appointed, one on a permanent basis 'to inspect the caution money account every three months' and the other on a temporary basis to examine the current state of the account.[201] From the investigations of the *ad hoc* group, it transpired that the apothecary, Mr John Skuse, had since 1779 'with the connivance of the late register interfered improperly in taking upon himself to keep the account of patients' caution money'. He owed the governors over £27, which had already been deducted from his salary. However, the weekly committee concluded that his continued employment was 'incompatible with the interests of this Hospital' and he was given notice to quit.[202] The payment of 'approved sureties' by each subsequent register was normally minuted,[203] the sum rising to 'five hundred pounds' in 1805.[204] From 1792, a treasurer assumed responsibility for vetting the caution money, both periodically[205] and when the register resigned.[206]

The Bath Hospital was less pedantic than some institutions in the measures that were taken to avoid conflicts of interest within the governing body. Whereas a number of infirmaries banned paid employees from becoming governors,[207] the General Hospital relied heavily on its first apothecary, John Morris, particularly for the crucial function of house visiting. From July 1742 until his retirement in 1757,[208] he became a 'perpetual' visitor, serving almost every week along with one of the other assistants in rotation. The House Visitors Books show that as the interest of other governors waned, Mr Morris assumed more importance. Between June 1742 and November 1743, he was the sole visitor on 116 days. His isolated calls peaked at 209 in the calendar year 1755, but they still totalled 121 in 1754 and 89 in 1756. John Morris enjoyed the confidence of his fellow governors and when the general court decided in 1750 that 'no person receiving a salary from this Hospital shall be a governor', they exempted him from this stricture.[209] Yet however valuable his knowledge of day-to-day administration, during the periods that he operated alone the weekly committee lost the independent perspective that house visiting was supposed to inject.

The position of governors who supplied goods and services to their institutions was also compromised. The Bath Infirmary neither denied contractors governor status nor favoured them with a share of the relevant orders or access to a system of rotating contracts.[210] Only the printing of *Annual Reports* rotated during the long eighteenth century; and though this job was farmed out to four local printers in sequence between 1822 and 1829, they were not all governors or annual subscribers.[211] Overall, clashes of interest were rare because the governors were men of high socio-economic status who were not generally engaged in the non-luxury trades from which the Hospital purchased. However, there were apparently no qualms about buying from supporters where appropriate. Mr James Leake and Mr Charles Harford respectively sold books and paper, and deals and scaffolding to the Infirmary when they were trustees,[212] and Mr Howse continued to supply linen cloth after his appointment as governor and assistant in 1756.[213]

If few governors won commercial contracts as a result of their connections with the Bath Infirmary, the structures and procedures created to prevent corruption by paid staff were slow to unearth discrepancies: both the steward and the register were able to escape detection for several years. But these incidents of fraud – the only two recorded for the Georgian period – were not embezzlement on the grand scale of

Anthony Wingfield, who by 1799 had swindled St Thomas' Hospital in London of more than £4 000.[214] In short, supervision by a bevy of part-time governors meant that Bath shared with many voluntary infirmaries a vulnerability to comparatively minor acts of dishonesty.[215] What the General Hospital did not become was a seedbed of corruption.

In this chapter, we have examined the Bath Infirmary as a response to the mercantile conditions of post-Restoration England. Associated philanthropy has been presented as a means of bending the economic concept of the joint-stock company to charitable ends and applying it to the moral regeneration of a nation anxious about the pervasiveness of vice. This aim was pursued through administrative structures and practices which were manned by governors appointed on the basis of financial sponsorship or election. From mid-century, general courts, weekly committees and house visiting were increasingly augmented by the use of specialist subcommittees. Expert advice was also more frequently sought, and bonds demanded of senior paid staff. Finally, in 1829 an annual statement was introduced, explaining the activities of the weekly committee to the governing body as a whole. This more formal 'bourgeois'[216] or 'business-like ethos',[217] evident in the civil service from the 1780s and extended to local government in the Municipal Corporations Act of 1835, reflected the new power and influence of the middling sort whose professional and meritocratic values encouraged both a wider role for administrative specialization and outside advice, and procedural mechanisms to reinforce the personal reputations of governors and paid officers. This evolution of managerial practice coincided with the deterioration in attendance at general courts and weekly committees, which reached its lowest point in the 1790s. Throughout the Georgian period, however, there was a hard core of supporters committed to running the Hospital and they provided an adequate level of supervision which was sufficient to avoid major abuses. Therefore, the image of administrative and financial propriety, which the governors strove to sustain, was generally justified. Good management served several ends: impeccable record-keeping helped the Hospital to weather professional, political and religious conflict; open accounting brought public acclaim to benefactors and enticed them to give again. Central to the promotion of civic virtue, however, was the defusion of the ethical tensions which afflicted a commercial economy.

Notes

1. Paul Slack, *The English Poor Law 1531–1782* (London: Macmillan, 1990), p. 52. See also Paul Slack, *Poverty and Policy in Tudor and Stuart England* (London: Longman, 1988), pp. 162–9.
2. Andrew, *Philanthropy and Police*, pp. 46–9; Paul Langford, *Public Life and the Propertied Englishman 1689–1798* (Oxford: Clarendon Press, 1991), pp. 490–94; David Owen, *English Philanthropy 1660–1960* (Cambridge, MA: Harvard University Press, 1964), pp. 74, 87; Porter, 'Gift Relation', pp. 156–7.
3. Jonathan Barry, 'Bourgeois Collectivism? Urban Association and the Middling Sort', in Jonathan Barry and Christopher Brooks (eds), *The Middling Sort of People: Culture, Society and Politics in England 1550–1800* (London: Macmillan, 1994), pp. 88–95; Slack, *English Poor Law*, p. 50; Peter Clark, *Sociability and Urbanity: Clubs and Societies in the Eighteenth-Century City*, Eighth H.J. Dyos Memorial Lecture (Leicester: University of Leicester Victorian Studies Centre, 1986), pp. 6–11.
4. Borsay, *English Urban Renaissance*, pp, 154, 179, 219–21, 332–49.
5. Andrew, *Philanthropy and Police*, pp. 49–53; Owen, *English Philanthropy*, pp. 3, 11–13.
6. *Gentleman's Magazine*, 1, 11 December 1731, p. 516.
7. *Gentleman's Magazine*, 1, 19 October 1731, p. 447–8; 2, 4 February 1732, pp. 626–7.
8. Ruth McClure, *Coram's Children: The London Foundling Hospital in the Eighteenth Century* (New Haven: Yale University Press, 1981), p. 20.
9. Langford, *Polite and Commercial People*, pp. 21–2; W.A. Speck, *Stability and Strife: England 1714–1760* (London: Edward Arnold, 1977), p. 228
10. Derek Heater, *Citizenship: The Civic Ideal in World History, Politics and Education* (London: Longman, 1990), pp. 23–4, 27–32.
11. Speck, 'Conflict in Society', p. 141.
12. Pocock, *Virtue, Commerce and History*, pp. 48–50, 107–10, 121; Speck, 'Conflict in Society', pp. 135–6. See also Dickinson, *Liberty and Property*, pp. 169–75; Langford, *Public Life*, p. 482; William Stafford, *Socialism, Radicalism and Nostalgia: Social Criticism in Britain 1775–1830* (Cambridge: Cambridge University Press, 1987), pp. 78–80.
13. Lawrence Stone, 'Introduction', in Lawrence Stone (ed.), *An Imperial State at War: Britain from 1689 to 1815* (London: Routledge, 1994), p. 11.
14. H.T. Dickinson, 'Radicals and Reformers in the Age Wilkes and Wyvill', in J. Black (ed.), *British Politics and Society from Walpole to Pitt 1742–1789* (London: Macmillan, 1990), p. 129; Langford, *Polite and Commercial People*, pp. 567–8; 633; W.D. Rubinstein, 'The End of the "Old Corruption": in Britain 1780–1860', *Past and Present* **101** (1983), pp. 57, 60–64, 72–3.
15. *Gentleman's Magazine*, **81**, 5 August 1811, pp. 125–7.
16. David Dabydeen, *Hogarth, Walpole and Commercial Britain* (London: Hansib Publications, 1987), pp. 11–13; Peter Linebaugh, *The London Hanged: Crime and Civil Society in the Eighteenth Century* (Harmondsworth: Penguin Books, 1991), p. 115.

17. Pocock, *Virtue, Commerce and History*, p. 147.
18. Kathleen Wilson, 'Urban Culture and Political Activism in Hanoverian England: The Example of Voluntary Hospitals', in Eckhart Hellmuth (ed.), *The Transformation of Political Culture: England and Germany in the Late Eighteenth Century* (Oxford: Oxford University Press, 1990), pp. 173–4.
19. J. Blomfield, *St George's 1733–1933* (London: Medici Society, 1933), p. 19; A.E. Clark-Kennedy, *The London: A Study in the Voluntary Hospital System*, 2 vols (London: Pitman Medical, 1962–63), vol. 1: *1740–1840* (1962), pp. 138–9.
20. Wood, *Bath*, pp. 286, 292.
21. Letter Book, T. Carew to W. Oliver, 10 April 1739.
22. Wood, *Bath*, p. 292.
23. McClure, *Coram's Children*, pp. vii–viii, 32.
24. Keith Jenkins, *Re-Thinking History* (London: Routledge, 1991), pp. 47–50.
25. Wood, *Bath*, pp. 278–9.
26. Ibid., pp. 286.
27. Minute Book, 16 February 1738, 'Plan and Elevation'; 12 Geo. II, p. 582.
28. The London Hospital asked 30 guineas of life governors; while in the provinces, Bristol, Liverpool, Manchester and Shrewsbury each adopted a threshold of 20 guineas. See Clark-Kennedy, *The London*, p. 30; G. Munro Smith, *A History of the Bristol Royal Infirmary* (Bristol: Arrowsmith, 1917), p. 10; McLoughlin, *Liverpool Infirmary*, p. 63; Brockbank, *Royal Infirmary, Manchester*, p. 202; W.B. Howie, 'The Administration of an Eighteenth-Century Provincial Hospital: The Royal Salop Infirmary, 1747–1830', *Medical History*, 5 (1961), p. 35.
29. 12 Geo. II, p. 573.
30. 12 Geo. II, p. 585.
31. See, for example, Brockbank, *Royal Infirmary, Manchester*, pp. 202–4; Clark-Kennedy, *The London*, p. 30; Hall, Stevens and Whyman, *Kent and Canterbury Hospital*, pp. 29–31; Howie, 'Royal Salop Infirmary', pp. 36–8; McLoughlin, *Liverpool Infirmary*, pp. 63–4; P.M.G. Russell, *A History of the Exeter Hospitals 1170–1948* (Exeter: Exeter Medical Post-Graduate Institute, 1976), pp. 22–3.
32. Abel-Smith, *Hospitals*, p. 32.
33. 12 Geo. II, pp. 580–82.
34. Minute Book, 15 November 1744; 1 May 1792; 1 May 1793.
35. Minute Book, 1 May 1750; 1 May 1751.
36. Minute Book, 14 November 1750; 3 July 1751; 1 May 1754.
37. Minute Book, 15 November 1744.
38. Minute Book, 2 August 1758
39. See, for example, Minute Book, 26 March 1760; 8 October 1760; 14 April 1770; 26 November 1800; 17 November 1824.
40. Minute Book, 22 October 1783.
41. Wood, *Bath*, pp. 300–301
42. See, for example, Minute Book, 12 June 1751; 20 December 1752; 9 November 1763; 29 October 1794; 13 January 1796; 10 March 1830; 7 July 1830.
43. See, for example, Minute Book, 1 May 1754; 31 July 1754; 26 January

1757; 27 July 1791; 25 January 1792; 1 May 1792; 1 January 1793; 1 May 1806; 1 May 1818; 26 November 1828.

44. Minute Book, 25 February 1829.
45. See, for example, Minute Book, 28 October 1778; 1 May 1793; 31 July 1793; 28 October 1818; 2 May 1825; 28 October 1829; 27 October 1830.
46. See, for example, Minute Book, 24 October 1781; 22 October 1783; 29 May 1797; 1 May 1802; 11 September 1811; 28 October 1830.
47. See, for example, Minute Book, 1 May 1760; 30 March 1774; 13 April 1774; 1 May 1789; 13 February 1828; 30 July 1828; 21 April 1831.
48. See, for example, Minute Book, 1 May 1762; 18 May 1775; 21 May 1783; 1 May 1812; 1 May 1826.
49. See, for example, Brockbank, *Royal Infirmary, Manchester*, pp. 203–5; Clark-Kennedy, *The London,* p. 142; Hall, Stevens and Whyman, *Kent and Canterbury Hospital*, pp. 84–5; Howie, 'Royal Salop Infirmary', pp. 44–5; George Haliburton Hume, *The History of the Newcastle Infirmary* (Newcastle upon Tyne: Andrew Reid, 1906), pp. 24–5; McLoughlin, *Liverpool Infirmary*, pp. 66–7, 69; Philip Shemilt et al., *Salisbury 200: The Bi-Centenary of Salisbury Infirmary 1766–1966* (Salisbury: Salisbury General Hospital, 1967), p. 25.
50. Wood, *Bath,* pp. 294–6.
51. Minute Book, 13 April 1774; 30 October 1782.
52. Rules and Duties of Staff Eighteenth Century Onwards, 'House Visitors'. Minute Book, 1 June 1750; 15 June 1750.
53. Over a hundred appeared at a quarterly court of the London Infirmary in 1751 to adjudicate between competing plans for a new building; whilst at Newcastle in 1802 a special court had to adjourn to the Assembly Rooms after 240 governors arrived to debate the merits of opening fever wards at the Infirmary. See Clark-Kennedy, *The London,* p. 119; Hume, *Newcastle Infirmary*, pp. 34–5.
54. Minute Book, 16 March 1768; 30 March 1768; 13 April 1768; 27 July 1791; 17 August 1791; 28 September 1791.
55. Minute Book, 18 May 1757; 18 May 1775; 1 May 1785.
56. 12 Geo. II, p. 574.
57. *Annual Report*, 1749/50; 1829/30.
58. McMenemey, *Worcester Royal Infirmary*, p. 53. For participants in the weekly committee at the Bath Hospital, see Appendix G.
59. Minute Book, 2 May 1748. [Bath General Infirmary], 'A Short Account of the Nature, Rise and Progress of the General Infirmary at Bath', in John Dalton, *The Religious Use of the Visitation of Sickness* (Bath: Thomas Boddely, 1746), pp. 21–2; [Bath General Infirmary], 'A Short Account of the Nature, Rise and Progress of the General Infirmary at Bath', in R. Leyborne, *Charity Conducive to God's Glory: A Sermon for the Benefit of the General Hospital in Bath* (Bath: Thomas Boddely, 1754), p. 38; [Bath General Infirmary], 'A Short Account of the Nature, Rise and Progress of the General Infirmary at Bath', in R. Olive, *The Particular Excellence and True State of the Bath Infirmary* (Bristol: E. Farley, 1759), p. 32.
60. Minute Book, 15 November 1744; 9 May 1759.
61. House Visitors Book 2, 29 May 1759. Minute Book, 6 June 1759; 7 February 1781; 19 August 1801.

62. Henry Bevan, *Records of the Salop Infirmary from the Commencement of the Charity to the Present Time* (Shrewsbury: Sandford and Howell, 1847) p. 11.
63. 11 Geo. IV, *An Act for Altering and Amending an Act Passed in the Twelfth Year of the Reign of his Majesty King George the Second for Establishing and Well-Governing an Hospital or Infirmary in the City of Bath; and for Constructing Baths Therein, and Supplying the Same with Water from the Hot Baths in the Said City* (London, 1830), p. 14.
64. McClure, *Coram's Children,* p. 169; Philip Rhodes, *Dr John Leake's Hospital: A History of the General Lying-In Hospital, York Road, Lambeth 1765–1971* (London: Davis-Poynter, 1977), p. 86; Barbara Carpenter Turner, *A History of the Royal Hampshire County Hospital* (Chichester: Phillimore, 1986), p. 56.
65. W.B. Howie, 'Complaints and Complaint Procedures in the Eighteenth- and Early Nineteenth-Century Provincial Hospitals in England', *Medical History*, 25 (1981), p. 361. Similarly, senior officers took seriously the regular inspection of naval hospitals. See N.A.M. Rodger, *The Wooden World: An Anatomy of the Georgian Navy* (London: Fontana, 1986), p. 111.
66. See, for example, Minute Book, 6 May 1742; 28 November 1770; 30 July 1800; 26 May 1830.
67. Minute Book, 25 July 1744.
68. See, for example, House Visitors Book 2, 5 January 1756; 4 October 1756; 2 September 1758; 12 July 1759; 18 August 1759.
69. House Visitors Book 2, 21 December 1758; 4 April 1759.
70. Minute Book, 15 April 1767; 29 March 1786; 10 January 1787; 31 January 1787.
71. Minute Book, 21 February 1787; 9 May 1792; 2 May 1796; 1 May 1800, 1 May 1810.
72. Minute Book, 21 February 1827.
73. Wood, *Bath* p. 275.
74. Minute Book, 9 February 1738.
75. See, for example, Minute Book, 6 May 1742; 28 November 1770; 28 May 1800; 28 October 1830.
76. See, for example, Minute Book, 22 April 1767; 23 April 1800; 14 April 1831.
77. Minute Book, 21 April 1773. See also Minute Book, 28 April 1779; 25 April 1787.
78. Minute Book, 7 October 1807. See also Minute Book, 7 May 1766; 14 May 1806.
79. Minute Book, 17 May 1769; 31 May 1769. See also Minute Book, 9 December 1767.
80. Minute Book, 22 July 1801.
81. Minute Book, 7 December 1738; 21 December 1738.
82. See, for example, *Annual Report*, 1744/45; 1770/71; 1800/01; 1830/31. Minute Book, 1 May 1755; 22 April 1789; 23 April 1800; 21 April 1830.
83. See, for example, *Annual Report*, January 1739–May 1740; 1741/42; 1743/44; 1780/81.
84. Similar methods also produced accurate financial records at the Bristol,

Northampton, and Devon and Exeter Infirmaries. See Berry, 'Patronage', pp. 117–22.

85. Minute Book, 29 April 1829; 1 May 1829; 28 April 1830; 1 May 1830.
86. Minute Book, 16 June 1762; 1 June 1763. In 1770/71 ratification of the minutes was noted on four occasions, in 1785/86 on nine, in 1800/01 on two and in 1815/16 on one. During 1830/31, however, minutes were 'read' at every meeting, though the term 'confirmed' was used only once.
87. Minute Book, 18 February 1829; 25 February 1829; 18 March 1829; 15 April 1829; 29 April 1829.
88. Minute Book, 1 May 1829.
89. Minute Book, 24 February 1830; 28 July 1830.
90. Minute Book, 25 February 1829.
91. See, for example, Clark-Kennedy, *The London*, pp. 56, 121–3; Ernest R. Frizelle and Janet D. Martin, *The Leicester Royal Infirmary 1771–1971* (Leicester: Leicester No. 1 Hospital Management Committee, 1971), pp. 37–8; Charles Haskins, *The History of the Salisbury Infirmary* (Salisbury: Salisbury and District Infirmary and Hospital League, 1922), p. 3; Rhodes, *Dr John Leake's Hospital*, pp. 24–8, 93.
92. *Dictionary of National Biography* [hereafter *DNB*], vol. 18, p. 249.
93. Minute Book, 9 March 1738.
94. Minute Book, 30 March 1738.
95. Minute Book, 15 June 1738. See also Minute Book, 9 November 1738.
96. Minute Book, 3 May 1739; 24 May 1739; 16 June 1739; 16 July 1739; 27 September 1739.
97. Minute Book, 16 October 1740; 30 October 1740.
98. Minute Book, 29 September 1739; 30 May 1740.
99. Minute Book, 1 May 1741.
100. Minute Book, 6 March 1793; 1 May 1793. See also Minute Book, 3 July 1793; 8 January 1794.
101. Minute Book, 2 January 1793; 6 March 1793; 1 May 1793; 29 May 1793.
102. Minute Book, 26 November 1828. See also Minute Book, 21 January 1829.
103. Minute Book, 25 February 1829.
104. Minute Book, 15 April 1829; 1 May 1829; 27 May 1829; 17 March 1830.
105. Minute Book, 1 May 1830.
106. Minute Book, 1 May 1829.
107. See, for example, Minute Book, 26 June 1745; 31 May 1749; 28 August 1751; 28 July 1762.
108. See, for example, Minute Book, 19 June 1745; 22 February 1749; 7 February 1753; 25 June 1760.
109. See, for example, Minute Book, 21 October 1742; 14 February 1759; 26 May 1773; 18 June 1783.
110. Minute Book, 8 May 1754; 29 February 1792.
111. Minute Book, 14 February 1753.
112. Minute Book, 15 August 1750.
113. House Visitors Book 2, 14 November 1757. See also House Visitors Book 2, 27 May 1756; 10 November 1757; 6 November 1758.
114. Minute Book, 26 October 1814; 29 August 1827.
115. Minute Book, 11 October 1826; 18 October 1826.

116. Minute Book, 13 January 1796; 11 August 1819.
117. Minute Book, 21 October 1742.
118. Minute Book, 13 May 1742.
119. Minute Book, 20 May 1742; 27 May 1742.
120. Minute Book, 18 May 1743; 25 May 1743; 15 May 1744; 23 May 1744.
121. Minute Book, 6 October 1819.
122. Minute Book, 4 November 1772; 6 November 1776; 28 April 1779; 21 March 1781; 18 September 1793; 30 March 1796; 11 November 1807; 26 April 1809; 4 December 1811.
123. Minute Book, 28 October 1747; 25 November 1747; 12 October 1803. See also Minute Book, 26 May 1824.
124. See, for example, Minute Book, 5 October 1743; 18 September 1745; 7 September 1748; 19 August 1752; 22 November 1756; 19 August 1761.
125. Minute Book, 1 June 1743.
126. Minute Book, 11 October 1752; 22 November 1756.
127. Minute Book, 11 October 1752; 22 November 1756; 29 November 1758.
128. Minute Book, 28 September 1748; 12 October 1757.
129. Minute Book, 26 June 1805.
130. Minute Book, 26 November 1741.
131. Minute Book, 18 March 1742; 3 August 1748.
132. Minute Book, 11 March 1742; 14 January 1747.
133. Minute Book, 7 November 1750; 20 November 1751; 4 July 1753; 11 December 1754; 8 September 1756.
134. Minute Book, 18 July 1753; 31 July 1745. See also Minute Book, 15 November 1747.
135. Minute Book, 30 September 1747.
136. Minute Book, 24 December 1741; 3 June 1742.
137. Minute Book, 19 August 1742; 14 October 1742; 2 May 1753.
138. House Visitors Book 1, 14 August 1742; 18 October 1742; 20 October 1742; 3 December 1742; 7 December 1742; 26 June 1743. House Visitors Book 2, 16 April 1755; 22 February 1756; 5 July 1756; 21 June 1758.
139. House Visitors Book 2, 4 July 1754.
140. House Visitors Book 2, 8 September 1755.
141. House Visitors Book 2, 7 May 1759.
142. Minute Book, 4 June 1794.
143. House Visitors Book 2, 20 June 1757.
144. See, for example, House Visitors Book 1, 2 September 1742; 2 March 1743; 27 September 1743. House Visitors Book 2, 1 May 1754; 16 April 1755; 7 January 1756; 4 May 1757; 5 August 1758; 8 May 1759.
145. See, for example, House Visitors Book 1, 14 August 1742; 29 March 1743; 26 June 1743. House Visitors Book 2, 21 November 1754; 16 October 1756.
146. See, for example, House Visitors Book 2, 26 July 1754; 28 February 1756; 28 December 1757; 15 August 1758; 14 February 1759.
147. See, for example, House Visitors Book 1, 23 July 1742; 29 November 1742; 30 March 1743. House Visitors Book 2, 21 August 1754; 4 February 1755; 27 April 1756; 14 March 1758.

148. House Visitors Book 1, 16 August 1742.
149. House Visitors Book 1, 29 April 1743.
150. Minute Book, 3 July 1751. See also Minute Book, 15 November 1757.
151. House Visitors Book 2, 12 October 1757. House Visitors Book 1, 26 February 1743.
152. Wood, *Bath*, p. 296. See also Clark-Kennedy, *The London*, p. 142; McLoughlin, *Liverpool Infirmary*, pp. 69–70.
153. House Visitors Book 1, 13 September 1742; Minute Book, 16 September 1742.
154. House Visitors Book 1, 6 September 1742.
155. House Visitors Book 2, 3 April 1759. See also House Visitors Book 1, 25 June 1742; 15 July 1742; House Visitors Book 2, 30 March 1754; 28 December 1757; 4 November 1758; 10 February 1759.
156. House Visitors Book 2, 16 November 1757; 30 March 1758.
157. House Visitors Book 1, 6 September 1742.
158. House Visitors Book 1, 13 January 1743.
159. House Visitors Book 1, 18 March 1743.
160. This appears to be the case at other hospitals too. See Blomfield, *St George's*, p. 42; Brian Frith, *The Story of Gloucester's Infirmary* (Gloucester: Gloucester, Stroud and the Forest Hospital Management Committee, 1961), pp. 9, 11; Alexander George Gibson, *The Radcliffe Infirmary* (Oxford: Oxford University Press, 1926), pp. 212–14; C. Bruce Perry, *The Voluntary Medical Institutions of Bristol* (Bristol: Bristol Branch of the Historical Association, 1984), p. 3; F.F. Waddy, *A History of Northampton General Hospital 1743 to 1948* (No place of publication or publisher, 1974), pp. 62–4.
161. House Visitors Book 1, 28 September 1742. House Visitors Book 2, 12 September 1757.
162. House Visitors Book 1, 21 June. 1743; 24 June 1743; 23 July 1743. See also House Visitors Book 2, 5 September 1756.
163. Minute Book, 12 May 1784; 26 May 1784; 12 January 1785.
164. House Visitors Book 1, 19 March 1743. Minute Book, 12 March 1766; 30 October 1811.
165. See, for example, Minute Book, 25 January 1739; 8 March 1739; 20 May 1742; 1 November 1749; 1 May 1764; 2 May 1785; 1 May 1800; 1 May 1830.
166. Bayly, *Sermon*, p. 15. See also [Bath General Infirmary], 'Short Account', in Dalton, *Religious Use*, p. 21; [Bath General Infirmary], 'Short Account', in Leyborne, *Charity Conducive*, p. 38; R. Olive, *The Particular Excellence and True State of the Bath Infirmary* (Bristol: E. Farley, 1759), p. ii.
167. [Bath General Infirmary], 'Short Account', in Olive, *Particular Excellence*, p. 31. See also [Bath General Infirmary], 'A Short Account of the Nature, Rise and Progress of the General Infirmary at Bath', in E. Bayly, *A Sermon Preached at the Abbey-Church at Bath* (Bath: Thomas Boddely, 1749), p. 24; [Bath General Infirmary], 'Short Account', in Dalton, *Religious Use*, p. 21.
168. [Bath General Infirmary], 'Short Account', in Bayly, *Sermon*, p. 26; [Bath General Infirmary], 'Short Account', in Dalton, *Religious Use*, p. 22; [Bath General Infirmary], 'Short Account', in Leyborne, *Charity*

Conducive, p. 40; [Bath General Infirmary], 'Short Account', in Olive, *Particular Excellence*, p. 33.

169. See, for example, *Annual Report*, 1747/48; 1759/60.
170. Minute Book, January 1738, 'A Copy of a Letter to be Inserted in the Public Papers'.
171. Minute Book, 16 February 1738, 'Plan and Elevation'.
172. *Bath Journal*, 30 May 1748. See also *Bath Journal*, 6 June 1748; 2 October 1752.
173. *Gentleman's Magazine*, **19**, 28 February 1749, pp. 90–91.
174. *Bath Journal*, 25 February 1745; *Gentleman's Magazine*, **15**, 14 March 1745, p. 162.
175. See, for example, *Bath Journal*, 19 July 1824; 10 May 1824; 9 May 1825.
176. Minute Book, 17 March 1743.
177. Minute Book, 2 February 1738, 'Copy of a Letter to Mr Benjamin Hoare, Banker in Fleet Street, London'; 13 December 1739.
178. *Gentleman's Magazine*, **9**, 28 February 1739, p. 105. Bath *Journal*, 7 January 1745; 7 April 1745.
179. *Bath Journal*, 4 April 1760; 8 May 1786; 10 May 1824.
180. See, for example, *Bath Journal*, 5 November 1744; 9 May 1748; 17 May 1756; 10 December 1759; 24 May 1762; 6 November 1762; 2 December 1765; 7 May 1770; 12 November 1770; 8 May 1786; 25 December 1786; 10 May 1824.
181. Smith, *Bristol Royal Infirmary*, pp. 88, 95–7, 111, 120–21, 152–3.
182. The Pauper Scheme was founded in 1747 to offer outdoor medical assistance to the sick poor of Bath who were excluded from the General Hospital. See Hembry, *English Spa*, p. 272.
183. Philip Thicknesse, *The New Prose Bath Guide for the Year 1778* (printed for the author), pp. 102–3.
184. R.E.M. Peach, *Bath, Old and New: A Handy Guide and a History* (London: Simpkin, Marshall and Co., 1888), p. 160. See also Rowland Mainwaring, *Annals of Bath from the Year 1800 to the Passing of the New Municipal Act*, (Bath: Meyler, 1838), p. 306.
185. *Report of a Committee Appointed by the Governors of the Bath General Hospital, to Examine a Statement Circulated by Mr Parish, Respecting the Finances and Administration of that Institution* (Bath: Cruttwell, 1819), pp. 3–4, 6–7.
186. Minute Book, 8 July 1819; 28 July 1819; 27 October 1819. *Report of a Committee*, pp. iii–iv, 16–22.
187. *Letter to the President and Governors of the Bath General Hospital from J. Parish, Esq.* (Bath: Wood, 1819), pp. 5–6.
188. *Report of a Committee*, p. 24.
189. Minute Book, 1 May 1747. See also Minute Book, 3 November 1762.
190. See, for example, Blomfield, *St George's*, p. 205; Brockbank, *Royal Infirmary, Manchester*, p. 205; Peter Eade, *The Norfolk and Norwich Hospital 1770–1900* (London: Jarrold and Sons, 1900), p. 215; W.B. Howie, 'Finance and Supply in an Eighteenth-Century Hospital' *Medical History*, 7 (1963), p. 135; McLoughlin, *Liverpool Infirmary*, p. 70.
191. See, for example, Brockbank, *Royal Infirmary, Manchester*, pp. 32, 205; Eade, *Norfolk and Norwich Hospital*, p. 215; McLoughlin, *Liverpool*

Infirmary, p. 68; Russell, *Exeter Hospitals*, p. 26; Turner, *Hampshire County Hospital*, p. 19; Waddy, *Northampton General Hospital*, p. 16.

192. See, for example, Brockbank, *Royal Infirmary, Manchester,* p. 205; McLoughlin, *Liverpool Infirmary*, p. 69.
193. See, for example, S.T. Anning, *The General Infirmary at Leeds*, 2 vols (Edinburgh: Livingstone, 1963–66), vol. 1: *The First Hundred Years 1767–1869* (1963), p. 57; Brockbank, *Royal Infirmary, Manchester,* pp. 17, 202; Clark-Kennedy, *The London*, p. 85; Eade, *Norfolk and Norwich Hospital*, p. 212; Frizelle and Martin, *Leicester Royal Infirmary*, p. 42; Howie, 'Royal Salop Infirmary', pp. 42, 43; McLoughlin, *Liverpool Infirmary*, pp. 26, 63–4; McMenemey, *Worcester Royal Infirmary*, pp. 58–9; Smith, *Bristol Royal Infirmary*, pp. 101, 145; Arthur Rook, Margaret Carlton and W. Graham Cannon, *The History of Addenbrooke's Hospital, Cambridge* (Cambridge: Cambridge University Press, 1991), p. 34.
194. Minute Book, 23 February 1738. See, for example, *Annual Report*, 1746/47; 1760/61; 1778/79; 1800/01; 1830/31.
195. Wood, *Bath*, p. 295. Minute Book, 1 June 1743; 2 August 1749.
196. Minute Book, 19 November 1777; 24 June 1778.
197. Minute Book, 26 April 1749.
198. Howie, 'Royal Salop Infirmary', p. 43. See also Hilary Marland, *Medicine and Society in Wakefield and Huddersfield 1780–1880* (Cambridge: Cambridge University Press, 1987), p. 139.
199. Letter Book, undated, E. Brett to T. Carew. Minute Book, 2 February 1738, 'Copy of a Letter to Mr Benjamin Hoare, Banker in Fleet Street, London'.
200. Minute Book, 29 October 1755; 6 January 1773; 24 February 1773; 6 April 1774.
201. Minute Book, 22 October 1783.
202. Minute Book, 3 March 1784.
203. Minute Book, 24 October 1792; 1 September 1802; 26 February 1812; 1 March 1826.
204. Minute Book, 13 February 1805.
205. See, for example, Minute Book, 28 November 1792; 1 May 1795; 29 January 1800; 6 February 1805; 17 October 1810; 28 August 1816; 21 November 1821; 20 December 1826; 31 March 1831.
206. Minute Book, 1 March 1826.
207. See, for example, Clark-Kennedy, *The London*, pp. 87, 141; Rhodes, *Dr John Leake's Hospital*, p. 43.
208. Minute Book, 2 May 1757.
209. Minute Book, 1 May 1750.
210. Contractors were excluded at Addenbrooke's Hospital, but governors who supplied the Salop and the Norfolk and Norwich Hospitals were given preferential treatment over their competitors. See Rook, Carlton and Cannon, *Addenbrooke's Hospital*, p. 34; Howie, 'Finance and Supply', p. 142; Eade, *Norfolk and Norwich Hospital*, p. 71.
211. Minute Book, 1 May 1822; 1 May 1823; 1 May 1824; 2 May 1825; 1 May 1826; 1 May 1827; 1 May 1828; 1 May 1829. The names of governors and subscribers were listed in the *Annual Reports*.
212. *Annual Report*, January 1739–May 1740. Minute Book, 8 February 1739.

213. Minute Book, 11 March 1742; 23 January 1754; 11 November 1760; 3 February 1761. *Annual Report*, 1749/50; 1755/56.
214. F.G. Parsons, *The History of St Thomas's Hospital*, 3 vols (London: Methuen, 1932–36), vol. 2: *From 1600–1800* (1934), p. 254. See also McMenemey, *Worcester Royal Infirmary*, p. 172; Hilary St George Saunders, *The Middlesex Hospital 1745–1948* (London: Max Parrish, 1949), p. 16.
215. Anning, *General Infirmary at Leeds*, p. 64; Brockbank, *Royal Infirmary, Manchester*, p. 45; Clark-Kennedy, *The London*, p. 84; Howie, 'Finance and Supply', p. 135; McMenemey, *Worcester Royal Infirmary*, pp. 58–9, 153, 195; Rook, Carlton and Cannon, *Addenbrooke's Hospital*, p. 75.
216. Langford, *Public Life*, p. 582.
217. Penelope J. Corfield, *Power and the Professions in Britain 1700–1850* (London: Routledge, 1995), pp. 193, 211–12.

CHAPTER THREE

The Achievement of Financial Solvency

In Chapter 2, we considered the ways in which the Georgian Bath Infirmary was able to allay fears of corruption by developing exemplary administrative structures and procedures. The upsurge in post-Restoration trade which commercialized the British economy and exposed the monied interest to moral disapprobation also ignited economic growth and prepared the ground for the Agricultural and Industrial Revolutions which were to forge increasing prosperity after 1700. If the long-term path was upwards, however, intermittent crises continued to intrude as war, and the economic consequences of peace, aggravated the effects of population growth and food shortages. Chapter 3 assesses the effectiveness with which the General Hospital responded to the financial as opposed to the ethical conditions of a commercial economy. First, the crude balance between revenue and expenditure is related to broad economic trends. Secondly, the Hospital's costs are broken down and strategies for their containment scrutinized. Finally, the changing pattern of income is teased out and the methods used to generate funds are investigated.

Balancing the books

The Bath Infirmary was a long time in gestation. First mooted in 1711, it was 1723 before a subscription opened and 1742 before patients were admitted. Finding a suitable site was a stumbling block: an increase in the projected size of the institution led to the abandonment of one conveyance; another offer was accepted, only to be decreed void for procedural reasons; and it was not until 1737 that the trustees decided to buy the former playhouse, together with adjacent properties. However, funds as well as land proved problematic. The 1723 subscription raised under £300. A second appeal was launched in 1731, but by the end of 1737 income had accumulated to just £379. 10s. Simultaneously, estimated costs were rising. The 1731 figure of £2 500 to purchase the ground and erect and furnish the Hospital had grown to £6 000 by the time the trustees fixed on the site; and even when the builders took up their tools in April 1738, a mere £2 000 had been collected.[1] Starting work was an act of faith. Since no archival sources survive for the early years of the Infirmary, we have to rely on John Wood's *Description of Bath*. Closely involved with the scheme, Wood attributed much to his own dynamism and claimed that the charity remained in a 'languishing state' until he settled in the city in 1727.[2] Yet not only did a decade lapse between his intervention and the commencement of building, but the initial stages of the Bath proposal were not dissimilar to the experience of other voluntary hospitals. Even the Westminster Infirmary – the founder member of the movement which dated from 1716 – allocated its initial funds to sick debtors in the London prisons and when patients were admitted in 1720, it was to rented premises. Many Georgian foundations likewise evolved gradually.[3] At Bath, however, the trustees were committed to a purpose-built infirmary and the small amount set aside in 1723 'for the use of poor people at that time in the city' had been incorporated into the construction fund when the first *Annual Report* appeared in January 1739. The plan for specially designed premises sat uneasily with the volatile early eighteenth-century economy, especially disrupted by bad harvests during the 1720s.[4] This economic instability, when combined with the experimental nature of voluntary hospitals, led the Bath trustees to share the fate of other medical philanthropists whose ambitions for dedicated facilities were frustrated by delay.[5]

The publication of *Annual Reports* from the late 1730s enables us to locate the finances of the General Infirmary more firmly within their economic context. In his study of Bristol, Martin Gorsky could find no unequivocal relationship between the economic histories of local charities and the trade cycle for the port.[6] There are no convenient serial indicators for the Bath economy. However, setting levels of income against levels of expenditure, at five-yearly intervals after 1745/46, suggests that financial problems of the General Hospital broadly coincided with crises in the national economy (Table 3.1). The deficits of the early 1740s may have been primarily due to construction costs and the 'teething problems' of running a brand new institution; certainly, the building programme stretched other voluntary hospitals to breaking-point, compelling them to take out loans or stop work altogether.[7] None the less, grain shortages, an extended national debt and the disruption of trade by almost a decade of war after 1739 meant that the nascent Infirmary was also working in a harsh economic climate.[8] Furthermore, revenue shortfalls did not disappear after the Hospital had found its feet. In May 1755, the general court revoked a previous decision to divert substantial benefactions to a capital fund, ordering instead that 'all sums whatsoever given or bequeathed to this Hospital be applied to the running cash unless particularly directed ... otherwise

Table 3.1 Bath General Hospital: income and expenditure, 1738–1830

Year	*Income* £	*Expenditure* £	*Balance* £
1738/39	3 554.90	1 725.75	+1 829.15
1739/40	1 305.50	1 859.85	–554.35
1740/41	362.85	1 488.65	–1 125.80
1741/42	2 979.40	950.00	+2 029.40
1742/43	1 629.25	2 001.35	–372.10
1743/44	1 305.85	1 815.35	–509.50
1744/45	2 443.30	1 059.05	+1 384.25
1745/46	1 864.20	1 002.80	+861.40
1750/51	1 710.25	1 302.75	+407.50
1755/56	1 871.10	1 554.35	+316.75
1760/61	957.55	1 189.80	–232.25
1765/66	1 833.05	1 553.60	+279.45
1770/71	2 956.55	1 511.30	+1 445.25
1775/76	1 524.60	1 648.60	–124.00
1780/81	1 704.50	1 967.20	–262.70
1785/86	3 013.45	1 952.50	+1 060.95
1790/91	2 907.30	2 160.55	+746.75
1795/96	2 674.95	2 741.70	–66.75
1800/01	3 386.50	3 620.55	–234.05
1805/06	2 716.15	3 271.60	–555.45
1810/11	3 258.35	3 609.15	–350.80
1815/16	5 199.25	3 427.05	+1 772.20
1820/21	3 573.00	3 281.30	+291.70
1825/26	3 362.65	3 507.15	–144.50
1830/31	4 227.05	4 747.55	–520.50

Note: The first set of Hospital accounts covers the period from foundation until 15 January 1738/39, and the second set runs from this date until 30 April 1740. Thereafter, the financial year begins on 1 May.

Source: *Annual Reports*.

... by the donor'.[9] By the later 1750s, the *Annual Report* was drawing attention to the depletion of existing capital funds, noting in 1757/58 that the sale of bonds and annuities to meet outgoings had 'reduced the capital near one thousand pounds in two years'.[10] These strains, visible in the annual deficit for 1760/61, coincided with a bad harvest and the Seven Years War, both of which struck in 1756. Though trade was less damaged than in earlier Hanoverian hostilities, the unprecedented demand for capital so inflated taxation and the cost of borrowing that the war has been blamed for the major depression of 1761/62.[11] Economic turbulence was a characteristic of the 1770s too. Food prices, high in 1766 and 1767, also rose in 1772 and 1774. Important London banks collapsed during the financial crisis of 1772, seriously undermining the nation's monetary stability. And in 1775 the American War of Independence broke out, temporarily derailing transatlantic trade and generating huge war loans.[12] In Bath wartime shortages and rocketing prices led to fears of mob violence, and encouraged the formation of a Provisions Committee during 1779 to buy food and coal for the poor with charitable subscriptions.[13] The General Hospital rode out the storm, but only by continuing to divert legacies from the capital to the revenue account when resources were tight. The sample years reveal annual deficits in 1775/76 and 1780/81. Thereafter, cash flow problems intensified. In December 1782, the treasurers were paid 'an interest of 5 per cent ... for what monies have been advanced by them since the 1st of May last for the use of the House'. The next spring, annuities worth over £500 were also sold 'to make good the arrears due to the treasurers'.[14]

Bath's financial history was not a unique one, cash crises being documented for other infirmaries after 1750.[15] Faced with the Napoleonic Wars, however, and their associated economic hardships, these difficulties paled into insignificance. To foot the colossal bill for military expenditure between 1793 and 1815, the government pushed up taxation to unprecedented levels and borrowed heavily. Industry, agriculture and trade were also thrown into disarray by the conflict, and grain prices fluctuated wildly, particularly when fears of a blockade were compounded by poor harvests between 1795 and 1800, and 1808 and 1812.[16] With economic upheaval of such magnitude, many voluntary hospitals were subjected to acute financial pressure and periodically became overdrawn.[17] At Bath, the General Hospital was being extended when war erupted. Both local banks and the property market went into crisis during the 1790s,[18] but extra patients were admitted to the Infirmary as planned in 1795 and only one of the two new wards was closed as an economy measure two years later.[19] During the first phase of the battle against Napoleon, shortfalls were tackled by the usual direction of bequests to current expenditure.[20] From 1795/96, the quinquennial sample of balance sheets registers a growing deficit, and between 1807 and 1811 the Minute Books record that the governors were forced to liquidize capital assets to settle outstanding debts, disposing of almost £4 000 in bank annuities.[21] However, the survival of the local tourist trade afforded a degree of protection from the financial ravages of the conflict[22] and by 1815 the Infirmary had accumulated a substantial surplus. The wars were ambivalent in their economic ramifications, depressing some sectors of the economy while stimulating others; and, therefore, the cessation of hostilities worked no miracles. A deep recession, triggered by a glut of production and plummeting prices, delayed recovery until 1820, and by the middle of the decade the Bath Infirmary, along with other institutions,[23] was sliding into deficit as the post-war return to prosperity was interrupted by a short-term slump and banking crisis. Economic depression was similarly a backdrop to the political turmoil that preceded the Great Reform Act of 1832.[24] But though the Bath Infirmary ended the long eighteenth century with annual costs outstripping income, the premises had recently undergone a major refurbishment. It was the governors' proud boast that the expense of this exercise, more than £2 800, was financed without 'encroaching upon the capital of the Hospital'.[25]

Patterns of expenditure

To understand how the Bath Infirmary weathered the vagaries of the Georgian economy, we must delve beyond the broad correlation of crises to unravel expenditure patterns and sources of income. After 1742/43, the *Annual Report* consistently divided expenditure into four main categories: Hospital expenses (e.g. construction, improvement and repair costs, furniture, insurance, ground and water rents); wages for the apothecary, register, steward, matron, nurses, chairmen, bath guides, and other 'menial servants'; drugs and spirits for the apothecary's shop; and House expenses (e.g. provisions, printing and stationery, legal services). The most substantial miscellaneous items were clothing for the porter and chairmen, and 'bathing apparel' for the patients and their guides. Hospital expenses, which explained the lion's share of expenditure up to 1742,[26] accounted for just 5 to 10 per cent of outgoings after the premises were finished – unless, as in the late 1820s, a special project was under way (Table 3.2). Conversely, the cost of wages, drugs and House expenses had a greater bearing on the Infirmary's vacillating financial fortunes because, whereas building and repair work could be scheduled according to the available resources, revenue elements within the budget were more open to blows from the economy.

Strategies for cost containment, and for the generation of additional income, were shaped both by the routine administrative structure,[27] and by special general courts[28] and specialized subcommittees.[29] Among the methods selected to clip revenue costs was the reduction of patient numbers. Since admission was by medical recommendation rather than by lay sponsorship, the governors were free to follow the common practice of opening and closing beds in response to funding[30] without upsetting donors by restricting their powers of patronage. In his *Description of Bath*, John Wood wrote of an Infirmary capable of holding 150 patients, but the Minute Books suggest that 112 beds were accommodated.[31] It is not clear how many inmates were originally admitted, but in 1744 financial exigency prompted a cut in the quota resident at any one time, first to 40 for the ensuing year and then to 45 following a benefaction from Francis Colston. Annual admissions gradually climbed until in 1751 the governors permitted a full House, comprising 63 male and 49 female patients. But this reprieve was temporary. In 1757 an upper limit of 90 patients was imposed, going down to 70 the next year and not again attaining the maximum for a decade. A subsequent decision to cut the intake was rescinded in 1783 after publicity about the Hospital's plight attracted the necessary funds. However, the governors were compelled to close between 20 and 30 beds as the Napoleonic Wars took their toll in the later 1790s,[32] although a full complement of patients was consistently authorized after 1800.[33] The closure of beds was not uniform in its impact upon revenue expenditure. As the governors themselves appreciated, wages were relatively inelastic and created diseconomies of scale; costs were high, argued an account of the Infirmary attached to a charity sermon of 1749, because with the small number of patients 'we can prudently admit ... the expense of servants will be very near the same ... as it would be if we had a much greater number'.[34] None the less, when running the new Hospital produced two consecutive deficits in the early 1740s, staff wages were included in the repertoire of responses. The nursing quota, pruned from nine to four in 1744, was again a target in 1758 when, after an enquiry by the physicians and surgeons, three of the nine nurses were discharged. The post of steward was also abolished in 1774 and his duties redistributed to the matron, apothecary and register.[35] But despite its popularity across the hospital sector,[36] the impact of rationalizing staff was limited. Not only were wage rates moving against the lower orders from the mid-eighteenth century,[37] but at Bath the wage bill absorbed a declining share of the annual budget after 1750 (Table 3.2). Of far more consequence were spiralling prices.

Both medical supplies and House expenses were exposed to inflation. Apart from an early burst of expenditure in the mid-1740s, the apothecary's shop ate up a steady 3 to 7 per cent of the yearly budget. Elsewhere, the figures were higher. At Edinburgh, with its prestigious medical school, 'drug-related expenses amounted to 22% of the total hospital outlays' in 1770, before inexplicably falling back to 8 per cent in 1800. At the Bristol, Northampton, and Devon and Exeter Hospitals – with no medical schools – spending on medical goods came second

Table 3.2 Bath General Hospital: patterns of expenditure, 1742–1830

Year	*Hospital expenses*		*Wages*		*Apothecary's shop*		*Household expenses*		*Other*		*Total*	
	£	%	£	%	£	%	£	%	£	%	£	%
1742/43	1 111.35	55.53	220.65	11.03	118.10	5.90	548.70	27.42	2.55	0.13	2 001.35	100.00
1743/44	391.35	21.56	328.85	18.12	60.90	3.36	1 034.25	56.97	—	—	1 815.35	100.00
1744/45	96.80	9.14	370.05	34.94	122.60	11.58	469.60	44.34	—	—	1 059.05	100.00
1745/46	60.00	5.98	317.95	31.71	29.60	2.95	568.70	56.71	26.55	2.65	1 002.80	100.00
1750/51	87.70	6.73	366.80	28.16	67.05	5.15	728.25	55.90	52.95	4.07	1 302.75	100.00
1755/56	118.95	7.65	389.55	25.06	89.00	5.73	908.00	58.42	48.85	3.14	1 554.35	100.00
1760/61	95.95	8.06	346.30	29.11	64.35	5.41	683.20	57.42	—	—	1 189.80	100.00
1765/66	98.20	6.32	364.60	23.47	58.95	3.79	1 031.85	66.42	—	—	1 553.60	100.00
1770/71	74.15	4.91	369.70	24.46	47.10	3.12	1 020.15	67.50	0.20	0.01	1 511.30	100.00
1775/76	90.00	5.46	389.20	23.61	63.25	3.84	1 105.70	67.07	0.45	0.03	1 648.60	100.00
1780/81	429.85	21.85	391.20	19.89	83.35	4.24	1 062.80	54.03	—	—	1 967.20	100.00
1785/86	225.60	11.55	390.70	20.01	136.60	7.00	1 199.60	61.44	—	—	1 952.50	100.00
1790/91	198.95	9.21	395.05	18.29	152.95	7.08	1 413.60	65.43	—	—	2 160.55	100.00
1795/96	180.75	6.59	447.45	16.32	182.30	6.65	1 931.20	70.44	—	—	2 741.70	100.00
1800/01	204.50	5.65	440.00	12.15	174.95	4.83	2 801.10	77.37	—	—	3 620.55	100.00

1805/06	262.45	8.02	460.95	14.09	195.90	5.99	2 352.30	71.90	—	—	3 271.60	100.00
1810/11	274.05	7.59	459.35	12.73	179.10	4.96	2 696.65	74.72	—	—	3 609.15	100.00
1815/16	338.55	9.88	492.20	14.36	177.90	5.19	2 417.40	70.54	1.00	0.03	3 427.05	100.00
1820/21	351.60	10.72	486.55	14.83	193.60	5.90	2 248.25	68.52	1.30	0.04	3 281.30	100.00
1825/26	326.65	9.31	504.40	14.38	203.10	5.79	2 406.75	68.62	66.25	1.89	3 507.15	100.00
1830/31	2 010.95	42.36	731.35	15.41	160.55	3.38	1 737.75	36.60	106.95	2.25	4 747.55	100.00

Notes:

1. Household expenses may have been inflated by staff taking items for their personal use and placing the money in the Hospital Box. See Minute Book, 24 Feb 1773.
2. Among the items in the 'other' category of expenditure were surgical expenses (1742/43); staff clothing (1745/46, 1750/51 and 1755/56); bathing apparel (1750/51); letters of attorney (1770/71 and 1825/26); unspecified profit and loss (1775/76); forged bank notes and base coins found in donations and subscriptions (1815/16, 1820/21 and 1825/26); payments to Economic Life Assurance Society (1825/26 and 1830/31); 'five annuities under the will of the late Dr. Perry' (1830/31); and legal and administrative costs incurred in running the Charmy Down Estate (1825/26 and 1830/31).
3. Percentages have been rounded up or down and so do not always total exactly 100.00.

Source: *Annual Reports*.

only to provisions, while the dispensary at the Salop Infirmary accounted for a fifth of total costs throughout the second half of the eighteenth century and the decadal average between 1747 and 1836 never dropped below 12 per cent.[38] Its small budgetary share may explain why the apothecary's shop at Bath was less prone to the retrenchment that many voluntary infirmaries imposed, particularly from the 1790s.[39] Only two such savings are minuted: an attempt in 1773 to reduce the cost of raisin wine by replacing inhouse distillation with outside purchase,[40] and a request, included in the *Annual Report* from 1785/86, for 'ladies, and others ... to send old linen ... for lint and rollers'. The modest bill which largely exempted the apothecary's shop from economy measures may reflect the role of spa therapy in complementing conventional remedies at Bath. But at neither Edinburgh nor the provincial hospitals did expenditure on drugs and surgery fit neatly with any intensification of clinical practice in the late eighteenth century.[41]

If the income devoted to drugs, spirits and appliances was atypical, Bath's experience of grappling with household costs was more representative of the hospital movement in general. Any financial honeymoon after the Infirmary opened was short-lived; for between 1743 and 1744, housekeeping costs plummeted from over £1 000 to under £500 – a fall disproportionate to the drop in staff and patient numbers.[42] With the outbreak of the Napoleonic Wars, the governors implemented emergency measures focusing on the shortage of grain. In January 1796, a general court agreed 'unanimously that the bread to be used ... for the ensuing month be made of two third parts of wheaten flour, and one third part of barley flour'. In April a new 'wheat mill and dressing machine ... [was] fixed up in the Servants' Hall'; and in September 'standard wheaten flour' became the sole ingredient of Hospital bread for the trial period of a fortnight. Finally, 1801 saw the governors requesting 'five barrels of American flour ... [for] an experiment to be made ... according to the usual mode of baking'. A few months before, the physicians and surgeons had approved a drop in the allocation of bread per patient, to be compensated by 'a small addition of potatoes'. It seems that throughout the wars economies at Bath were confined to corn-based products with no switch from high to low protein foods. In the late 1820s, however, weekly ceilings were prescribed for the consumption of meat which other hospitals had included in their rationing strategies during the conflict.[43]

Apart from these isolated efforts to deal with exceptional circumstances, governors at Bath apparently left the management of household costs to their routine procedures. This does not imply a static position. On the contrary, House expenses shot up during the second half of the long eighteenth century, to peak at almost 80 per cent of annual outgoings in 1800/01 before dropping back to two-thirds in the 1820s (Table 3.2). Relating housekeeping costs to the incidence of inflation confirms that the Napoleonic Wars were a point of crisis. Figure 3.1 compares Tucker's consumer goods index with household expenditure, controlling for the size of the patient body but not for resident staff. When 1745 is taken as the base line, we find that after falling in the 1750s at a time when overall prices were rising, the Hospital's house expenses index broadly followed the trend line for consumer goods and by 1790 had exceeded its original value. At its highest in 1800, the house expenses index came close to the Tucker index and the two indices virtually touched again during the peacetime troubles of the mid-1820s. Wartime inflation aggravated an established and continuing pattern of accelerating Hospital expenses.

Yet although household costs were mounting at the General Infirmary, their rate of increase was generally slower than the overall rate of inflation. Consumer prices grew by almost 60 per cent between 1745 and 1830, house expenses per Bath patient by less than 40 per cent, and whereas the house expenses index had almost returned to its 1790 level by 1830, the consumer goods index rose by over 20 per cent. A shortage of equivalent published data makes comparison with other institutions difficult. At the Edinburgh Infirmary, where household costs consumed a similar proportion of the annual budget between 1770 and 1800, house expenses per patient more than doubled in line with the increase at Bath during the same period (Table 3.3). With such a narrow time scale, however, neither the long-term effects for inflation nor the short-term effects of the Napoleonic Wars can be properly assessed. Technical problems in measuring the movement of prices likewise dictate caution. Tucker's index, while encompassing the long eighteenth century (and beyond), is dated; and his basket of consumer goods, while using the prices paid for supplies at the Greenwich, Chelsea and Bethlem Hospitals,[44] may better replicate the structure of domestic than institutional expenditure. Nevertheless, even after these reservations have been borne in mind, there are grounds for concluding tentatively that, with isolated exceptions, the Bath Infirmary was successful in holding household expenses below the rate of inflation. Given evidence that the city experienced particularly high prices,[45] this was no mean achievement.

Generating income

If the Georgian economy exerted inflationary pressure on the costs of the Bath Infirmary, its steady growth released surplus income and dispersed it in the direction of the middling sort. The trustees and governors

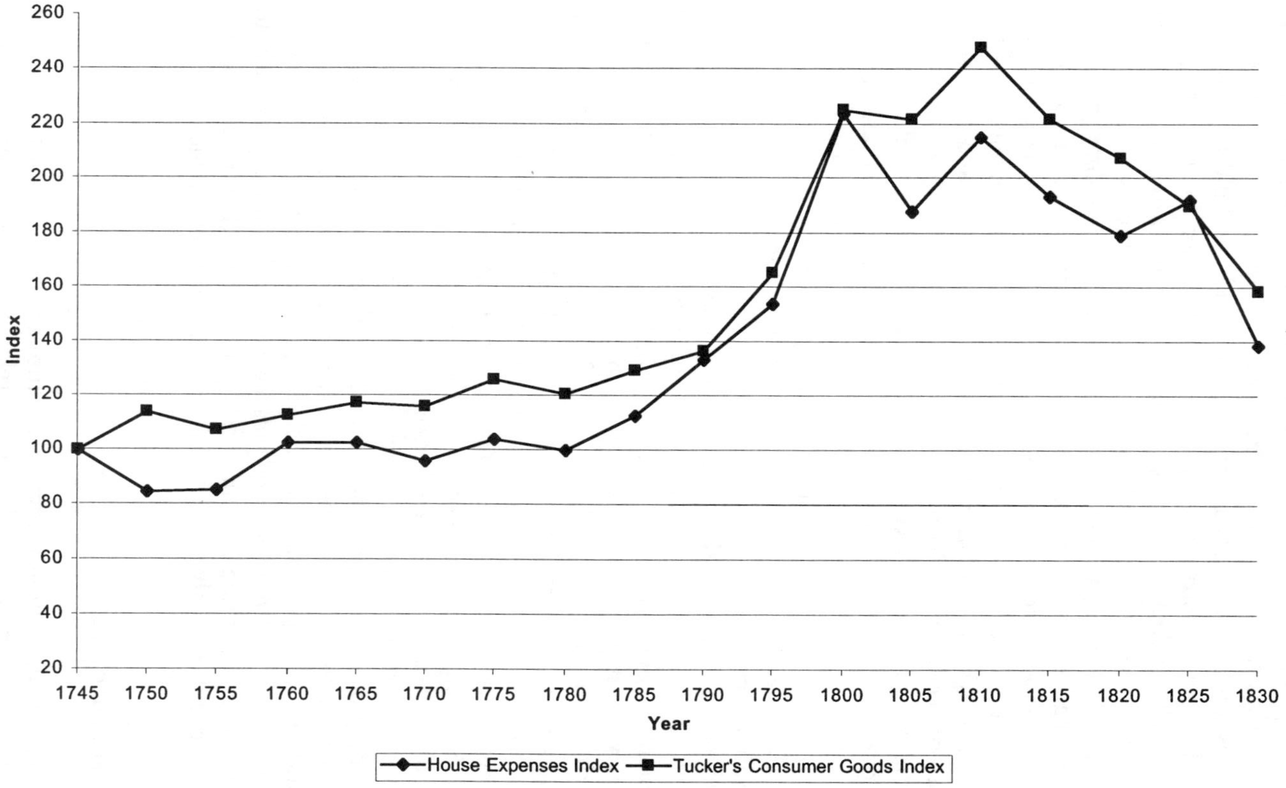

3.1 Bath General Hospital: a comparison of house expenses and the price of consumer goods, 1745–1830

Notes:

1. The annual quota of patients was determined at the May general court and recorded in the Minute Book. In 1750/51 a gift of Old South Sea annuities from Lord Coleraine permitted an additional admission (Minute Book, 2 August 1749; 1 May 1750); and an improving financial situation led to a mid-year increase of 20 patients (Minute Book, 31 October 1750), which has been incorporated into the annual figure. The quota rise in 1795/96 reflects the opening of the attic storey (Minute Book, 4 February 1795; 4 November 1795).
2. 1745/46 has been taken as the base year for the house expenses index and the values for subsequent years stated in proportion to the value of the base year i.e.

$$\text{house expenses index} = \frac{he_1}{he_0} \times 100$$

Sources: *Annual Reports*. R.S. Tucker 'Real Wages of Artisans in London, 1729–1935', in Arthur J. Taylor (ed.), *The Standard of Living in Britain in the Industrial Revolution* (London: Methuen, 1975), pp. 27–9. The consumer goods index has been recalculated with 1745 as the base year.

were energetic in attempting to tap these resources and quick to develop marketing tactics to generate income. Unhappy with an early 'Address to the Public' which appeared in the national press in 1738, the trustees transmitted precise directions as to its subsequent layout and location, using one of their number – Bath Master of Ceremonies, Richard Beau Nash – who was in London:

> the public notice of this charity, instead of being inserted in a small letter among the public advertisements, may for the future be the first article after the foreign news, for we are apprehensive that as it now stands 'twill be slightly passed over by some and not read by others.[46]

Such attention to detail was vital because coverage was intensive and the announcement occurred 'every other day in three ... papers for three months'.[47] In addition to carrying proposals,[48] the press reported news of voluntary hospitals[49] which included the foundation-stone ceremony for the Bath Infirmary, held in July 1738: an occasion of sufficient country-wide interest to merit an item in the *London Evening Post* as well as the *Gentleman's Magazine*,[50] which was editorially committed to the movement.[51] The press was also valuable for highlighting financial pressure. Therefore, when the governors were forced to close beds in 1797, they ordered that 'the resolution ... stating the reasons for reducing the number of patients be inserted in the ... Bath papers, in the Salisbury, Gloucester, Sherborne, one of the Bristol papers and in the *Sun*, and *Star*, once in each'.[52] But even the publication of routine administrative information – the charter,[53] reports of meetings and

Table 3.3 Edinburgh Infirmary and Bath General Hospital: a comparison of house expenses and the price of consumer goods, 1770–1800

Year	*Edinburgh Infirmary*						*Bath house expenses index*	*Tucker's consumer goods index*
	Total annual expenditure	*Total house expenses*		*Annual quota of places*	*House expenses per patient*	*House expenses index*		
	£	£	%					
1770	2 283.45	1 277.60	55.95	132	9.68	100.00	100.00	100.00
1775	2 479.00	1 501.55	60.57	167	8.99	92.90	108.30	108.60
1780	2 416.70	1 496.40	61.92	168	8.91	92.10	104.20	103.80
1785	2 713.35	1 849.45	68.16	170	10.88	112.40	117.60	111.10
1790	3 137.85	2 165.50	69.01	128	16.92	174.80	138.50	117.60
1795	3 374.40	2 406.75	71.32	146	16.49	170.40	160.60	142.40
1800	5 079.80	3 953.70	77.83	169	23.40	241.70	232.90	193.80

Notes:

1. 1770 has been taken as the base year for the house expenses indices of both institutions and the values for subsequent years stated in proportion to the value of the base year i.e.

$$\text{house expenses index} = \frac{he_1}{he_0} \times 100$$

2. The house expenses total used for the Edinburgh Infirmary includes the following categories: 'plenishing and utensils'; 'coal and candles'; and 'maintenance', which is assumed to cover food, clothing, and other supplies and services not itemized in the accounts. The annual quota relates to the number of in-patients on 1 January in each year.

Sources: *Annual Reports*. Guenter B. Risse, *Hospital Life in Enlightenment Scotland: Care and Teaching at the Royal Infirmary of Edinburgh* (Cambridge: Cambridge University Press, 1986), p. 40, table 1.3; pp. 46–8, table 1.4. Tucker, 'Real Wages of Artisans in London, 1729–1935', pp. 27–9.

personnel,[54] and details of contributions – had publicity spin-offs, especially if there was a human touch; in 1762, for instance, the *Bath Journal* noted in relaying the sum deposited in the Pump Room Box, that it 'included five guineas, as a very small, but grateful return, for the great care and tenderness shown in this Hospital, during a long troublesome illness to a gentleman reduced to narrow circumstances'.[55]

The press was not the only medium with publicity potential; medical texts, guidebooks and local histories also lauded the General Infirmary and touted for contributions.[56] Furthermore, the governors followed the practice of other hospitals in producing and circulating their own material.[57] No fewer than 6 000 copies of the 'Address to the Public' were printed in 1738, together with 1 000 copies of the more elaborate 'Plan and Elevation', both of which outlined the objectives of the charity and instructed contributors on how to donate.[58] The Act of Parliament, incorporating the Hospital, was also run off in tranches – 500 each in 1739, 1749 and 1788 'for the use of the governors',[59] and the specific clauses relating to patients reproduced still more prolifically – 12 000 in 1742, another 1 000 soon afterwards and 5 000 in 1750.[60] Financial pressures in the mid-1780s stimulated the production of 1 000 copies of an inscription for the Pump Rooms, commissioned from the poet, Christopher Anstey, to inform 'the public in general of the real state of the Hospital'.[61] But although a sharp rise in income followed the promotional package of which this broadsheet was a part (Table 3.1), it was routine rather than occasional publicity which dominated the bid to stay in the public's gaze and milk its purse. Of central importance was the *Annual Report*, which became increasingly sophisticated. After the Infirmary opened in 1742, the condition of patients at discharge was added to the accounts and the lists of benefactors and subscribers. More changes were introduced in the late 1740s, when advice on methods of donation and an annual list of governors were appended; and from the later eighteenth century, a relief of the Hospital was printed at the head of the *Report*.

Yet despite this marketing strategy aimed at the prospering charitable classes, the Bath Infirmary did not enjoy reliable financial support. Crude annual income more than doubled between 1745 and 1830, but it was erratic during the middle quarters of the eighteenth century, dipping to as low as half the base value in 1760 and not rising consistently above that level until 1785 (Table 3.1). This fickle financial predicament was closely tied to the Hospital's sources of income, ascertainable from the annual accounts. The first set up to January 1739 simply recorded the sums contributed by casual benefactors or deposited in the Pump Room Box. Profit and loss on South Sea stock appeared in 1740/41, and annual subscriptions a year later. After 1742 a more

Table 3.4 Bath General Hospital: patterns of income, 1738–1830

	£	%	£	%	£	%	£	%	£	%	£	%
Source	*1738/39*		*1739/40*		*1740/41*		*1741/42*		*1742/43*		*1743/44*	
Personal Donations	3 497.90	98.7	1 284.75	98.4	288.20	79.4	2 922.35	98.1	932.25	57.2	573.05	43.9
Revenue Account												
Capital Fund												
Annual Subscriptions	—	—	—	—	—	—	40.45	1.4	232.90	14.3	303.65	23.3
Hospital Box	—	—	—	—	—	—	—	—	21.50	1.3	16.55	1.3
Pump Room Box	47.00	1.3	20.75	1.6	3.60	1.0	10.60	0.4	10.40	0.6	16.50	1.3
Left at Pump Rooms	—	—	—	—	—	—	—	—	—	—	—	—
Left at Libraries	—	—	—	—	—	—	—	—	—	—	—	—
Social Events	—	—	—	—	—	—	—	—	2.10	<0.1	16.90	1.3
Church Collections	—	—	—	—	—	—	—	—	287.85	17.7	346.35	26.5
Interest	—	—	—	—	71.05	19.6	6.00	0.2	99.00	6.1	32.85	2.5
Rent	—	—	—	—	—	—	—	—	—	—	—	—
Other	—	—	—	—	—	—	—	—	43.25	2.7	—	—
Total	3 544.90	100.0	1 305.50	100.0	362.85	100.0	2 979.40	100.0	1 629.25	100.0	1 305.85	100.0
	1744/45		*1745/46*				*1750/51*		*1755/56*		*1760/61*	
Personal Donations												
Revenue Account	697.75	28.6	428.70	23.0			445.30	26.0	545.80	29.2	259.55	27.1
Capital Fund	852.10	34.9	538.85	28.9			18.90	1.1	307.35	16.4	—	—
Annual Subscriptions	345.00	14.1	281.40	15.1			278.60	16.3	267.75	14.3	216.45	22.6
Hospital Box	29.45	1.2	27.55	1.5			32.65	1.9	16.90	0.9	—	—
Pump Room Box	2.15	<0.1	52.85	2.8			9.45	0.6	13.45	0.7	10.80	1.1
Left at Pump Rooms	—	—	—	—			—	—	—	—	—	—

Left at Libraries	—	—	—	—			—	—	—	—	—	—
Social Events	113.65	4.7	25.35	1.4			124.85	7.3	83.70	4.5	—	—
Church Collections	329.20	13.5	409.50	22.0			452.85	26.5	346.20	18.5	196.25	20.5
Interest	50.00	2.0	97.00	5.2			347.65	20.3	124.95	6.7	82.00	8.6
Rent	—	—	—	—			—	—	165.00	8.8	192.50	20.1
Other	24.00	1.0	3.00	0.2			—	—	—	—	—	—
Total	2 443.30	100.0	1 864.20	100.0			1 710.25	100.0	1 871.10	100.0	957.55	100.0

	1765/66		*1770/71*		*1775/76*		*1780/81*		*1785/86*		*1790/91*	
Personal Donations					385.85	25.3	291.75	17.1			1 042.10	35.8
Revenue Account	371.60	20.3	449.80	15.2					671.0	22.3		
Capital Fund	508.25	27.7	1 390.00	47.0					677.50	22.5		
Annual Subscriptions	264.05	14.4	284.95	9.6	380.25	24.9	311.90	18.3	446.75	14.8	467.80	16.1
Hospital Box	25.90	1.4	28.55	1.0	42.55	2.8	15.90	0.9	19.90	0.7	15.60	0.5
Pump Room Box	29.65	1.6	36.10	1.2	8.25	0.5	26.85	1.6	17.10	0.6	27.05	0.9
Left at Pump Rooms	—	—	—	—	—	—	—	—	2.1	<0.1	29.95	1.0
Left at Libraries	—	—	—	—	—	—	—	—	—	—	5.25	0.2
Social Events	—	—	—	—	—	—	—	—	—	—	—	—
Church Collections	407.40	22.2	412.85	14.0	188.25	12.4	377.85	22.2	597.60	19.8	525.85	18.1
Interest	166.00	9.1	224.30	7.6	336.25	22.1	320.25	18.8	341.50	11.3	322.60	11.1
Rent	60.00	3.3	130.00	4.4	181.70	11.9	360.00	21.1	240.00	8.0	411.10	14.1
Other	—	—	—	—	1.5	0.1	—	—	—	—	60.00	2.1
Total	1 832.85	100.0	2 956.55	100.0	1 524.60	100.0	1 704.50	100.0	3 013.45	100.0	2 907.30	100.0

Table 3.4 concluded

	£	%	£	%	£	%	£	%	£	%	£	%
	1795/96		*1800/01*		*1805/06*		*1810/11*		*1815/16*		*1820/21*	
Personal Donations	909.00	34.0	1 131.10	33.4	403.15	14.8	397.50	12.2	2 250.35	43.3	1 092.45	30.6
Revenue Account												
Capital Fund												
Annual Subscriptions	369.35	13.8	386.00	11.4	465.90	17.2	507.75	15.6	405.85	7.8	445.1	12.5
Hospital Box	15.40	0.6	16.65	0.5	14.60	0.5	17.80	0.6	17.05	0.3	17.2	0.5
Pump Room Box	9.20	0.3	55.40	1.6	12.40	0.5	13.75	0.4	5.45	0.1	1.2	<0.1
Left at Pump Rooms	—	—	29.15	0.9	33.60	1.2	17.95	0.6	22.65	0.4	16.60	0.5
Left at Libraries	—	—	4.20	0.1	34.65	1.3	8.30	0.3	8.25	0.2	9.20	0.3
Social Events	—	—	—	—	—	—	—	—	—	—	—	—
Church Collections	566.75	21.2	787.65	23.3	898.2	33.1	923.60	28.4	992.05	19.1	818.55	23.0
Interest	529.65	19.8	580.45	17.1	654.55	24.1	811.30	24.9	784.10	15.1	809.20	22.7
Rent	263.45	9.9	273.45	8.1	199.10	7.3	556.75	17.1	713.50	13.7	363.50	10.2
Other	12.15	0.5	122.45	3.6	—	—	3.65	0.1	—	—	—	—
Total	2 674.95	100.0	3 386.50	100.0	2 716.15	100.0	3 258.35	100.0	5 199.25	100.0	3 573.00	100.0

	1825/26		*1830/31*	
Personal Donations	250.25	7.4	1 091.35	25.8
Revenue Account				
Capital Fund				
Annual Subscriptions	346.75	10.3	454.50	10.8
Hospital Box	17.35	0.5	15.40	0.4
Pump Room Box	6.40	0.2	3.75	<0.1
Left at Pump Rooms	23.40	0.7	2.10	<0.1

Left at Libraries	11.20	0.3	5.15	0.1
Social Events	—	—	—	—
Church Collections	887.30	26.4	310.75	7.4
Interest	850.50	25.3	1 668.10	39.5
Rent	938.50	27.9	463.50	11.0
Other	31.00	0.9	212.45	5.0
Total	3 362.65	100.0	4 227.05	100.0

Notes:

1. Only one charity collection was included in 1760/61, 1775/76 and 1830/31.
2. No separate sum for the Capital Fund appeared in the accounts until 1744/45 and this item was also missing in the following sample years: 1775/76, 1780/81, 1790/91, 1795/96, 1800/01, 1805/06, 1810/11, 1815/16, 1825/26 and 1830/31.
3. After 1790/91, rental income included a moiety/moieties from Siddington Manor in Gloucestershire.
4. After 1795/96, interest included dividend income on shares in the New Assembly Rooms at Bath.
5. Between 1810/11 and 1825/26, interest included the yield from turnpike deed poll/s.
6. The small amount in the 'other' category for 1775/76 arose from the sale of an old malt mill.
7. In 1790/91 and 1830/31, the 'other' category included profits from the sale of the late Miss H.M. Bowdler's essays and poems, printed for the benefit of the General Hospital. An additional £235 were raised in non-sample years.
8. In 1795/96, the 'other' category included the 'profits of a late publication' by Christopher Anstey Esq.
9. In 1800/01, the 'other' category comprised the 'residue of a subscription made for other purposes in the county of Wiltshire' and 'the remainder of a subscription raised in Gloucester for an orphan deceased'.
10. In 1810/11, the 'other' category comprised the 'further produce of the profit arising from the sale of a poem, called "The Months"' by Peter Sherston Esq.
11. In 1810/11, the 'other' category included refunded property tax.
12. In 1815/16, income from interest included arrears on the account from the previous year.
13. In 1825/26, the 'other' category included a returned power of attorney and a donation from the Bath Knot of Friendly Brethren.
14. In 1830/31, the 'other' category included a 'compensation' from the resident apothecary for boarding his apprentice.
15. Percentages have been rounded up or down and do not total exactly 100.00.

Source: *Annual Reports*.

detailed breakdown was adopted which included, in addition to casual donations and yearly subscriptions, gifts to the capital fund, investments, and the collection box at the Infirmary as well as the Pump Room. The lists of contributors published in the *Annual Reports* permit a refinement of these categories: in particular, the heading 'casual benefactions' can be disaggregated to distinguish personal donations from church collections and money raised at social events and venues. So analysing the accounts, again at five-yearly intervals after 1745/46, indicates that the income structure of the Bath Infirmary departed from that of other voluntary hospitals in three key respects: medical education was not a money spinner; annual subscriptions were relatively unimportant; and given only a gradual accumulation of permanent investments, casual benefactions remained crucial to financial solvency for much of the long eighteenth century (Table 3.4).

Medical education was a lucrative activity for hospitals which specialized in training and at the Edinburgh Infirmary the sale of tickets to students netted from 15 to 30 per cent of annual income between 1770 and 1800.[62] At provincial institutions, profits reflected the more circumspect scale of lectures and recruitment. But by 1830 even the Bath United Hospital, formed in 1823 from the merger of the Casualty Hospital and the City Infirmary and Dispensary, had 11 pupils on the books and was hosting lecture courses approved by the professional bodies for surgeons and apothecaries.[63] In contrast, the General Infirmary had no students. Indeed, only in 1830 was the apothecary authorized to take a single apprentice, for whom he was required to pay 'one hundred pounds dowry ... as a compensation for his maintenance in the Hospital for a period of five years'.[64] However, more significant to the financial profile of the Bath Hospital than the absence of medical education was the balance between annual subscriptions, casual benefactions and investment income.

Annual subscriptions

Amanda Berry has shown that at the Bristol, Northampton, and Devon and Exeter Infirmaries subscriber loyalty delivered a high degree of income stability.[65] At the Bath Hospital, however, the level of annual subscriptions was depressed by its special terms of reference; not only did a ban on the city's residents weaken ties with the local community but medical recommendation removed the right to sponsor patients, a privilege which contributors to other infirmaries enjoyed.[66] Neither individual nor corporate benefactors were unable to use their donations to 'buy' medical care for employees, and dispense patronage and power.[67]

Without these fillips, therefore, the incentives to offer support on an ongoing basis were fewer. The governors tried to triumph over this impediment by embarking upon a series of campaigns to win new annual subscribers and to chase up delinquents with lapsed payments. Soon after the subscription scheme was set up late in 1741, high initial running costs prompted the weekly committee to commission a team from within their ranks 'to go from house to house to solicit annual subscriptions'.[68] The recruitment drive extended outside Bath itself. Recommendatory letters from the diocesan bishop, urging local clergy to collect subscriptions, were not used as they were at Shrewsbury and Worcester, but the General Infirmary did imitate the system of agents adopted at these institutions[69] when in 1785 the governors wrote to 'respectable ... persons in ... the principal cities and towns in Great Britain and Ireland ... requesting them to receive such benefactions, or subscriptions as well disposed persons may chose to give for the benefit of this charity'. Parishes as well as individuals were a target of publicity. In June 1783, 500 copies of a representation of the Hospital were printed for patients returning to parishes which were not subscribing. Moreover, in January 1831, the governors decided to alert overseers in the parish of Walcot to the powers that they had acquired under the 1830 Hospital Act to contribute to funds from the poor-rate.[70] The *Annual Report* for 1830/31 broadened this attack; the governors wished

> to impress on parishes, that, as this Hospital admits patients from all parts of the kingdom, and is continually the means of relieving parishes from expense in the maintenance of paupers, it has a claim to parochial subscriptions ... wherever its benefits are extended. Those persons who have the management of parochial affairs will, therefore, it is hoped, see the propriety of contributing somewhat to its support, and thus assist in enabling it to continue the widely extended relief which it has afforded to the suffering poor ... for nearly a century.

The appeal to parishes went beyond in-house propaganda. In 1812, *The Improved Bath Guide* was singing the praises of a charity nation-wide in its scope, and recommending that 'the nobility and gentry ... promote a permanent annual subscription from the respective parishes in which they have an influence'.[71]

As well as seeking new subscribers, the governors attempted to pursue defaulters and kept non-payment under regular review. Since annual subscribers had neither sponsorship rights nor automatic governor status, the General Infirmary lacked the penalties for non-renewal imposed by other infirmaries.[72] From 1748/49, however, the *Annual Reports* 'earnestly desired' delinquent subscribers 'to pay ... within the year, it being one considerable part of the income on which the governors depend for the subsistence of the Hospital'. Though the rules were not specific about when payment was due and made no provision for the 'monitory letters' that were prescribed at Norwich, Shrewsbury, Manchester and Liverpool,[73] the weekly committee did periodically decide to send written reminders in 1761, 1774, 1779, 1797, 1802 and 1814.[74] The tone of such correspondence was tactful, begging the recipient 'to excuse this application, it being the constant custom of other infirmaries'.[75] In 1785, the wording of an advertisement destined for the local and national newspapers was equally diplomatic, the governors trusting that 'those ladies and gentlemen, who have had the goodness to become annual subscribers, and whose donations happen, through inadvertency, to be in arrears, will see the necessity of apprizing them of the [situation] ... with all deference and respect'.[76] None the less, there were occasions when discretion was cast to the wind. The Hospital stopped short of publishing names in the press,[77] but in 1765 it did adopt the more common practice of including in the *Annual Report* 'an additional column of subscribers in arrears ... in the same manner as is at present done in the Gloucester Infirmary'.[78] The strategy was justified as a means of preventing future errors and enabling the subscriber to 'see all his payments publicly acknowledged'.[79] But such use of disclosure was controversial. Dropped in 1769 because of the 'great offence [given] to many well-wishers of this charity', it was reintroduced two decades later and survived a challenge in 1803 when the general court resolved to continue printing arrears for four years, after which time negligent subscribers would be struck off the annual list and informed of the reason.[80]

The campaign to support the subscription scheme met with some success at Bath and the crude list of annual subscribers to the Infirmary grew from 111 individuals and two parishes in 1743/44 to 264 individuals and 118 parishes in 1830/31.[81] However, progress elsewhere was more impressive, the number of annual subscribers increasing tenfold at the Bristol Infirmary and fivefold at Leeds and Manchester between foundation and 1820.[82] Moreover, the modest rate of expansion at Bath was further undercut by high arrears. In 1802, for example, it was estimated that overdue individual and parish subscriptions together exceeded £750,[83] whereas at Winchester five years later actual payments fell short of promised payments by only £300.[84] The limitations of the Bath subscription scheme were carried through to its share of annual income. For whereas the generality of Georgian voluntary hospitals obtained between a half and three-quarters of their revenue from annual subscriptions,[85] the proportion at the General Infirmary in the sample years never exceeded a quarter and most commonly fell between 10 and 15 per cent (Table 3.4).

Casual benefactions

Revisionist readings of associated philanthropy play down the significance of the subscription principle and emphasize the continuing importance of endowment income.[86] At the Bath Hospital, however, the deficiency in annual subscribers was made good not by investment moneys from legacies and bequests but by meeting current expenditure from the casual benefactions of the affluent and fashionable Company who flocked to the city during the season. This *ad hoc* income was derived from three main sources: social events, church collections and personal donations. Sociability and philanthropy were interlocked during the Georgian age. The link was clearest where charities directly organized social events, running music festivals, balls and art exhibitions.[87] At Bath this rarely happened. In the spring of 1758, the Infirmary was approached by a group of musicians who offered their services gratis for an ambitious programme of sacred music in Bath Abbey. The weekly committee became intimately involved in planning the performance, supplying stewards and erecting scaffolding for the artists and the audience. After this first festival, the general court ordered a continuation of 'the musical collections ... every autumn and spring season' and a second series of concerts was held in May 1759. Assistants were also appointed for a performance in 1761, but there is no evidence of any further musical extravaganzas. That these events were short-lived was predictable, given the narrow profit margins of £162 in 1758 and £133 in 1759.[88] Yet though the Bath Infirmary did not usually stage-manage its own social occasions, the indigenous leisure industry was exploited. During the 1740s and 1750s, surpluses from balls and concert breakfasts were transmitted to the governors, most frequently by Richard 'Beau' Nash.[89] Benefit plays too were mounted on its behalf, as in 1756 when over £30 was collected at a 'masque given by Mr Brown and company'. These proceeds were gratefully received and one of the assistants was delegated 'to return the thanks of the governors to Mr Brown and to the proprietors of the house and to Mr Palmer for the candles'.[90] However, the sums involved, though typical of contemporary events in the provinces,[91] were disappointing in comparison with London. Thus when in 1747 the Foundling Hospital arranged a single 'breakfast for the ladies' to mark the laying of the foundation-stone for its chapel, over £700 was raised, representing 10 per cent of average annual income between 1739 and 1756.[92]

Like the social events organized by the General Infirmary itself, benefit concerts were reported only during the 1750s. Throughout the long eighteenth century, however, boxes and subscription books were placed at key venues. In addition to the Hospital Box installed to encourage gifts from visitors, the receptacle for donations in the Pump Room was fitted in 1738 and its purposes were spelt out some six months later in a printed handout 'given at the door'.[93] Boxes were not deposited in local taverns or in other towns,[94] but at an early stage books were acquired 'to lye at the public places to receive the subscriptions of the company'. Their use may have ceased. In any event, the Hospital again resolved in 1785 that 'subscription books ... be opened at the several coffee houses, booksellers' shops, rooms and pump rooms; and that a particular account of the nature of the charity be printed at the head of each page'.[95] The amounts left at the pump rooms and libraries were never large; and those collected from the two boxes were, in the words of the *Bath Journal*, 'very inconsiderable'.[96] Consequently, these types of donation did little to boost income from social events; and when all five categories are conflated, we find that they normally explain under three per cent of annual income. Only in the sample year 1750/51 did social gatherings and venues account for almost a tenth of total revenue (Table 3.4).

For infirmaries which combined religious observances with a feast and/or concert, social glitter was an integral part of the anniversary celebrations.[97] At Bath the general court which began the financial year may have been accompanied by a regular dinner,[98] but there was no other social event and the church services held on behalf of the General Hospital were chronologically separate. These religious gatherings – the second source of casual benefactions – were a considerable administrative commitment. The Infirmary did not possess its own chapel; nor did it sell seats for services.[99] Nevertheless, dates were routinely fixed for charity sermons, clergy commissioned to preach,[100] and unreserved pews made available to the public.[101] Publicity was also set in motion.[102] Gentleman were appointed to take up the collection.[103] And new churches and chapels in the expanding city were drawn in as they were completed; in 1773, for example, the 'obliging offer' of the first collection from the proprietary chapel in Brock Street was warmly accepted, while in 1820 the Rector of Bathwick was asked permission for the sermons usually preached in other local parishes to be allowed at his recently opened church.[104] Moreover, 1783 saw the governors acquainting charity preachers with the Hospital's parlous financial state; and two years later 5 000 copies of a leaflet describing its functions were printed specifically for distribution at charity services.[105] Such investment of time and effort was justified, given the unusually high levels of income raised through church collections. At the Salop Infirmary, anniversary sermons yielded from £32 to £319 between 1747 and 1829, the average falling between £70 and £90.[106] At Bath, on the other hand, the lowest figure for the sample years (where only two Sundays were included in the annual accounts) was in excess of £300, and the upper ceiling approached £1 000. Sermon income was substantial in relative as well as absolute terms. Until reduced from two to one in 1827, church collections regularly generated at least a fifth of the Hospital's annual revenue (Table 3.4). By way of comparison, preaching on behalf of the Northampton General Infirmary raised an average 3.5 per cent of yearly income between 1743 and 1844.[107]

Voluntary hospitals typically obtained only a small proportion of their incomes from *ad hoc* gifts so that benefactions, legacies and the anniversary meeting in combination were responsible for only a fifth of the Salop Infirmary's total revenue during the Georgian period.[108] At Bath, however, personal donations alone – the third type of casual contribution – only fell below 20 per cent on four occasions during the sample years and were normally in excess of a third (Table 3.4). The methods used to extract these incidental donations were both bizarre and conventional. Master of Ceremonies, 'Beau' Nash, was renowned for his flamboyant style, captured by Oliver Goldsmith's tale of his exchange with the Duchess of Queensberry whom he encountered whilst collecting at the assembly room:

> not being able to pass by him unobserved, she gave him a pat with her fan, and said, 'You must put down a trifle for me, Nash, for I have no money in my pocket.' 'Yes, madam,' says he, 'that I will with pleasure if your grace will tell me when to stop'; then taking an handful of guineas out of his pocket, he began to tell them into his white hat – 'One, two, three, four, five – ' 'Hold, hold!' says the duchess, 'consider what you are about'. 'Consider your rank and fortune, madam,' says Nash, and continues telling – 'six, seven, eight, nine, ten.' Here the duchess called again, and seemed angry. 'Pray compose yourself, madam,' cried Nash, 'and don't interrupt the work of charity – eleven, twelve, thirteen, fourteen, fifteen.' Here the duchess stormed, and caught hold of his hand. 'Peace, madam,' says Nash, 'you shall have your name written in letters of gold, madam, and upon the front of the building madam. Sixteen, seventeen, eighteen, nineteen, twenty.' 'I won't pay a farthing more,' says the duchess. 'Charity hides a multitude of sins,' replies Nash; 'twenty-one, twenty-two, twenty-three, twenty-four, twenty-five.' 'Nash', says she, 'I protest you frighten me out of my wits. L-d, I shall die!' 'Madam, you will never die with doing good; and if you do, it will be the better for you,' answered Nash ... and agreed to stop his hand, and compound with her grace for thirty guineas.[109]

This story speaks volumes for the social and moral springs of philanthropy. For all his swashbuckling, however, Nash was capable of more sober fund-raising. A report in the *Gentleman's Magazine* is said to describe him 'as complaisant and diligent with the basin at the Abbey to collect alms for the hospital and the charity children'.[110] Furthermore, in a society where personal application still predominated over the embryonic mass media, the 'Beau's' social connections allowed him to serve as an effective 'charitable conduit'.[111] Consequently, in the late 1730s, when the Infirmary project was in its infancy, he was able to communicate 'our design to many' and pass on their approval.[112]

With or without the agency of Nash, the personal donations received by the Bath Hospital were of diverse origins. In 1800, for example, Benjamin Price made a benefaction of one guinea, 'being part of a premium adjudged to him by the Bath and West of England Society for an essay on the most profitable and practicable manner of employing the poor in parish workhouses'.[113] Bets and fines were also received,[114] as they were by other charities,[115] and under legislation passed in 1740, the Hospital acquired a moiety of the penalties for excessive gambling levied in Somerset.[116] Complementing these types of gift were donations in lieu of a peal of bells to mark the arrival of wealthy visitors[117] and, like other towns and cities,[118] Bath forewent a display of illuminations to celebrate the Peace of Amiens in 1802, preferring to divert the subscription to philanthropic projects which included the General Infirmary.[119] Finally, sums intended for other good causes – such as 'the remainder of a subscription raised in Gloucester for an orphan deceased'[120] – found their way to the coffers. For all this variety, however, the majority of personal benefactions were donated by individuals in the customary manner. Sampling at 15-year intervals suggests that though contributions made during the donor's lifetime were more numerous than posthumous gifts, their average value was considerably lower and fell from almost £22 in 1741/42 to under £3 in 1830/31. Consequently, legacies comprised a larger portion of personal donations throughout the long eighteenth century (Table 3.5).[121] But financial pressures necessitated both the diversion of these legacies to revenue costs and the sale of existing capital investments. Thus far from enjoying the secure endowment income of the older charitable trust, this particular example of associated philanthropy endured until the late 1820s persistent financial insecurity.

The problem of inconstancy was compounded by inflation. Berry's comparative study indicates that there was not a clear positive or negative correlation between the Schumpeter–Gilboy index and subscription income, and that institutions were not consistent in their response to price rises.[122] The Bath Infirmary also reveals a volatile reaction to inflation (Figure 3.2). When total hospital income is converted into an index with 1745 as the base year, we see that it trailed the cost of consumer goods – almost without remission – until 1830. Categorizing income identifies a series of retrospective knee-jerk reactions to the cash flow crises which hit the General Infirmary with

Table 3.5 Bath General Hospital: personal donations, 1741–1830

Year	*All personal donations*	*Legacies*				*Other donations*			
	Overall value £	No.	*Total value £*	*Average value £*	*% of all personal donations by value*	No.	*Total value £*	*Average value £*	*% of all personal donations by value*
1741/42	2 917.60	1	2 000.00	2 000.00	68.55	42	917.60	21.85	31.45
1755/56	841.28	5	490.25	98.05	58.27	35	351.03	10.03	41.73
1770/71	1 737.80	4	1 540.00	385.00	88.62	30	197.80	6.59	11.38
1785/86	1 326.05	4	860.40	215.10	64.88	91	465.65	5.12	35.12
1800/01	1 162.22	7	804.60		69.23	55	357.62	6.50	30.77
1815/16	2 244.78	3	1 860.00	620.00	82.86	28	384.78	13.74	17.14
1830/31	1 084.35	7	1 002.75	143.25	92.48	30	81.60	2.72	7.53

Note: There is some discrepancy between the overall values for all personal donations given above and those in Table 3.4. The reason is that although both sets of figures rely on the *Annual Reports*, this table uses the list of casual benefactions whereas Table 3.4 uses the annual accounts.

Source: *Annual Reports*.

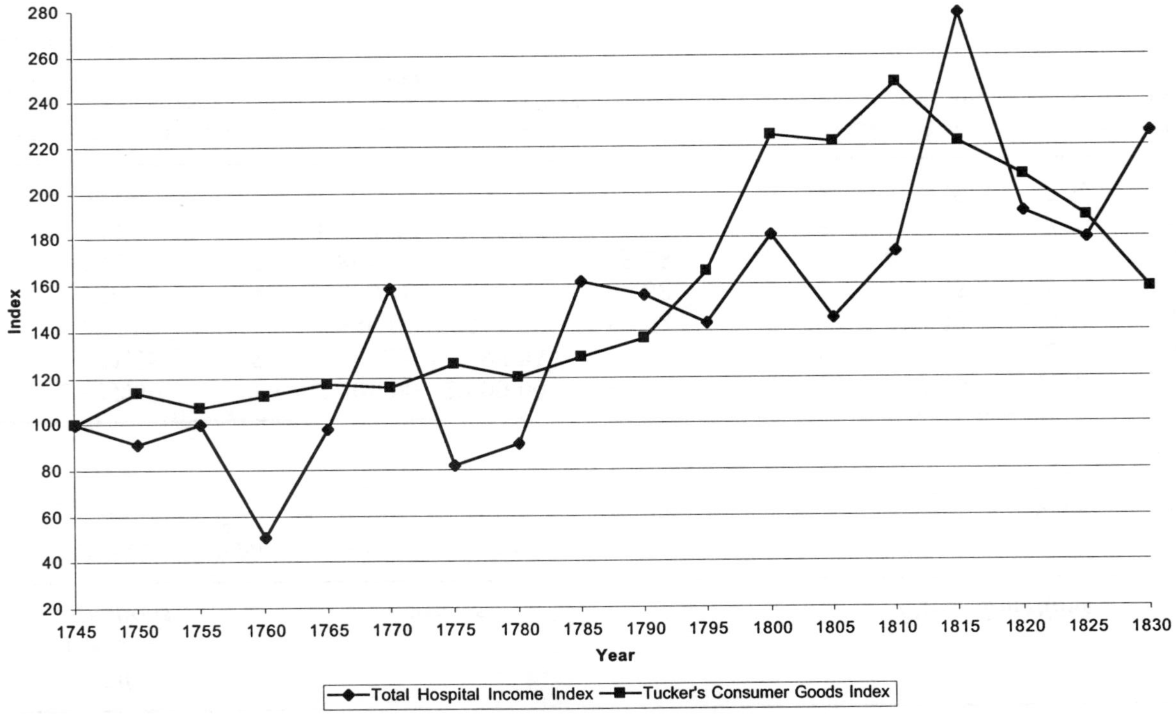

(a) Total hospital income

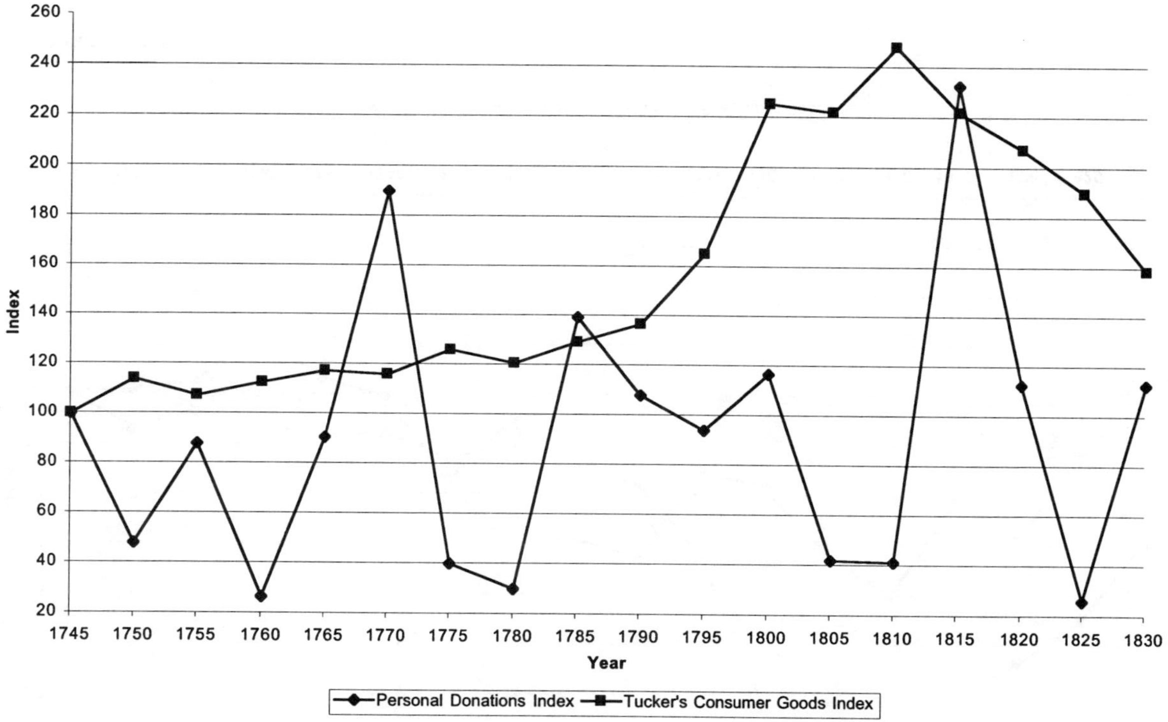

(b) Personal donations

3.2 Bath General Hospital: a comparison of sources of income, consumer prices and money wages, 1745–1830

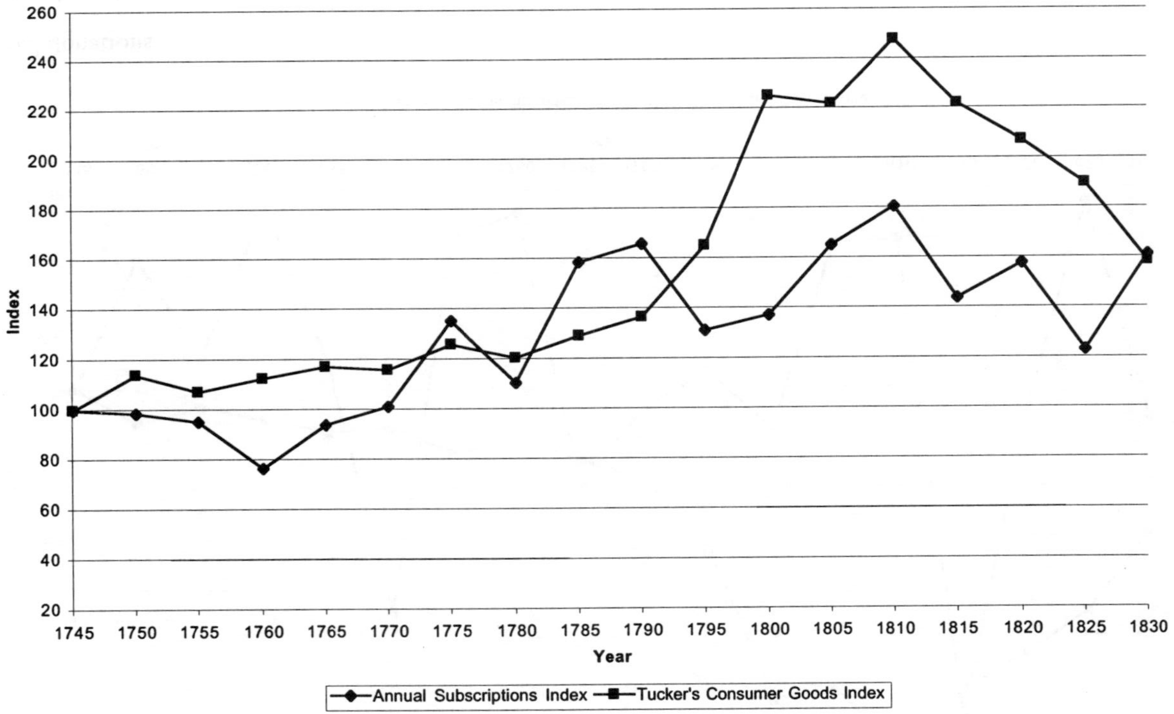

(c) Annual subscriptions

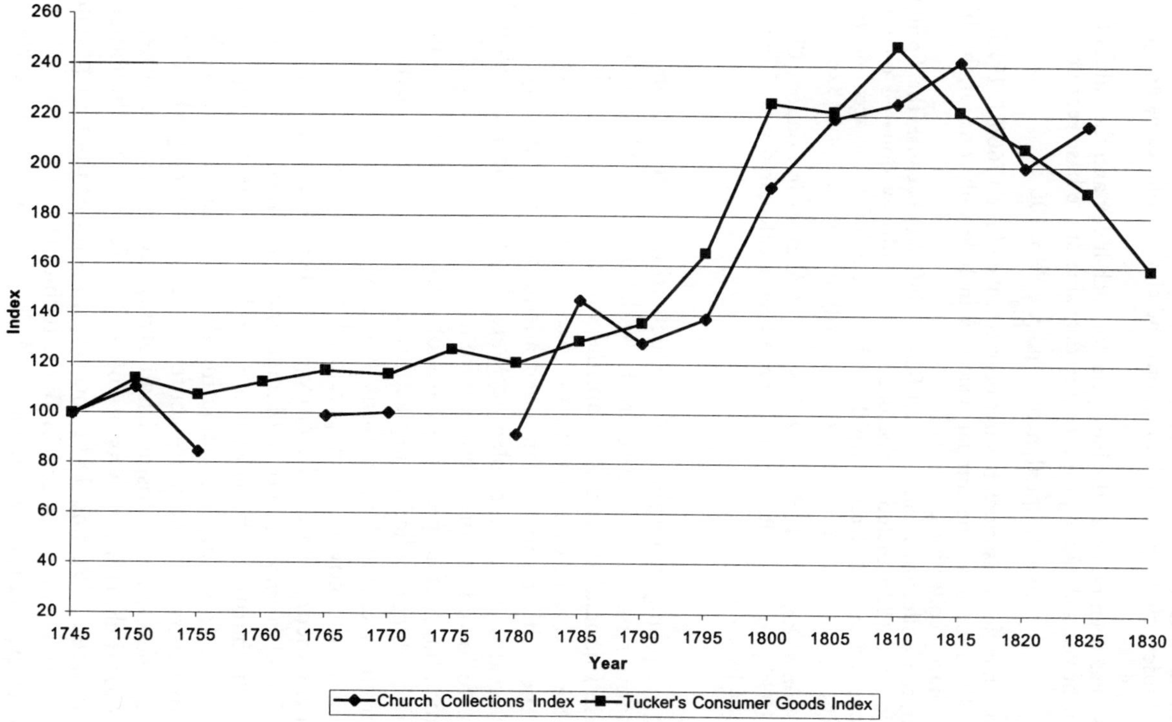

(d) Church collections

3.2 continued

Notes:
1. The total income of the General Hospital and the amounts obtained from annual subscriptions, personal donations and church collections are given in table 3.4.
2. 1745/46 has been taken as the base year for each index and the values for subsequent years stated in proportion to the value of the base year i.e.

$$\text{total hospital income index} = \frac{hi_1}{hi_0} \times 100$$

3. The church collections index has not been calculated for 1760/61, 1775/76 and 1830/31 because the annual accounts include only one of the bi-annual charity collections.
4. The church collections index is artificially inflated because the Spring collection for 1825 included one date in May. Money donated on this occasion, and on two dates in April has been included in the accounts for 1825/26, together with the proceeds of charity services in April 1826.

Sources: *Annual Reports*. Tucker, 'Real Wages of Artisans in London, 1729–1935', pp. 27–9. Both indices have been recalculated with 1745 as the base year.

increasing frequency from the 1770s. Fluctuating in the extreme, personal donations may have rallied in the wake of the 1780s campaign to advertise financial shortfalls. If annual subscriptions – steadier but still variable – were affected by the same campaign, the rise was more delayed. And neither source responded adequately and quickly to the economic strains of the Napoleonic Wars.[123] Only the later church collections followed the price index with any proximity, sermons having an immediacy of appeal at points of national and international tension. Though compelled to neglect investment by their dependence upon capricious casual benefactions which were insensitive to economic trends, the governors appreciated the dangers posed by an impermanent income base. Therefore, when beds were left empty in the late 1740s, *Annual Reports* blamed the smallness of the capital fund,[124] with charity sermons of this period – and the accompanying accounts of the Infirmary – articulating the same theme.[125] Paradoxically, the difficulty became more acute as the volume of philanthropy intensified. The General Hospital had always competed for benefactions with local charities such as the Blue-Coat School and the Pauper Scheme. Between 1790 and 1811, however, no fewer than 14 philanthropic societies were founded in Bath, including the City Infirmary and Dispensary, and the Eye Hospital.[126] These too may have suffered from lack of regular commitment; certainly, the City Infirmary and Dispensary drew only 27 per cent of its income from annual subscriptions in the early 1790s.[127] For the General Hospital, however, the explosion of new charities, catering for the local population and more in tune with the contemporary mood, meant an aggressive fight for funding. It may be for this reason that the capital fund surfaced as an issue again in the early nineteenth century, when *Annual Reports* began to emphasize the financial precariousness caused by the gap between 'certain annual income' and expenditure.

Investment income

Though casual benefactions remained the bread and butter of the Bath Infirmary until the very end of the Georgian era, steps were taken earlier to develop a more stable revenue from rent and investments. In 1764 there was a desperate but abortive attempt to raise money by letting vacant wards;[128] and from the 1790s small moieties were received from Siddington Manor in Gloucestershire.[129] The Infirmary's principal rental income, however, was derived from the Charmy Down Estate. The initial rent was fixed at £165 per annum and increased at a pace favourable to that for private landlords. Between 1750 and 1790, for example, the Duke of Kingston's rental income grew by 48 per cent, whereas that from Charmy Down increased by 62 per cent – twice the rate for estates in the hands of Guy's Hospital. There was a time lag before the Bath Infirmary caught up with the inflationary effects of the Napoleonic Wars,[130] but in 1810 the governors more than doubled the 1801 rent to £700 annually.[131] This increase proved unsustainable during the subsequent agricultural depression. In July 1822, a general court 'Resolved that an abatement of £200 of the rent in arrears ... be made to the tenant of Charmy Down Estate in consequence of the reduced prices of provisions between the past and present times'.[132] Moreover, by 1830 the annual rent, reduced to £550 in 1825, was down by a further £100.[133] The financial benefits of the estate were additionally undermined by persistent arrears. *Annual Reports* from the 1760s show successive tenants behind with their payments and in 1771, three years after he proposed 'quitting Charmy Down Estate at Lady Day next', the governors were threatening legal action against Mr Thomas Phillips to extract his outstanding rent.[134] Arrears were not the only problem. Like the endowed hospitals and other charities with substantial property holdings, the Bath Infirmary found its administrative resources severely taxed by maintenance and improvement.[135] Both the lease for lives and tenancies at will were rejected in preference for a medium-term let of seven or 14 years, which was believed to encourage occupiers to invest in the property.[136] With the approval of the general court, Benjamin Bathurst, a treasurer of the Hospital, became the first tenant; but his conduct was far from exemplary and in 1761 poor management of the estate prompted the appointment of three governors to acquaint him with 'the terms of his lease, particularly that part relating to the repairing of the buildings'. When Bathurst's term had almost expired, a new tenant was sought, not on the grapevine but through public advertisement and the submission of sealed bids.[137] However, the governors continued to face bills for repairs and upgrading,[138] as well as becoming embroiled in timber rights[139] and negotiations with the owners of adjacent land.[140] Given these frustrations, it is perhaps not surprising that the General Infirmary bought no further estates. Therefore, unless total income dropped significantly or a backlog of accumulated arrears was settled, under 10 per cent of annual revenue was usually acquired from rent (Table 3.4); the Hospital was a small-time landlord, choosing to invest its surpluses in stocks and shares.

When the proposal for a Bath Infirmary was revived in the late 1730s, the trustees tried hard to track down earlier assets. Humphrey Thayer, who had held these funds, was deceased, but his executor eventually located the sum, conceding that it had been 'a little unkind ... letting the money lye dead so long without placing it out at interest'.[141] A wiser investment strategy was subsequently adopted for the stocks and shares acquired by donation and by purchase. In 1749 Lord Coleraine, during his lifetime, transferred in trust £500 of Old South Sea annuities as a 'deed of gift' to support from the interest one patient extra to the established complement. Shares in the new Bath Assembly Rooms were similarly bequested by the Primate of All Ireland in the 1790s to maintain two supernumerary patients in the Hospital.[142] Later legacies also included deed polls in the Bath and Southampton Turnpikes,[143] and from 1800 the straightforward bequest of stocks became more commonplace.[144] Windfalls such as the £1 000 from the Guildhall Subscription – recompense for admitting soldiers who had helped to suppress the 1745 Jacobite Rebellion[145] – enabled the Infirmary to purchase its own investments, but the endeavour to earmark larger benefactions for a capital fund was interrupted by revenue difficulties which necessitated the deflection of all income to current expenditure. None the less, a stock market portfolio was gradually put together which, until the preference switched to bank annuities or consols in the 1770s, was dominated by the South Sea Company.[146]

Although amassing a capital base remained a primary objective for much of the long eighteenth century, there was a temporary revolt in the early 1790s when, prior to the construction of the attic storey, a group of governors argued publicly for 'extending the benefits of the charity, rather than apply[ing] the surplus income ... towards an accumulating fund'; the Hospital, they declared, 'should avoid being rich, as well as poor'.[147] The greater threat to a permanent income from stocks and shares was financial emergency, which impelled the Bath governors to dispose of their capital assets when the economy too was in a state of crisis and hence stock market prices depreciated. In 1807, for instance, the sale of bank annuities costing over £600 produced only £387[148] – a predicament repeated across the voluntary hospital sector.[149] In the long term, however, the build-up of capital assets far outweighed this short-term disadvantage. The Infirmary's *Annual Reports* show that stocks, valued at under £3 000 in 1760/61, had increased step by step to over £20 000 by 1825/26, and then nearly doubled in value during the next five years. Income from both interest and dividends grew correspondingly from around £100 before the mid-1760s to over £1 600 by 1830/31 (Table 3.4). With almost 40 per cent of its yearly income now derived from the stock market and a further 10 per cent from rent, the General Hospital achieved an enviable level of financial security. Not all provincial institutions were so fortunate.[150]

In this part, we have related the administrative and financial history of the Georgian Bath Infirmary to the commercial economy. The focus of Chapter 2 was the development of structures and practices to outlaw corruption and promote the ideal of civic virtue. This exemplification of propriety aided the financial management of the Hospital which, in Chapter 3, we have placed within its national economic context. Years of crisis in the economy were often years of crisis for the Infirmary, as annual revenue failed to match expenditure commitments. The cumulative effect of war and peace, population growth and food shortages was the persistent climb of inflation. Throughout the long eighteenth century, household costs remained below the inflation rate for consumer goods, thereby suggesting that everyday procedures were successful in controlling outgoings. Although annual subscriptions showed some reaction to these rising costs, they formed a comparatively small proportion of receipts. Repeated deficits from the 1770s stirred the governors into a vigorous publicity campaign. However, participation in Hospital government was at its lowest ebb in the 1790s and the test of the Napoleonic Wars was met by depleting capital assets rather than generating additional funds. Never large, these assets failed to yield a substantial investment income until the late 1820s. Consequently, despite the prosperity unleashed and diffused by the commercial economy, the Bath Infirmary had to achieve financial solvency by staying afloat on a sea of casual benefactions which were variable and not always in tune with economic trends. The need to win so many *ad hoc* contributions afresh each year left the Hospital highly vulnerable to the changing attitudes and aspirations of Georgian society, and so its experiences illuminate well the values and the behaviour of those élites who patronized Bath as a centre for recreation or residence. Especially relevant was the diversion of the civic virtue used for sanitizing the business ethos to the formulation of new moral economies of giving, and the affording of opportunities to acquire social status and to appease political and religious tensions through uniting around policing the poor. But this playing out of ethics, sociability and conflict at the General Infirmary occurred within a context where physicians, surgeons and apothecaries also functioned in a clinical capacity. Therefore, before probing the moral and religious, social and political functions which were performed for all patrons and governors, whether lay or medical, we must turn to the motivations of the Hospital's honorary physicians and surgeons, and to its role in the professionalization of medicine in Bath.

Notes

1. Wood, *Bath*, pp. 275–90.
2. Ibid., p. 283.
3. Humble and Hansell, *Westminster Hospital*, pp. 6–9, 14; T.G. Davies, *Deeds Not Words: A History of the Swansea General and Eye Hospital 1817–1948* (Cardiff: University of Wales Press, 1988), p. 17; K.J. Lowson, *The Hull Royal Infirmary* (no place of publication, publisher or date), p. 6; Marland, *Medicine and Society*, pp. 100–101; Eoin O'Brien, *The Charitable Infirmary, Jervis Street 1718–1987: A Farewell Tribute* (Dublin: Anniversary Press, 1987), p. 3; Francis W. Steer, *The Royal West Sussex Hospital: The First Hundred Years 1784–1884* (Chichester: Chichester City Council, 1960), pp. 1–2; Turner, *Hampshire County Hospital*, p. 6.
4. Wilson, *England's Apprenticeship*, p. 280.
5. See, for example, John Thackray Bunce, *A History of the Birmingham General Hospital and Musical Festivals* (Birmingham: Cornish Brothers, 1873), pp. 10–12.
6. Martin Gorsky, 'Charity, Mutuality and Philanthropy: Voluntary Provision in Bristol 1800–1870' (unpublished doctoral thesis, University of Bristol, 1995), chs 2 and 9.
7. Eade, *Norfolk and Norwich Hospital*, p. 34; McLoughlin, *Liverpool Infirmary*, pp. 43–4.
8. Langford, *Polite and Commercial People*, p. 632; Wilson, *England's Apprenticeship*, pp. 278, 280, 313.
9. Minute Book, 1 May 1750; 1 May 1755.
10. See also *Annual Report*, 1756–57. Minute Book, 6 April 1757; 14 December 1757; 30 August 1758.
11. Wilson, *England's Apprenticeship*, pp. 277–8, 280.
12. R.B. Outhwaite, *Dearth, Public Policy and Social Disturbance in England 1550–1800* (London: Macmillan, 1991), p. 20; Andrew, *Philanthropy and Police*, p. 136; Langford, *Polite and Commercial People*, p. 543.

13. Hembry, *English Spa*, p. 272.
14. Minute Book, 29 October 1766; 29 July 1767; 4 May 1768; 3 June 1772; 4 December 1782; 1 May 1783.
15. See, for example, Berry, 'Patronage', pp. 126, 129; Howie, 'Finance and Supply', pp. 128–9; Turner, *Hampshire County Hospital*, p. 38; Clark-Kennedy, *The London*, p. 169; McLoughlin, *Liverpool Infirmary*, pp. 44–5.
16. Briggs, *Age of Improvement* , pp. 161–72; Eric J. Evans, *The Forging of the Modern State: Early Industrial Britain 1783–1870* (London: Longman, 1983), pp. 79, 81, 83–5, 144.
17. See, for example, Haskins, *Salisbury Infirmary*, p. 12; Russell, *Exeter Hospitals*, p. 64; Saunders, *Middlesex Hospital*, p. 18; Smith, *Bristol Royal Infirmary*, pp. 150–51, 153.
18. Hembry, *English Spa*, p. 273.
19. Minute Book, 4 February 1795; 4 March 1795; 24 May 1797.
20. Minute Book, 29 October 1794.
21. Minute Book, 28 October 1807; 30 August 1809; 29 August 1810; 6 November 1811.
22. Hembry, *English Spa*, p. 276.
23. See, for example, Davies, *Deeds Not Words*, p. 38.
24. Briggs, *Age of Improvement*, pp. 162, 211; Evans, *Forging of the Modern State*, pp. 181, 191–4, 206.
25. Minute Book, 1 May 1830.
26. *Annual Report,* 1739/40; 1740/41; 1741/42.
27. Minute Book, 1 May 1758; 1 May 1797.
28. Minute Book, 1 May 1744; 15 May 1744.
29. Minute Book, 1 May 1802; 1 May 1812.
30. See, for example, Anning, *General Infirmary at Leeds,* p. 11; Bevan, *Salop Infirmary*, p. 9; O'Brien, *Charitable Infirmary*, p. 17; Russell, *Exeter Hospitals*, p. 64; Saunders, *Middlesex Hospital*, p. 16; Waddy, *Northampton General Hospital*, p. 12. Admission procedures are discussed more fully in Chapter 5.
31. Wood, *Bath*, p. 285. Minute Book, 29 May 1751.
32. Minute Book, 15 May 1744; 15 November 1744; 1 May 1745; 1 May 1746; 2 May 1748; 1 May 1749; 1 May 1750; 31 October 1750; 1 May 1751; 2 May 1757; 1 May 1758; 2 May 1768; 1 May 1783; 21 May 1783; 1 May 1797; 1 May 1798; 1 May 1799.
33. See, for example, Minute Book, 1 May 1800; 1 May 1810; 1 May 1820; 1 May 1830.
34. [Bath General Infirmary], 'Short Account', in Bayly, *Sermon*, p. 26. See also [Bath General Infirmary], 'Short Account', in Olive, *Particular Excellence*, p. 33.
35. Minute Book, 1 May 1744; 15 May 1744; 7 June 1758; 14 June 1758; 30 March 1774; 6 April 1744.
36. See, for example, Clark-Kennedy, *The London*, p. 171; Hall, Stevens and Whyman, *Kent and Canterbury Hospital*, pp. 12, 35; Humble and Hansell, *Westminster Hospital*, pp. 29–30, 55; Waddy, *Northampton General Hospital*, p. 17.
37. Daniel A. Baugh, 'Poverty, Protestantism and Political Economy: English Attitudes toward the Poor, 1660–1800', in S. Baxter (ed.), *England's Rise to Greatness 1660–1763* (Berkeley: University of California, 1983), p. 90.

38. Risse, *Hospital Life*, p. 39; Berry, 'Patronage', p. 138; Bevan, *Salop Infirmary*, No. 3, 'Comparative Average Statement'; No. 4, 'Statement of Receipts and Disbursements'.
39. For example, medical staff were exhorted to buy in bulk from cheaper London sources and to prepare small quantities of drugs internally to avoid expensive local chemists; the use of dressings, and alcohol for medicinal purposes, was more rigorously controlled; and at St George's Hospital in the capital, surgeons were required to 'make trial of poultices without oil' in order to save money. See Blomfield, *St George's*, p. 35; Clark-Kennedy, *The London*, pp. 72–3; Eade, *Norfolk and Norwich Hospital*, p. 60; Frizelle and Martin, *Leicester Royal Infirmary*, pp. 55–6; Haskins, *Salisbury Infirmary*, p. 15; Howie, 'Finance and Supply', pp. 138–9.
40. Minute Book, 24 February 1773.
41. Treatment regimes at the Bath Infirmary and the general development of hospital medicine are discussed in Chapter 4.
42. *Annual Report*, 1743/44; 1744/45.
43. Minute Book, 21 January 1796; 13 April 1796; 7 September 1796; 5 November 1800; 11 March 1801; 4 April 1827; 11 April 1827; 8 July 1829. See also Blomfield, *St George's*, pp. 34–5; Clark-Kennedy, *The London*, pp. 198–9; Hume, *Newcastle Infirmary*, p. 27; McMenemey, *Worcester Royal Infirmary*, p. 124; Saunders, *Middlesex Hospital*, p. 18.
44. R.S. Tucker, 'Real Wages of Artisans in London, 1729–1935', in Arthur J. Taylor (ed.), *The Standard of Living in Britain in the Industrial Revolution* (London: Methuen, 1975), pp. 24–5.
45. Neale, *Bath*, p. 86, table 3.6.
46. Letter Book, R. Allen to R. Nash, 20 February 1738.
47. Minute Book, January 1738, 'Copy of a letter to be inserted in the public papers'. Letter Book, R. Nash to R. Allen, 16 February 1738.
48. See also Brockbank, *Royal Infirmary, Manchester*, pp. 6–7; Frizelle and Martin, *Leicester Royal Infirmary*, p. 27; Hume, *Newcastle Infirmary*, pp. 4–5.
49. Clark-Kennedy, *The London*, pp. 123, 124, 137–8; Gibson, *Radcliffe Infirmary*, pp. 78–9.
50. *Gentleman's Magazine*, 8, 13 July 1738, p. 378; *London Evening Post*, 8 July 1738.
51. *Gentleman's Magazine*, 6, 18 October 1736, p. 618; 7, 31 October 1737, p. 636; 11, 31 August 1741, p. 441; 13, 20 September, 17 November 1743, pp. 496, 610–11.
52. Minute Book, 14 June 1797. See also Minute Book, 23 May 1744.
53. Minute Book, 19 May 1739; 31 May 1749; 16 January 1788.
54. Minute Book, 16 June 1739; 30 May 1740. *Bath Journal*, 7 May 1744; 4 May 1747
55. *Bath Journal*, 29 November 1762.
56. See, for example, Rice Charleton, *Three Tracts on the Bath Waters*, 2nd edn (Bath: R. Cruttwell, 1774), p. iii; *Improved Bath Guide*, p. 2; Richard Warner, *The History of Bath* (Bath: R. Cruttwell, 1801), p. 296.
57. See, for example, Clark-Kennedy, *The London*, p. 112; Frizelle and Martin, *Leicester Royal Infirmary*, p. 18; Rook, Carlton and Cannon,

Addenbrooke's Hospital, pp. 30–31; Turner, *Hampshire County Hospital*, pp. 10, 63.

58. Minute Book, January 1738, 'Copy of a letter to be inserted in the public papers'; 16 February 1738, 'Plan and Elevation'. Letter Book, R. Allen to R. Nash, 20 February 1738. Wood, *Bath*, pp. 285–9.
59. Minute Book, 17 May 1739; 31 May 1749; 16 January 1788.
60. Minute Book, 4 March 1742; 18 May 1742; 6 June 1750.
61. Minute Book, 14 December 1785.
62. Risse, *Hospital Life*, p. 36, table 1.1. See also H.C. Cameron, *Mr Guy's Hospital 1726–1948* (London: Longmans, Green and Co., 1954), pp. 145–8.
63. Jack Lloyd, *The Royal United Hospital, Bath: A Short History* (Bristol: Redcliffe, 1982), p. 11. Royal United Hospital, Minute Book, 26 July 1830. *Bath Journal*, 22 February 1830; 5 April 1830. See also Davies, *Deeds Not Words*, p. 23; Smith, *Bristol Royal Infirmary*, p. 51.
64. Minute Book, 24 February 1830.
65. Berry, 'Patronage', pp. 52–6.
66. At the London Hospital, the initial right of subscribers to recommend an indefinite number of in-patients soon had to be limited to one at a time. Elsewhere, sponsorship was specified from the outset. At Shrewsbury and Worcester, one guinea bought one recommendation; at Manchester and Liverpool, the price was two guineas. See Clark-Kennedy, *The London*, pp. 31–2; Howie 'Royal Salop Infirmary', p. 50; McMenemey, *Worcester Royal Infirmary*, p. 52; Brockbank, *Royal Infirmary, Manchester*, p. 206; McLoughlin, *Liverpool Infirmary*, p. 71.
67. Langford, *Polite and Commercial People*, pp. 136–8; John V. Pickstone, *Medicine and Industrial Society: A History of Hospital Development in Manchester and its Region 1752–1946* (Manchester: Manchester University Press, 1985), p. 11; Roy Porter, *Disease, Medicine and Society in England 1550–1860* (London: Macmillan, 1987), p. 39; Risse, *Hospital Life*, p. 99.
68. Minute Book, 26 November 1741; 25 November 1742.
69. Minute Book, 2 May 1785. Howie, 'Finance and Supply', pp. 129–30; McMenemey, *Worcester Royal Infirmary*, p. 58, 124.
70. Minute Book, 4 June 1783; 11 June 1783; 2 May 1785; 13 January 1831. See also Haskins, *Salisbury Infirmary*, p. 12; Steer, *West Sussex Hospital*, p. 20.
71. *Improved Bath Guide*, pp. 46–7.
72. See, for example, Brockbank, *Royal Infirmary, Manchester*, p. 206; Eade, *Norfolk and Norwich Hospital*, p. 217; Frizelle and Martin, *Leicester Royal Infirmary*, p. 41; Harold W. Hart, 'Some Notes on the Sponsoring of Patients for Hospital Treatment under the Voluntary System', *Medical History*, 24 (1980), p. 449; McLoughlin, *Liverpool Infirmary*, p. 72.
73. Wood, *Bath*, pp. 294–9; Eade, *Norfolk and Norwich Hospital*, pp. 214–15; Howie, 'Finance and Supply', p. 133; Brockbank, *Royal Infirmary, Manchester*, pp. 204–5; McLoughlin, *Liverpool Infirmary*, p. 67.
74. Minute Book, 29 July 1761; 2 May 1774; 1 May 1779; 11 October 1797; 28 July 1802; 18 May 1814.
75. Subcommittee Book, 8 May 1802.

76. Minute Book, 2 May 1785; 25 May 1785. See also Minute Book, 7 December 1761.
77. This happened at Worcester in the late 1790s. See McMenemey, *Worcester Royal Infirmary*, p. 125.
78. Minute Book, 1 May 1765. See also Howie, 'Finance and Supply', pp. 133–4; Turner, *Hampshire County Hospital,* p. 60.
79. *Annual Report,* 1764/65.
80. Minute Book, 10 May 1769; 1 May 1787; 2 May 1803.
81. *Annual Report*, 1743/44, 1830/31. Virtually all subscriptions fell into one of these two categories.
82. Steven Cherry, 'The Role of English Provincial Voluntary General Hospitals in the Eighteenth and Nineteenth Centuries', 2 vols (unpublished doctoral thesis, University of East Anglia, 1976), vol. 1, pp. 123–4.
83. Subcommittee Book, 8 May 1802.
84. Turner, *Hampshire County Hospital,* p. 61. See also Howie, 'Finance and Supply', pp. 128–30; Hume, *Newcastle Infirmary*, p. 16; Langford, 'History of Hereford General Hospital', p. 151.
85. See Owen, *English Philanthropy*, p. 48; Bevan, *Salop Infirmary*, No. 4, 'A Statement of Receipts and Disbursements'; Brockbank, *Royal Infirmary, Manchester*, p. 13; Marland, *Medicine and Society*, p. 114; McMenemey, *Worcester Royal Infirmary*, pp. 51, 177; Smith, *Bristol Royal Infirmary*, p. 43.
86. Martin Gorsky, 'Medicine and Charity: Some Evidence from Bristol Infirmary, 1780–1870' (unpublished paper, Hospital Finances Seminar, Wellcome Institute for the History of Medicine, London, January 1995).
87. See, for example, Blomfield, *St George's*, p. 41; Bunce, *Birmingham General Hospital,* p. 17; Clark-Kennedy, *The London,* pp. 111–12; Edward Copeman, *Brief History of the Norfolk and Norwich Hospital* (Norwich: Charles Muskett, 1856), pp. 36–9; Frizelle and Martin, *Leicester Royal Infirmary*, p. 76; Haskins, *Salisbury Infirmary*, p. 12; McClure, *Coram's Children*, pp. 66–71; Rook, Carlton and Cannon, *Addenbrooke's Hospital,* p. 55; F.G. St Clair Strange, *The History of the Royal Sea Bathing Hospital, Margate 1791–1991* (Rainham, Kent: Meresborough Books, 1991), p. 44.
88. Minute Book, 15 February 1758; 29 March 1758; 1 May 1758; 31 January 1759; 28 February 1759; 18 April 1759; 29 April 1761. Annual oratorios for the Norfolk and Norwich Hospital were likewise discontinued (and replaced with a grander triennial affair in the 1820s) because the organizational effort out-stripped the financial return. Copeman, *Norfolk and Norwich Hospital,* p. 36. See also Leader, *Sheffield General Infirmary*, p. 39.
89. See, for example, *Annual Report*, 1743/44; 1746/47; 1749/50; 1754/55.
90. Minute Book, 4 February 1756. See also Minute Book, 25 December 1751; 15 November 1752; 28 November 1753; 12 April 1758; 1 November 1758.
91. See Frith, *Gloucester's Infirmary*, pp. 4, 14; Smith, *Bristol Royal Infimary*, p. 90.
92. *Gentleman's Magazine*, 17, 1 May 1747, p. 245; McClure, *Coram's Children,* p. 265, Appendix V. See also Andrew, *Philanthropy and Police*, p. 80; Humble and Hansell, *Westminster Hospital*, p. 46.

93. Minute Book, 16 February 1738; 23 February 1738; 21 September 1738.
94. Such boxes were used at Leicester, Shrewsbury, Worcester and Northampton. See Frizelle and Martin, *Leicester Royal Infirmary*, p. 68; Howie, 'Finance and Supply', p. 135; Joan Lane, *Worcester Infirmary in the Eighteenth Century* (Worcestershire Historical Society, 1992), p. 5; Waddy, *Northampton General Hospital*, p. 103.
95. Minute Book, 16 March 1738; 19 October 1738; 26 January 1785; 9 February 1785.
96. *Bath Journal*, 6 May 1754.
97. See, for example, Clark-Kennedy, *The London*, pp. 51–3, 123, 124–6, 137–8; Eade, *Norfolk and Norwich Hospital*, pp. 42, 51, 55, 62, 64, 65, 70; Frizelle and Martin, *Leicester Royal Infirmary*, p. 76; Rook, Carlton and Cannon, *Addenbrooke's Hospital*, p. 55.
98. *Bath Journal*, 30 April 1759; 20 April 1761.
99. This practice was followed at the Lock Hospital in London, and at the Leicester and Nottingham Infirmaries. See Andrew, *Philanthropy and Police*, p. 81; Frizelle and Martin, *Leicester Royal Infirmary*, p. 47; Jacob, *Nottingham General Hospital*, p. 51.
100. See, for example, Minute Book, 12 October 1743; 19 October 1743; 9 April 1755; 18 April 1770; 20 April 1785; 26 November 1800; 15 March 1815; 4 November 1830.
101. Wilfred J. Jenkins, 'A History of the Proprietary Chapels of Bath' (unpublished typescript, Bath Central Library, 1948), p. 18. Minute Book, 1 May 1804.
102. Minute Book, 12 October 1742; 27 November 1745. See also *Bath Journal*, 17 October 1748; 29 October 1770.
103. See, for example, Minute Book, 2 May 1753.
104. Minute Book, 4 August 1773; 22 March 1820.
105. Minute Book, 1 May 1783; 2 May 1785.
106. Howie, 'Royal Salop Infirmary', p. 41; Howie, 'Finance and Supply', p. 134. See also *Gentleman's Magazine*, **61**, 7 July 1791, p. 669; Hume, *Newcastle Infirmary*, pp. 127–8; Leader, *Sheffield General Infirmary*, p. 23; McLouglin, *Liverpool Infirmary*, p. 105, Appendix XI; McMenemey, *Worcester Royal Infirmary*, pp. 54, 62; Smith, *Bristol Royal Infirmary*, p. 61; Thomas Sympson, *A Short Account of the Old and of the New Lincoln County Hospitals* (Lincoln: James Williamson, 1878), pp. 56–7.
107. Waddy, *Northampton General Hospital*, p. 175.
108. Bevan, *Salop Infirmary*, No. 4, 'Statement of Receipts and Disbursements'. See also McMenemey, *Worcester Royal Infirmary*, p. 114; Waddy, *Northampton General Hospital*, p. 175.
109. Oliver Goldsmith, *The Miscellaneous Works of Oliver Goldsmith*, introduced by David Masson, first pub. 1868, repr. (London: Macmillan, 1908), p. 542; William Addison, *English Spas* (London: Batsford, 1951), p. 65; Falconer, *Mineral Water Hospital*, pp. 31–2. Addison claims that the woman in question was the Duchess of Marlborough; Falconer argues more convincingly that she was the Duchess of Queensberry.
110. Quoted in Falconer, *Mineral Water Hospital*, p. 32. I have been unable to trace this reference in the volume for 1745 which Falconer cites.
111. Andrew, *Philanthropy and Police*, p. 84.
112. Letter Book, R. Nash to R. Allen, 16 February 1738.

113. Minute Book, 24 December 1800.
114. Minute Book, 22 January 1755; 6 July 1757; 20 May 1767. *Annual Report*, 1770/71; 1785/86; 1815/16; 1830/31.
115. See, for example, Andrew, *Philanthropy and Police*, pp. 81–2; Blomfield, *St George's*, p. 35; Davies, *Deeds Not Words*, p. 22; McMenemey, *Worcester Royal Infirmary*, pp. 117, 151, 178, 186; John Patrick, *A Short History of the Glasgow Royal Infirmary* (Glasgow: Glasgow Royal Infirmary, 1940), pp. 15–16.
116. Falconer, *Mineral Water Hospital*, pp. 34–5.
117. Minute Book, 27 March 1745; 1 September 1756; 11 February 1761. *Annual Report*, 1770/71.
118. See, for example, McMenemey, *Worcester Royal Infirmary*, p. 147; Rook, Carlton and Cannon, *Addenbrooke's Hospital*, p. 79.
119. Mainwaring, *Annals*, p. 13.
120. *Annual Report*, 1800/01.
121. Similar trends have emerged from Amanda Berry's work, although the values of benefactions and legacies – averaged over three sample decades – were higher. See Berry, 'Patronage', pp. 75–9.
122. Berry, 'Patronage', pp. 84–5.
123. A not dissimilar trend has been plotted for annual subscriptions at the Bristol, Exeter and Northampton Infirmaries, using the Schumpeter–Gilboy index. See Amanda Berry, 'Patterns of Patronage: English Voluntary Hospitals in the Eighteenth Century', (unpublished paper to the Annual Conference of the Society for the Social History of Medicine, University of Southampton, July 1993).
124. *Annual Report*, 1747/48; 1748/49; 1749/50; 1750/51.
125. Bayly, *Sermon*, p. 17; [Bath General Infirmary], 'Short Account', in Bayly, *Sermon*, p. 26; [Bath General Infirmary], 'Short Account', in Leyborne, *Charity Conducive*, p. 40; [Bath General Infirmary], 'Short Account', in Olive, *Particular Excellence*, p. 33.
126. Peach, *Bath*, pp. 139, 157; Hembry, *English Spa*, p. 273; John Kirkup, 'A Pioneer Accident Service: Bath Casualty Hospital, 1788–1826', in Roger Rolls, Jean Guy and John R. Guy (eds), *A Pox on the Provinces: Proceedings of the 12th Congress of the British Society for the History of Medicine* (Bath: Bath University Press, 1990), p. 56; Mainwaring, *Annals*, p. 114.
127. *State of the Bath City Infirmary and Dispensary ... from the 1st of October 1792 to January 1st 1794* (Bath: Cruttwell, 1794), p. 20.
128. Minute Book, 5 December 1764; 19 December 1764.
129. See, for example, *Annual Report*, 1790/91, 1810/11; 1830/31.
130. Minute Book, 21 April 1751; 14 November 1764; 19 August 1778. *Annual Report*, 1759/60; 1795/96. B.E.S. Trueman, 'The Purchase and Management of Guy's Hospital Estates, 1726–1806', in C.W. Chalklin and J.R. Wordie (eds), *Town and Countryside: The English Landowner in the National Economy 1660–1860* (London: Unwin Hyman, 1989), p. 73; F.G. Parsons, *The History of St Thomas's Hospital*, 3 vols (London: Methuen, 1932–36), vol. 3: *From 1800 to 1900* (1936), p. 34.
131. Minute Book, 8 April 1801. Subcommittee Book, 10 July 1810.
132. Minute Book, 31 July 1822. See also Parsons, *St Thomas's Hospital*, vol. 3, p. 43.
133. Minute Book, 2 March 1825. *Annual Report*, 1830/31.

134. Minute Book, 13 April 1768; 17 April 1771.
135. Owen, *English Philanthropy*, p. 73; Trueman, 'Guy's Hospital Estates', p. 52.
136. Trueman, 'Guy's Hospital Estates', p. 71.
137. Minute Book, 24 April 1751; 1 May 1751; 28 October 1761; 1 May 1764.
138. Minute Book, 21 May 1766; 12 November 1766; 8 November 1769; 25 June 1783; 10 September 1828.
139. Minute Book, 11 June 1750; 14 February 1753; 30 January 1754; 1 January 1755; 6 January 1762; 26 April 1769; 1 December 1773.
140. Minute Book, 1 December 1773.
141. Minute Book, 2 February 1738, 'Copy of a letter to Nathaniel Gould'; 9 February 1738; 2 March 1738. Letter Book, E. Brett to T. Martin, 24 December 1737; T. Martin to E. Brett, 31 December 1737; T. Martin to E. Brett, 5 January 1738.
142. Minute Book, 2 August 1749; 10 June 1752; 4 November 1795; 18 November 1795; 2 May 1796.
143. Minute Book, 12 July 1809. *Annual Report*, 1825/26.
144. Minute Book, 1 October 1800; 20 April 1803; 5 September 1804; 24 April 1805; 27 August 1817; 1 May 1826. See also *Annual Report*, 1763/64; Minute Book, 17 April 1771.
145. Minute Book, 18 March 1748. *Gentleman's Magazine*, 18, 28 January 1748, p. 41.
146. *Annual Report*, January 1739–1830/31.
147. *An Address to the Governors of the Bath Hospital on the Propriety of Extending the Benefits of that Humane and Laudable Institution* (Bath: R. Crutwell, 1792), p. 26. See also Subcommittee Book, 26 January 1792.
148. Minute Book, 9 December 1807. See also Minute Book, 12 November 1794; 20 September 1809; 20 November 1811.
149. See, for example, Howie, 'Finance and Supply', p. 136; McLoughlin, *Liverpool Infirmary*, pp. 45–6.
150. At the Salop Infirmary, for instance, income from interest and dividends rose steadily, but had only reached approximately 20 per cent of total receipts by the 1820s. Bevan, *Salop Infirmary*, No. 3, 'A Comparative Average Statement'.

PART THREE

The Medical Profession

CHAPTER FOUR

The Rewards of Service

In his meticulous study of Augustan England, the late Geoffrey Holmes argued that physicians, surgeons and apothecaries experienced 'momentous changes' between the 1660s and 1740s; these years, he insisted, saw 'the rise of a true medical profession, and one that already had a measure of homogeneity by contrast with the motley collection of professionals, quasi-professionals, tradesmen and skilled craftsmen which had uneasily occupied the world of legitimate medicine at the time of the Restoration'.[1] Other historians have likewise identified an early convergence of specialisms, with some examples dating back to the late sixteenth century.[2] But although the legal right of apothecaries to dispense advice with their drugs was confirmed in 1704, they acquired no new powers; and the advances in medical education and community standing, to which Holmes attributed so much significance, were more clearly a feature of the second half of the eighteenth century.[3] By 1783, the movement towards integration was well established. Over 80 per cent of practitioners listed in the *Medical Register* for that year were described as 'surgeon apothecaries' and with the subsequent 'spectacular rise in [Georgian] surgery', even the physician lost his 'traditional superiority ... within the hierarchy of medicine'.[4] In this part, we explore how these changes were worked through at the Bath Infirmary. Confronting the view that charitable motives alone inspired hospital service, Chapter 4 examines the participation of doctors in the government of the institution and relates their levels of interest to the more worldly economic, socio-cultural and medical rewards on offer. Chapter 5 then considers the extent to which clinical autonomy was limited by the interface with the local medical community and by the interaction between physicians, surgeons and governors within the Infirmary. The part concludes with an assessment of the contribution of the General Hospital to the professional development of medicine in Bath. As a preliminary to these issues, however, we must turn to the roles which doctors undertook inside the Infirmary.

Medical roles, foundation and government

Although the voluntary hospital has been portrayed as a positive force for professional assimilation,[5] at Bath the roles of physician, surgeon and apothecary hardened rather than softened the historical division of labour.[6] At the bottom of the hierarchy was the apothecary, a mere paid employee. The incumbents of this post were typically long-serving and between 1742 and 1832, only five appointments were made, each lasting an average of almost 20 years (Table 4.1). Despite the apothecary's expertise in dispensing drugs, the set of rules included in John Wood's *Description of Bath* required only that he accompany the physicians and surgeons on their ward rounds. This occupational subordination was underlined by the regular inspection of the shop by governors who were medically qualified.[7] In 1774 the written responsibilities of the apothecary were expanded after the scandal which led to the dismissal of the house steward and a reallocation of tasks. Reference to dispensing skills was scant. Over and above discharging 'the several duties of his profession', however, the apothecary was to 'buy in all the provisions, coals and spirits'; maintain proper financial records of purchases; and ensure discipline amongst patients and servants.[8] Such a wide-ranging agenda, allied to the apothecary's daily presence, made him the 'keystone' of the Hospital's administration,[9] but the mix of medical and non-medical duties served to clinch his low status. In the third decade of the nineteenth century, a more autonomous clinical role was formally recognized. When the other medical staff were absent, the apothecary was permitted 'to afford such assistance as the urgency of ... cases may require'.[10] Nevertheless, not only did the administrative jobs remain but, under normal circumstances, the directions of the physicians and surgeons were still to be followed. Like other medical institutions,[11] therefore, the Bath Infirmary was slow to adjust to the growing professional stature of apothecaries.

Whereas the apothecary was usually on the payroll of voluntary hospitals, physicians and surgeons normally offered assistance gratuitously. Their functions were differentiated. Surgeons applied their manual

Table 4.1 Bath General Hospital: dates of service for apothecaries, 1740–1830

Name	*Dates of service*
John Morris	1740–57
Edward Cole	1757–63
John Skuse	1763–84
William Balne Farnell	1784–1829
George Fredrick Bush	1829–32

Source: Minute Books.

skills to the treatment of external conditions, carrying out operations but more commonly dealing with wounds and fractures. Physicians, conversely, dealt with internal disorders, tying their diagnoses to case histories which included observation of the patient as well as information about his or her constitution and lifestyle.[12] Given their honorary status, relatively little was asked of medical staff deploying these skills within a voluntary hospital. Thus at Bath the rules in Wood's *Description of Bath* specified only two requirements: one physician and one surgeon were expected to be present at the weekly committee in order to admit patients, and all the honorary medical men were to attend together on two days each week to visit the wards and single out patients for discharge.[13] Throughout the Georgian period, a physician and a surgeon were nominated each week on a rota basis to handle admissions,[14] but in the late 1820s the level of clinical supervision was increased when the medical staff replaced bi-weekly with daily visits.[15] As well as making a clinical contribution, medical men have traditionally received much of the credit for the foundation of voluntary infirmaries, whether as financial benefactors or as campaigners and organizers.[16] Roy Porter has contested the importance assigned to physicians and surgeons, arguing that 'the medical professions were perhaps less conspicuous in the launching of infirmaries than one might have supposed'.[17] In the case of Bath, however, his reservations are unjustified. When earlier attempts to create a hospital were rekindled in the late 1730s, two of the trustees who survived from the committee of 1728 were physicians, including the famous Dr George Cheyne, author of a popular *Essay on Health and Long Life*. A further nine were added, so that by the time the Hospital became a corporation in 1739 10 per cent of trustees were physicians. A strong medical presence was retained under the new charter: of the 91 governors named, eight were 'Doctors of Physic', one was a surgeon and three were apothecaries.[18] Surgeons and apothecaries are more difficult to pick out in subsequent lists of governors. However, physicians, visible as a result of the MD label, lost ground in the second half of the eighteenth century and in the *Annual Report* for 1830/31 they constituted only 3.4 per cent of the governing body. Initial interest was not sustained.

The willingness to be associated with hospital administration has been linked to the pursuit of honorary medical posts; it is suggested that practitioners became governors in the hope that they would be appointed physician or surgeon when a vacancy arose.[19] At Bath the connection was more complex. In May 1740, the governors elected three physicians and one surgeon.[20] The surgeon, Jeremiah Peirce, a long-standing supporter, was a governor of the Hospital, but surgeons subsequently appointed worked an average of 2.6 years in an honorary

Table 4.2 Bath General Hospital: dates of service for honorary physicians and surgeons, 1740–1830

Name	*Governor*	*Physician*	*Name*	*Governor*	*Surgeon*
William Oliver	1739	1740–61	Jeremiah Peirce	1739	1740–61
Edward Harington	1739	1740–50	Archibald Cleland	—	1742–43
Alex Rayner	1739	1740–50	Thomas Palmer	1749	1742–62
David Hartley	1742	1744–48	Henry Wright	1750	1742–94
Richard Bostock	1744	1744–45	John Donne	1748	1742–67
Thomas Brewster	1742	1744–57	Giles Jones	1751	1744–55
Prof. William Woodford	1746	1747–57	Philip Ditcher	1751	1744–81
Abel Moysey	1747	1747–80	Joseph Phillott	1768	1767–1820
John Summers	1749	1748–52	Harry Atwood	1778	1781–1806
Rice Charleton	1752	1757–81	Morgan Nicholls	1795	1794–1817
Robert Gusthart	1752	1761–80	William Tudor	1806	1806–36
Henry Harington	1763	1780–99	George Kitson	1810	1817–42
Daniel Lysons	1771	1781–1800	J.G. Elkington	—	1820–21
John Staker	1781	1781–84	William Terry	1825	1821–27
William Falconer	1784	1784–1819	Richard F. George	1828	1827–60
Caleb Hillier Parry	1783	1799–1817			
James Holman	1799	1800–04			
Sir George Smith Gibbes	1804	1804–18			
John Ford Davis	1809	1817–34			
Charles Henry Parry	1817	1818–22			
Edward Barlow	1819	1819–44			
James Muttlebury	1825	1822–30			
John Bampfylde Daniell	1832	1830–44			

Source: Minute Books.

Table 4.3 Bath General Hospital: the ages of appointment and resignation/death for honorary physicians, 1740–1830

Name	*Dates of birth and death*	*Age at appointment*	*Age at resignation*
William Oliver	1695–1764	45	66
Edward Harington	1696–1757	44	54
David Hartley	1705–57	39	43
Thomas Brewster	b. 1705	39	52
Abel Moysey	1716–80	31	64
Rice Charleton	1710–89	47	71
Henry Harington	1727–1816	53	72
Daniel Lysons	1727–1800	54	73
William Falconer	1744–1824	40	75
Caleb Hillier Parry	1755–1822	44	62
Sir George Smith Gibbes	1771–1851	33	47
John Ford Davis	1773–1864	44	61
Charles Henry Parry	1779–1860	39	43
Edward Barlow	1779–1844	40	65

Note: For dates of appointment, see Table 4.2

Sources: *DNB*; *Alumni Cantabrigienses: Part I to 1751*, 4 vols (Cambridge: Cambridge University Press, 1922–27; *Alumni Cantabrigienses: Part II 1751–1900*, 6 vols (Cambridge: Cambridge University Press, 1940–54; *Alumni Oxoniensis: The Members of the University of Oxford 1715–1886*, 4 vols (London: Joseph Foster, 1888); Randle Wilbraham Falconer, *History of the Royal Mineral Water Hospital, Bath*, rev. by Anthony Beaufort Brabazon (Bath: Charles Hallett, 1888); Irvine Loudon, *Medical Care and the General Practitioner 1750–1850* (Oxford: Clarendon Press, 1986).

capacity before winning election to the governing body. As Table 4.2 shows, only Harry Atwood and George Kitson became governors prior to being appointed surgeons and the length of professional apprenticeship was particularly extended pre-1750. The personal details of surgeons are not easy to trace, but their prolonged service – over 50 years for Henry Wright and Joseph Phillott – imply that they gained posts at a comparatively young age when their careers were at a formative stage. With physicians this was not the case.[21] Of the 14 Georgian 'doctors of physic' for whom dates of birth have been obtained, only two were significantly below 40 when he joined the honorary staff and the average age of appointment was 42 years (Table 4.3). Therefore, these men were established rather than up and coming physicians. Until the 1820s,

Table 4.4 Bath General Hospital: average attendance at weekly committees by honorary physicians and surgeons, 1742–1830

Year	*Total attendance: all assistants*	*No. of assistants*	*Average attendance per assistant*	*Total attendance: all honorary physicians*	*No. of honorary physicians*	*Average attendance per honorary physician*	*Total attendance: all honorary surgeons*	*No. of honorary surgeons*	*Average attendance per honorary surgeon*
1742/43	577	37	15.60	96	3	32.00	18	1	18.00
1745/46	386	34	11.35	96	6	16.00	8	1	8.00
1750/51	452	35	12.91	71	5	14.20	75	5	15.00
1755/56	316	36	8.78	63	4	15.75	79	6	13.17
1760/61	289	35	8.26	69	3	23.00	72	5	14.40
1765/66	315	35	9.00	13	3	4.33	49	3	16.33
1770/71	277	34	8.15	1	3	0.33	70	3	23.33
1775/76	339	34	9.97	1	3	0.33	77	3	25.67
1780/81	356	34	10.47	32	5	6.40	81	4	20.25
1785/86	307	34	9.03	54	3	18.00	48	3	16.00
1790/91	311	36	8.64	43	3	14.33	37	3	12.33
1795/96	235	33	7.12	40	3	13.33	45	3	15.00
1800/01	173	32	5.41	10	3	3.33	14	3	4.67
1805/06	105	32	3.28	2	3	0.67	2	3	0.67

1810/11	226	32	7.06	0	3	0.00	2	3	0.67
1815/16	188	32	5.88	0	3	0.00	0	3	0.00
1820/21	191	33	5.79	3	3	1.00	0	2	0.00
1825/26	193	33	5.85	4	3	1.33	0	3	0.00
1830/31	291	32	9.09	5	3	1.67	2	3	0.67

Notes:

1. For most of the Georgian period, there were three honorary physicians and three honorary surgeons in post. In 1744, however, the governors formally agreed to increase the quotas to six. Four years later, it was decided to reduce them to their original level by natural wastage.
2. Only medical staff who were governors and hence eligible for election to the weekly committee are included. The surgeon, Philip Ditcher, became a governor early in 1751. In 1780/81, two physicians and one surgeon were appointed during the course of the administrative year, thereby inflating the annual number in post. In 1820/21, the new surgeon had no governorship.

Source: Minute Books.

moreover, they generally served an administrative rather than a professional apprenticeship, acting as governors for an average of three years before achieving a medical post (Table 4.2). After the quota, raised to six in 1744, was cut back to three in 1750,[22] governor physicians tended to wait longer for an appointment. Length of service also reduced opportunities. Although their mean of 14 years fell short of the quarter of a century notched up by surgeons, turnover was not rapid.[23] David Hartley resigned 'on account of his ill state of health' and Sir George Smith Gibbes resigned just before being elected to attend Queen Charlotte[24] but, on the whole, physicians continued into old age (Table 4.3). The resulting stagnation may explain the relative decline of physicians within the governing body; with few new openings for medical staff, there was less incentive to become a governor.

The physicians and surgeons who held honorary medical posts at Bath were not always financial supporters of the General Hospital and by 1830 only three of the six incumbents paid annual subscriptions.[25] Their administrative commitment was also variable. Governors who served in a clinical capacity were automatically appointed to the weekly committee. Table 4.4 sets out their participation at five-yearly intervals. It shows that in 1742/43 – the first year in which the wards were open – average attendance by honorary physicians ran at double the rate for all assistants. The 1760s and 1770s apart, they continued to engage more intensively in administration, as did honorary surgeons once elected to the governing body. But medical staff were not equally or consistently active.[26] Moreover, the resurgence of interest on the part of physicians, following the marked lull post-1760, was due largely to the efforts of Daniel Lysons. By 1800, the attendance of both physicians and surgeons had dropped to below the average, within the context of a general decline. Overall participation was back to its 1785 pitch in 1830, but the honorary doctors did not return. Medical staff were not excluded from governor status in the way that they were at other new[27] and established[28] institutions. Rather, they chose to concentrate on their clinical roles, effectively abandoning the administration of the Hospital to lay control. Therefore, just as management strategies became more specialized in the later Georgian period, so did management personnel.

The satirical attack

The rise and fall of doctors' administrative interest in the Bath Hospital reflected the rewards to be reaped from philanthropic service. Physicians and surgeons enjoyed a mixed press during the eighteenth century. Whereas in the *Gentleman's Magazine* they escaped universal condemnation, the

Spectator sniped that 'When a Nation abounds in Physicians, it grows thin of people'.[29] Bath's reputation as the frivolous playground of Georgian England left its medical practitioners highly susceptible to satirical attack. Particularly biting was a pamphlet called *The Diseases of Bath*, published in 1737. Not only was the city lambasted as a cesspit of infection; but its leading doctors were ridiculed, including a number connected with the General Infirmary:

> But lo a long Procession nigh – make room:
> Five bred Physicians! bred to fix our doom.
> Sad Evils these for one poor town to bear:
> Five Plagues than Egypt's seven far more severe.
> Say, florid Florister, if you can tell:
> How many Patients you've dispatched to Hell?
> Say Harrington of not inferior skill!
> How many Church-yards thy Prescriptions fill?
> Procus has laid his thousands on the Floor;
> And modest Bostick his ten thousands more.
> Big blust'ring Cheyne, not the last in fame,
> Tho' the Muse lead up in the rear his Name,
> Has sent such Colonies to Pluto's land;
> The God was forced to beg he'd stop his hand.[30]

Satire of this ilk was remorseless in Georgian Bath. In his novel, *The Adventures of Peregrine Pickle* (1751), Smollett has the leading character poking fun at the contradictory diagnoses revealed when he arranged for a bevy of doctors to visit an elderly colonel with gout: 'The first who gave his opinion said, the distemper was an obstinate arthritis; the second affirmed, that it was no other than a confirmed pox; and the third swore that it was an inveterate scurvy.' Upon waking, the patient was not impressed:

> seeing himself beset with such an assemblage of solemn visages and figures, which he had always considered with the utmost detestation and abhorrence, [he] was incensed to a most expressible degree of indignation; and so inspirited by his rage, that though his tongue denied its office, his other limbs performed their function; he disengaged himself from the triumvirate, who had taken possession of his body, sprung out of bed with incredible agility, and seizing one of his crutches, applied it so effectually to one of the three, just as he stooped to examine the patient's water, that his tye-periwig dropped into the pot, while he himself fell motionless on the floor.[31]

Christopher Anstey's *New Bath Guide*, reprinted many times after its first edition in 1766, was no less caustic. Having witnessed a gaggle of physicians talk more about politics and economics than medicine whilst visiting her sick brother, Jenny likewise took the law into her own hands:

'I'll teach them,' she said, 'at their next consultation,
To come and take fees for the good of the nation.'
I could not conceive what the devil she meant,
But she seiz'd all the stuff that the doctor had sent,
And out of the window she flung it down souse,
As the first politician went out of the house.
Decoctions and syrups around him all flew,
The pill, bolus, jule, and apozem too;
His wig had the luck a cathartic to meet,
And squash went the gallipot under his feet.
She said, 'twas a shame I should swallow such stuff,
When my bowels were weak, and the physic so rough';
Declared she was shock'd that so many should come
To be doctor'd to death such a distance from home,
At a place where they tell you that water alone,
Can cure all distempers that ever were known.[32]

Greed joined with incompetence in the satirical dissection of doctors. Peregrine Pickle, for example, complained that 'among the secret agents of scandal none were so busy as the physicians, a class of animals who live in this place, like so many ravens hovering about a carcass, and even ply for employment, like scullers at Hungerford Stairs'.[33] Exorbitant bills were an enduring feature of the assault on Bath doctors. Indeed, Granville in 1841 went so far as to blame the town's eclipse as a spa on the accelerating cost of treatment: 'visits were multiplied; the interference of the Doctor with the action of the Bath waters became incessant; and the patients soon found that they might as well have staid at their own homes; for, instead of mineral water and fair play, they had nothing but physic and to pay!'[34]

It is important not to take this unremitting censure at face value. Medical practitioners had long been represented textually and visually as 'dangerous charlatans'.[35] Moreover, though their very public squabbles made Georgian doctors easy fodder for satirists, these disputes were themselves the product of an emergent profession grappling with its own internal conflicts and competing for business in a society which was itself in a state of flux. Medical men were caricatured so astringently under these changing conditions not because they were vulnerable but because they were increasing their 'cultural influence and ... potential power over individual lives'. At the same time as paying tribute to professional authority, however, satire also reined it in by warning patients of the 'discrepancies between high claims and base reality', and by mocking practitioners for their 'generic faults and foibles'.[36] Physicians and surgeons, anxious to win and retain public belief in their services, saw charity as a valuable mechanism for counteracting satire, and this may be why the revival of the General Hospital scheme quickly followed the poisonous invective on *The Diseases of Bath*.[37] But philanthropy exercised through a medical institution bestowed additional rewards. Of course, charitable motives for service – a genuine desire to help the sick poor – cannot be ruled out; but nor are they incompatible with a shrewd calculation of the likely returns. More specifically, voluntary infirmaries offered three main prizes to physicians and surgeons anxious to advance their careers: economic gain, social capital, and clinical knowledge and autonomy. As the *Edinburgh Medical and Surgical Journal* advised young practitioners in 1809: 'Endeavour to establish a hospital or dispensary by the voluntary subscription of your friends; for many men have wriggled themselves into notice by professions of charity, and have qualified themselves for genteel practice, by sharpening their wits upon the carcasses of the poor.'[38]

Money, status and culture

The economic attractions of honorary posts derived from their capacity to enhance private practice, especially in the provinces where attracting paying patients was more difficult; hospital physicians and surgeons not only acquired prominence in the community from their charitable activity, but also the chance to socialize with the local élites who were their prospective clientele.[39] The growing prosperity, which medical practitioners shared with the middling orders,[40] alerts against overstating financial motivation, particularly in a cosmopolitan city like Bath where doctors were central to the use of the spa waters. Founder-governor, William Oliver, ran one of the leading local practices well before the Hospital opened and he obtained a post. Similarly, the annual income of Dr Caleb Hillier Parry rose from £39 in 1780 to £1 600 in 1790, yet he was not made an honorary physician until 1799.[41] The financial circumstances of surgeons are more difficult to trace, but there is evidence that at least some were prosperous: Joseph Phillott, in post from 1767 to 1820, belonged to a local banking family, while Philip Ditcher, an early appointment who served for almost 40 years, speculated in property and left an estate worth £9 000.[42] If the practitioners attached to the General Hospital were often rich, however, they were also operating in an aggressive market-place. Bath was a magnet for physicians, its position as the premier English watering-place luring highly qualified men with impressive publications and experience of honorary posts elsewhere.[43] According to one estimate, the ratio of physicians to population in Bath during the 1740s was between 1:900 and 1:1 000, whereas the comparable figure for Great Britain as a whole was only 1:5 200. By 1810, the gap had almost closed,[44] and although collectively physicians, surgeons and apothecaries increased from 50 in 1747 to 75 in 1830, this rise was far outstripped by demographic expansion. The growth of Bath's medical community, largely a phenomenon of the later Georgian period, was dominated by surgeons, whose ranks were augmented by an influx of retired military practitioners and by the gravitation of apothecaries towards surgery.[45] This advent of general practice may have catered mainly for the exploding residential population. But even among the visiting company, neither physicians nor surgeons enjoyed a primacy in medical care. So when a niece fell ill during a stay in 1807, Katherine Plymley first applied her own remedies and then wrote to the family doctor in Shrewsbury before calling in a local apothecary, and only as a last resort did she summon the prestigious Dr William Falconer.[46] Given such commercial rivalry, therefore, the extra exposure offered by an honorary post at the Bath Infirmary was a valuable weapon in the armoury of the most oppulent physician or surgeon.[47]

The economic benefits of a hospital appointment were compounded by the social capital which accrued. Despite their growing affluence, Georgian medical practitioners retained an affinity with trade which undermined their professional or gentlemanly status.[48] Irvine Loudon has correctly emphasized the dangers of polarity: the 'young practitioner who "set up a business"', he argues, 'was likely to say [that] he did so in order to "practise his profession"'.[49] In the provinces, the boundaries were generally dissolving, but early eighteenth-century Bath may have borne more resemblance to London, where the profusion of doctors made the distinction between the profession of physic and the business or trade of surgery more resilient. It is for this reason that the majority of honorary surgeons were elected to governorships of the Hospital only after a spell of voluntary service; their occupation lacked the kudos to guarantee immediate access to a social élite. The cachet of medical charity was not confined to marginal men. Established practitioners also sought to deny 'the commercial roots of medical enterprise, and ... [adopt] instead the demeanour of the gentleman philanthropist'.[50] Bath felt this pressure acutely, given the exceptional wealth of its doctors and their role in a city which profited from the relentless pursuit of leisure and luxury. The Hospital countered these tensions in several ways. Both *Annual Reports* and occasional publications advertised that the physicians and surgeons gave their services gratuitously;[51] from 1773 the May general court formally passed a vote of thanks for the 'great care and attention' of the medical staff;[52] and when a resignation or death occurred, there was fullsome praise for the 'long and valuable', 'faithful' and 'constant and able' attendance rendered.[53] The accolades continued in obituaries: thus when Dr David Hartley died in 1757, having been a short-term but enthusiastic governor and physician, the *Bath Journal* described his loss as 'much lamented by the poor'.[54] Local histories and guidebooks have since added their voice, immortalizing the contribution of Bath doctors to the General Hospital.[55] However, nowhere is this process clearer than in the address which marked the unveiling of a memorial tablet to William Oliver in 1935, itself a commemoration of his Hospital role. 'We say in common parlance', advised the speaker, a consulting physician from London, that 'Dr Oliver is dead. But I say he is not dead, but lives in the walls of his beloved Hospital which is sanctified by 200 years of service to sufferers from rheumatism'.[56] The fruits of benevolence extended beyond the grave, conferring upon medical practitioners an antidote to their commercialism.

Throughout the long eighteenth century, physicians and surgeons at the General Infirmary continued to net social capital from their honorary posts, not always limiting themselves to one charity. In 1747, the medical staff became involved in a Pauper Scheme to supply the sick poor in the city with free medicines. Subsequently, multiple appointments were held: Henry Harington simultaneously served Bellot's Hospital; Daniel Lysons the Casualty Hospital; John Ford Davis and James Muttlebury the Bath Eye Infirmary; and Edward Barlow the United Hospital.[57] Philanthropy, however, was not the only source of the social prestige so essential to successful practice; cultural refinement was also a prerequisite. Like doctors elsewhere,[58] Bath practitioners were renaissance men, with wide-ranging interests and aptitudes. William Oliver was described by contemporaries as a 'civilized personality', fascinated by books, painting and architecture.[59] David Hartley was a respected philosopher of the materialist school.[60] Caleb Hillier Parry, highly regarded as a natural historian and agriculturalist, was also accomplished in art, music, literature, modern languages and the classics.[61] Finally, his son, Charles – 'disgusted' by the 'obnoxious' work of the physician – enjoyed more distinction in literature than in medicine and was acquainted with the poets, Coleridge, Southey and Wordsworth.[62]

The embodiment of these personal pastimes within organizational structures was to affect the social role of the Bath Infirmary. Although this development dated from the late eighteenth century, Roy Porter has rightly dismissed any utilitarian alliance with the Industrial Revolution and coupled the blossoming of provincial science with cultural Enlightenment and the ambitions of the growing middling sort for status and differentiation.[63] However, his thesis that in Bath doctors played little part in nurturing literary and scientific ventures requires qualification because the hospital physicians were to the forefront of cultural initiatives. William Falconer and Caleb Parry were early members of the Bath and West Society, founded in 1777 (as the Bath Society) to promote 'Agriculture, Arts, Manufactures, and Commerce'. Dr Henry Harington co-founded the Bath Harmonic Society; and both he and Falconer attended the local Literary Club. Finally, when in 1825 earlier versions of the Bath Philosophical Society evolved into the Literary and Scientific Institution – thanks partly to the efforts of Edward Barlow – a former Hospital doctor, Sir George Smith Gibbes, delivered the inaugural address.[64] Porter attributes the cultural commitments of doctors in other urban centres to their insecure professional status. Identification with an old-fashioned spa water hospital may have predisposed the honorary physicians to assert their occupational credentials by joining organizations dedicated to the advance of scientific knowledge. However, these doctors were not peripheral members of the local medical fraternity or of Bath society. Quite the opposite, they were professional and social leaders. Their engagement in the new cultural diversions thus intimates a reorientation of sociability. As Bath became less of a resort and more of a residential town, running a hospital which barred native patients yielded fewer social returns. Therefore, the physicians, and surgeons, began to restrict their administrative input, seeking to integrate with the community, and tap future customers, through the exclusive cultural organizations by which a more permanent population of middle men sought prestige and hierarchy.

In stressing the social capital which flowed from honorary appointments, it is tempting to reduce Georgian physicians and surgeons to 'status professionals', only 'able to maintain a foothold among the ranks of ... gentlemen by glossing over their work responsibilities and emphasizing ... [their] leisured and honourable life-style'.[65] The appeal of such an interpretation is strengthened by the failure of those Bath cultural clubs with a scientific orientation to contribute to the medical debate; within five years of its foundation, for example, Charles Parry was complaining that the Institution was 'chiefly sought as a place for newspapers and pamphlets and easy chairs and heated air'.[66] This deficiency was not offset by the kind of local medical society that had been emerging in the provinces from the third decade of the eighteenth century.[67] In 1788, Caleb Parry did present a seminal paper on heart disease to the Gloucestershire Medical Society, whose membership included his lifelong friend, Edward Jenner, of vaccination fame.[68] However, it was not until 1836 that a local branch of the Provincial Medical and Surgical Association was founded with the assistance of Edward Barlow.[69] In contrast, Leeds had a medical society from 1768, five years before John Coakley Lettsom founded the Medical Society of London.[70] Yet despite the lack of a forum for clinical discussion, physicians and surgeons in Georgian Bath were more than just 'status professionals'. Complementing their social competences were claims to an 'occupational professionalism', based on an assumed command of medical knowledge and a desire for clinical control in its implementation. During the course of the nineteenth century, this bid for technical expertise 'came to be seen as an alternative and increasingly important' root of prestige.[71] However, occupational proficiency was also a powerful objective before 1800, and one which the voluntary infirmary was able to further. Therefore, practitioners were enticed to honorary posts by the opportunity to enhance their professional knowledge and autonomy.

Medical knowledge: evaluating the spa waters

In his 'Essay Towards the Improvement of Physic', published in 1714, John Bellers put forward an early case for hospital construction, arguing that medical knowledge would be greatly assisted by gathering patients in infirmary wards where they could be conveniently watched and the success of their treatments monitored.[72] The suitability of institutionalized patients for 'experimental practice' was reiterated later in the eighteenth century.[73] However, the historical emphasis on Parisian medicine has distracted attention from the clinical implications of the first infirmaries both in Britain and on the continent of Europe.[74] Drawing on the work of Ackerknecht, radical scholars from a range of disciplines have diminished eighteenth-century medicine to the 'bedside' model and contrasted it with the 'clinic', which allegedly emerged in post-Revolutionary Paris and signalled the birth of proper 'hospital' medicine.[75] This crude bifurcation overlooks significant developments in Georgian medicine which stemmed from the Scientific Revolution. By the seventeenth century, the 'new science', enshrined in the Royal Society after 1660, was transforming both methodology and theory. Newton's scientific method, which he defined as 'making experiments and observations and ... drawing general conclusions from them by induction',[76] was combined with a revolutionary theoretical approach, in which matter was conceptualized as 'particles ... of different sizes, shapes and motions'.[77] Medicine was slow to react to the theoretical thinking of the Enlightenment. Although the 'basic entities of the humoral system were redefined in terms of material entities, such as corpuscular flow or excitement of the muscles, the general conception of the bodily system' remained loyal to the ideas of Hippocrates and Galen; good health consisted of a stable balance of blood, phlegm, yellow and black bile, 'in proportions appropriate to the age and personality of each individual'.[78] None the less, by the mid-eighteenth century, military and civilian hospitals were providing a context well suited to the methodology of observation and experiment.[79] Voluntary infirmaries in search of funds latched on to this epistemological function.[80] Therefore, when the

Bath trustees drew up their 'Plan and Elevation' in 1738, the progress of medical expertise was a principal theme: 'a few years will furnish more histories of cases, which may be depended upon ... than any man's private practice could have done in an age'. Moreover, 'if the knowledge of the nature and efficacy of these waters could still be rendered more extensive and certain, it would be doing great service to every individual person, who may hereafter, in any country or age, have occasion for their use'.[81]

This confidence in the clinical possibilities of the Bath springs survived virtually unchallenged for most of the Georgian period.[82] In the mid-1750s, however, trouble broke out over the composition of the waters when an Irish physician called Charles Lucas refuted the presence of sulphur to which their curative properties were historically credited.[83] The resuscitation of this dispute, dating back to the late seventeenth century,[84] was a threat to the whole city and not just to its doctors. Lucas professed puzzlement at 'how a solution of brimstone could mix with water ... [and] why this ... "principle of sulphur" ... was necessary for hot baths'. Their clinical value he did not repudiate, but he attributed it to 'the ability of the water to induce evacuation in the body, and thereby restoration of proper balance of the humours'. Consequently, the springs held no unique qualities. Instead of the 'bitumen, sulphur, nitre, and ... fixed alcali' customarily used by chemists to explain the healing properties, he found only small quantities of iron, marine salt and 'a calcarious, or sparry stone'. The implications were threatening to the local community and to its doctors because, as Lucas concluded, 'Whatever warm water, charged with these like ingredients can do, that, and that alone is to be expected from Bath water'.[85] These arguments were soon to be regurgitated by another physician, William Baylies from Evesham in Worcestershire. But his indictment went further. Whereas Lucas posited only that the physicians of the General Infirmary published inaccurate patient histories to hide the ineffectiveness of their treatments, Baylies proclaimed a wider conspiracy in which both the Bath Corporation and the local medical establishment actively discouraged the analysis of the waters, and the Hospital – as a vehicle for their self-interest – deliberately suppressed clinical information.[86] This revival of the sulphur controversy has been read by G.S. Rousseau as a Galenist, iatromechanical attack on Paracelsian chemistry.[87] However, Lucas himself not only claimed a superior grasp of chemistry, but also put the case for a more sophisticated analysis of the waters. Therefore, the episode is better understood as a conflict between medical practitioners rather than medical theories.[88]

The 'bedside' model of Georgian medicine has emphasized the divisive impact of competition for patients, which mitigated against the 'free exchange' of ideas; in Jewson's words, 'medical innovators sought occupational advancement by utilizing their discoveries in private practice, where they were often kept as trade secrets, rather than by sharing them with professional rivals'.[89] At Bath, however, professional status joined with commercial pressures to fracture the medical community along several axes. It is no coincidence that Lucas and Baylies were 'outsiders' trying to break into a competitive market, that neither held Oxbridge degrees and, critically, that both had worked previously as lowly apothecaries.[90] As Lucas observed, his Bath protagonists were 'pretty unanimous ... in pronouncing my name with a "The Apothecary" – a terrible stigma!' But he went on, 'I proudly own the charge. I was, and hope I still am an apothecary ... since it is more plain, that he who is not an Apothecary and a Chirurgeon, cannot deserve the name of a physician'.[91] In short, the vitriolic discourse about the sulphur content of the spa waters became a vehicle for the expression of commercial and professional frictions.

Being the medical showcase of the city and publicly committed to the promotion of medical knowledge, the General Infirmary was inevitably sucked into this 'balneological war'.[92] Even before Lucas went into print, Robert Leyborne used his charity sermon to defend the Hospital's research record. 'Already have the physicians of this place been enabled ... to confute some dangerous mistakes of the most experienced in other places ... and with unparalleled disinterestedness and benevolence, they engage not to confine what other knowledge they gain ... but to publish it throughout the world.'[93] But how justified were the complaints of concealment? The honorary physicians of the General Infirmary were among the Bath doctors who analysed the springs.[94] For much of the eighteenth century, however, chemistry remained rudimentary with a confused terminology, unreliable methods and hence inconsistent outcomes.[95] These problems legitimated scepticism towards the 'very imperfect view'[96] provided by chemical analysis; the case for spa therapy had to rest on its results. This position was articulated by Bath physicians throughout the Georgian period. Consequently, Daniel Lysons, in post at the General Infirmary for the last two decades of the century, spoke for many when he wrote in 1783 that:

> Since ... the impregnation of our hot baths are so subtle as to baffle the inquiries of the most curious, and their virtues depend not upon one, but all the materials of which they are composed, blended together in an unimitable manner; we must necessarily have recourse to experience of their effects for ascertaining the propriety of their use.[97]

Such firm commitment to clinical empiricism demonstrates that physicians to the Bath Infirmary had rejected the abstract, theoretical accounts of illness characteristic of traditional Galenism and embraced the observational (if not the experimental) criteria of Enlightenment science.[98] The Hospital was ideally placed to implement this empiricism and document the application of the waters. An Admissions Register was duly set up listing the names and parishes of patients, together with 'their ages and distempers', dates of stay, and condition at discharge.[99] This information was then compiled into yearly statements for the *Annual Reports*. But these bald statistics were not enough to quench the professional thirst of those without an honorary post, who grumbled that the categories of disorder were so broad that 'little light' was shed on 'any ... particular disease'.[100] The appearance of more detailed clinical material was sporadic, prompting Smollett to impute 'a shameful laziness in those who belong to the hospital, in a medicinal capacity; or ... a reserve in the directors, which ... very ill becomes the trustees of a voluntary subscription'.[101] Nevertheless, several studies were undertaken.[102] A 1760 volume of William Oliver's cases, stimulated by the tirade from Lucas and Baylies, was simply a collation of 15 case histories, detailing previous treatment, the patient's condition at admission, and the regimen followed.[103] Critics were not impressed by this 'one six-penny number', which was a highly selective coverage of 'eighteen years of hospital practice'.[104] Almost a decade before, however, John Summers had been more systematic, taking the Hospital Register as the basis for commenting on the advanced age of many paralytic patients whose impairment had improved by the time they were discharged. A 1787 *Narrative*, produced under the auspices of the Hospital, likewise relied on the Register, using its statistics to preface a selection of cases.[105] But it was in the research of Rice Charleton and William Falconer that the Infirmary records were used with most imagination and effect.

Charleton and Falconer were representatives of a group of 'arithmetic observationist clinicians' who from the mid-century, as part of their campaign for public health and institutional hygiene,[106] picked up the 'political arithmetic' of John Graunt and William Petty and began to complement the acute observation of patients with a numerical manipulation of medical statistics.[107] Charleton had responded quickly to Lucas in a riposte which drew a dubious line between 'sulphur' – the chemical element – and 'sulphureous' – a conveniently loose term that was 'applicable to any oily or greasy substance'.[108] In the 1770s, however, he published a more innovative investigation of paralytic cases, which aimed to discover whether the spa waters were 'useful or detrimental in palsies'. After tabulating the fate of patients admitted with this condition between 1751 and 1764, he concluded that they were indeed helped since over 800 'received benefit' and only '240 little or none'. More specific questions were also posed and answered with greater sophistication. For instance, Charleton tested the common assumption that warm bathing aggravated apoplectic strokes and was able to reject the hypothesis after a comparison of mortality ratios: the hemiplegic category was slightly less likely to die than the patient body as a whole, despite containing a number of smallpox fatalities.[109] The arithmetic analysis of spa water therapy was extended by William Falconer. One of his most elaborate studies was an examination of rheumatic cases, published in 1795. Over 400 patients were divided into five groups, according to their state at discharge. Each group was then classified by age and sex, and the average length of stay was calculated for cases admitted in each month and in each season. From these foundations, Falconer argued that women were no more liable to the disease than men. Furthermore, by adjusting for the sex ratio, and projecting a success rate for men from the rate achieved by women, he was able to suggest that male patients responded more effectively to treatment. Similar techniques were applied to the impact of age and seasonality.[110] By the late eighteenth century, therefore, the General Hospital was playing host to a new specimen of clinician who subjected his cases to arithmetic analysis as well as observation.

The activities of Charleton and Falconer enable us to discredit the view that clinical statistics were an invention of post-Revolutionary Parisian medicine. Yet these arithmetic clinicians had no successors at Bath. This is significant but not unexpected. From the late eighteenth century, the General Hospital did appoint fewer physicians with a classical Oxbridge education and more with qualifications from Edinburgh University which was at the forefront of medical training.[111] However, doctors with an interest in quantification were a small if vocal minority, whose concern about epidemic diseases predisposed them to locate in the industrializing areas and not in elegant resort-cum-residential towns.[112] Moreover, even Charleton and Falconer were conservative in outlook, the parameters of their clinical research confined by chemical experiments in which they were content to confirm the sulphur orthodoxy.[113] Therefore, the Bath Infirmary was a halfway house between 'bedside' and 'hospital' medicine; it was a 'proto-clinic', in which existing knowledge was ratified but never fundamentally challenged.[114]

Clinical autonomy: the doctor–patient relationship

The conservative nature of clinical work at the General Infirmary is corroborated by the relationship between doctors and patients. The connection between spas and popular healing encouraged an early assertion of medical orthodoxy at Bath,[115] as doctors sought to cash in on the social differentiation which accompanied the emergence of a polite society. Thus Edward Jorden, writing in 1631, argued that only the physician could recommend the best way to drink and bathe in the waters due to the 'many cautions and observations ... drawn from the particular constitutions of bodies; from the complications of diseases, and from many other circumstances which cannot be comprehended in general rules, or applied to all bodies alike'.[116] From the 1740s, the Bath Infirmary buttressed this position because its very existence articulated the importance of medical practitioners in determining treatment programmes: 'Is not the physician's aid most essentially requisite for the proper and effectual application of the fountains of health?' asked the Reverend Mr Olive in a charity sermon of 1759. Without this, and the 'collateral medicines' of food and care, 'what advantage is it to the poor Lazar that he is brought even to the brink of the pool, if at last he cannot get down to partake of its virtues? This, methinks, does but aggravate his misery!'[117] As for the poor, so for the rich. If wealthy visitors to Bath were financing professional advice for indigent Hospital patients, should they not impart the same blessing upon themselves?

Voluntary infirmaries further rarefied medical expertise by providing a context in which physicians and surgeons could exercise clinical autonomy. 'Bedside' medicine construes the Georgian patient as all-powerful, dispensing patronage and payment to practitioners emasculated by the rigours of the market-place.[118] In reality, the micro-politics of the consultation were more subtle. Doctors, themselves increasingly wealthy, were not inevitably intimidated even by their aristocratic clientele, and although patients in control of the purse strings were free to ignore advice, illness created a dependency that the practitioner was able to exploit in his own interests. At the same time, however, both parties to the encounter shared a common medical culture, heavily indebted to the classical theory of humours; and, therefore, orthodox opinions – of which there were many – exercised no monopoly over lay or 'fringe' remedies.[119] The net effect of these cross-currents was 'a rough and ready parity' between doctor and patient, rather than the 'quasi-monopolistic professional control' that was to thrive in the second half of the nineteenth century.[120] The merits of an environment in which the inmate had no such power were regularly expounded in hospital publicity. As the Bath trustees noted in their initial 'Plan and Elevation':

> persons of higher rank are too often negligent of their own health; and, by no means, so exact in taking their medicines ... and staying a due time ... in order to give the physician a sufficient opportunity either of doing them all the service their case would admit of, or making observations for the future benefit of others.

> Whereas in this Hospital every person will be under his government and direction in all circumstances regarding his health ... [121]

When the Infirmary opened, the authority of the medical staff was duly enforced; and patients like James Shepherd were promptly 'discharged for not complying with the physician's orders'.[122] The creation of such a strict regime had far-reaching implications for medical knowledge as well as medical control. Taking Bristol as her example, Mary Fissell has posited that voluntary infirmaries so increased medical power over the lower orders that the patient's narrative vanished from hospital consultations. On the basis of manuscript and published case notes, she suggests that from the 1750s doctor and patient began to inhabit different conceptual worlds of illness. Increasingly, the doctor came to rely on 'signs and symptoms' which were conducive to 'a disease-orientated diagnosis' and to 'the demands of hospital practice'. Alien labels were, therefore, attached to patients' conditions, the treatment of which was no longer negotiable. The consequence was not a stampede into major surgery; for the most part, hospital medicine, like private medicine, did not become dominated by operations such as amputation, herniotomy, trephining and lithotomy. However, a rigid therapeutic routine was imposed, which at Bristol normally meant 'an anti-phlogistic regimen [of] bleeding, purging, blisters, and a bland diet'. The upshot was a widening gulf between clinical knowledge and patient perception, which gradually spilt over from the hospital to medical practice at large.[123]

There is a risk of overgeneralizing these changes. Not all provincial infirmaries adopted so enthusiastically the Latin terminology used at Bristol,[124] and even London practitioners at the forefront of clinical training engaged in 'safe' science which 'conformed to cultural sensibilities' about how medical experiments should be conducted.[125] Nevertheless, the therapeutic regime at the Bath Infirmary offers qualified backing for the Fissell hypothesis. Bathing, and drinking the waters, were the mainstay of treatment and some cases received little else besides.[126] However, the physicians and surgeons were prepared to admit that the spa was 'by no means a panacea'[127] and other therapies were used. In 1795, for instance, Lobbs machines 'for the extension of contractions' were ordered for two newly opened wards.[128] Although surgical intervention was tried where the spine was distorted,[129] major surgery was apparently an exceptional event: the Minute Books up to 1830 contain only one reference to a serious operation when in 1807 the weekly committee, on being informed that a patient required amputation above the knee, left the matter 'to the discretion of the medical faculty'.[130] Electrotherapy, the subject of a rapid growth in interest from the 1750s,[131] was also sparingly applied. Practitioners at Bath were sceptical, despite – or perhaps because – of its popularity for patients with the rheumatic and paralytic conditions considered most appropriate for the spa.[132] Dr Oliver's 1760 volume includes no case of electrical treatment, and the 1787 *Narrative* just one. Moreover, even this single example conveys ambivalence. The medical staff acknowledged that electricity was used 'with some appearance of success' for Susanna Bruner, whose arm was in a constant state of involuntary motion following an injury from bleeding; but the entry goes on to record that 'the patient often declared she thought the ... pump afforded the greatest relief'.[133]

The published patient histories imply that throughout the eighteenth century bathing and drinking were most commonly mixed with medicines and/or minor surgical interventions. Mary Scriggins was prescribed one such package when admitted in 1758 with 'scorbutic rheumatism'. Upon her arrival, wrote Dr Oliver:

> we took nine ounces of blood from her arm; the next day purged her gently; then she began to drink three half pints of the Bath water a day, and bathed twice a week. By this course her pains gradually abated; the gummy swellings at her joints were dispersed; she could turn her head, and neck without any uneasiness, and her ankles grew so strong that she could walk almost as well as ever.[134]

Establishing how treatments changed over time is difficult because even where the diagnosis was the same, the nature and severity of the symptoms may have differed. However, juxtaposing two cases of painters who had fallen victim to lead poisoning hints at an intensification of the non-water treatments over time. When John Stevens was admitted with this condition in the mid-1750s, balneology was his sole therapy: 'by drinking the waters, and bathing, his bowels were brought into a good state; his stools became regular; he recovered the motion of his arms, hands, and fingers; the muscles of the thumbs grew much plumper, and he was discharged cured'.[135] Thirty years later James Lewis Markes was subjected to more aggressive management.

> After taking a gentle dose of purging physic, he was directed to drink the waters, to bathe twice a week, and to pump the hands daily. He also took ten grains of the aromatic pill occasionally to keep the body regular, and had blisters to his arms and hands ... he also rubbed his hands occasionally with an embrocation of tincture of cantharides.

After 12 months, he too was discharged, '*much better*, being able to use his hands very well for the common purposes of life, but not for any laborious operation'.[136]

By the end of the Georgian period, an invasive therapeutic regime closer to that at Bristol was evolving. Not only did physicians and surgeons start to visit daily rather than just twice a week; but in 1830 they recommended 'the full services of an assistant' for the apothecary on the grounds that medicine had forged ahead:

> an improved knowledge of the symptoms and treatment of several diseases (particularly of some formerly comprehended under the general name of rheumatism, but now distinguished as inflammatory afflictions of the hip joint ... muscle, and ... spinal cord) has led to a more extensive use of auxiliary remedies, as bleeding, cupping, leeches, +c, requiring much personal attention from the apothecary and assistant.[137]

Embedded within both Dr Oliver's *Cases* and the 1787 *Narrative*, however, were early signs of the shift that was occurring in clinical practice and perception. First, standardized treatment programmes were implemented. When Elizabeth Jordan was admitted with 'a leprous complaint' in 1758, for example, she was 'prepared by bleeding and purging' on account of her 'full habit, and sanguine complexion'. Similarly, William Smith 'was put upon the dry diet' because 'he was of a lax habit' after arriving with distorted vertebrae in 1781.[138] Secondly, physicians were careful to flag any lay narrative, William Oliver making clear that it was the patient who 'supposes that his disease arose from lying on the cold wet ground' when George Pope entered the Infirmary with rheumatism.[139] This self-conscious distancing from non-medical perspectives was reflected in the application of a technical language to clinical conditions and their bodily locations: sacrum and sternum, os pubic and os coccygis, were terms foreign to patients, who were also unlikely to describe themselves as having a 'peripneumonic complaint', 'debility in the urinary passages', or 'paralysis of the muscles of deglutition'.[140] Finally, by the later eighteenth century, doctors at the Bath Hospital were beginning to record their use of diagnostic techniques so that when Anne Chalacombe was admitted with acute lead poisoning in 1785, the fact that her 'pulse [was] low and weak, but not too quick' was judged worthy of note.[141]

In decoding these changes, we must avoid exaggeration because the Bath case notes kept aspects of the patient narrative alive. Take William Toop of Frome 'ill two months with the loss of his lower limbs by going into the water to gather watercresses'. Or David House, a Bristol cooper whose condition 'terminated in a paralytic stroke' when he 'was seized with a violent cold after remaining several hours in a cold, damp cellar, whilst he was bottling wine'.[142] People like these were not entirely reduced to their bodily ailments, for if refused the authority to interpret their own symptoms, their individual identities survived the medical gaze. In the 1820s work of Edward Barlow, there is movement towards the impersonal case history: 'Susanna Ponting, aged 36; admitted 7th February, 1821. Ill a month; cough, dyspnoea; great swelling of legs and thighs; urine copious; pulse 90; subject for years to complaints of chest.' This example of 'inflammatory oedema', however, was drawn from Barlow's practice at the Bath City Infirmary and Dispensary. When he quoted from the journals of the General Hospital, the style was less detached; pulse was measured numerically and drug intake logged in a technical format, but there was still reference to occupation and the account of symptoms upheld the patient's voice. Thus, a publican called Henry Southern was said to have 'complained of pain and stiffness of the right ankle, knee, and hip' after being admitted with gout in 1821, whilst a year later Edward Medcraft, also a victim of gout, was described as presenting 'a sallow sickly aspect, with blanched lips, and every appearance of extensive constitutional disease'.[143]

Comparison with the Bristol Infirmary helps us to comprehend why the patient perspective persisted at the Bath General Hospital. Early nineteenth-century British medicine had not absorbed the tissue pathology of Bichat which served as an 'intellectual cement' for physicians and surgeons in France, and encouraged the former to view the interior as well as the exterior of the body as a suitable object for surgical intervention. None the less, Enlightenment surgery did enjoy enhanced status and power across the channel, which enabled its practitioners at Bristol to seize control of the Infirmary and profit from the fees which students were willing to pay for the hands-on experience of patients. This surgical dominance fostered the development of an impersonal, localized pathology which, though based on individual organs and hence at variance with the Paris school, represented a significant departure from the humoral tradition.[144] At the Bath Hospital, conversely, the devotion to spa therapy precluded the adoption of the new surgery and required fidelity to the holistic approach despite the gradual decline of humoralism.[145] As Edward Barlow wrote in 1822:

> In the various forms and degrees of chronic rheumatism, an essential object is to have a clear conception of the accompanying constitution; for without first rectifying its derangements, we shall in vain endeavour to cure those local ailments which form the most painful and troublesome part of this formenting malady.[146]

For patients, the effect of this framework was to preserve a degree of meaningful consultation because the lay narrative still had relevance to a holistic therapeutic regime.

The durability of the patient narrative, when allied to the still birth of clinical statistics, suggests that by the early nineteenth century the Bath Hospital was beginning to trail behind mainstream medicine. Up to 1800, the Infirmary functioned as a medical laboratory for those doctors who chose to puts its records to statistical effect. From the mid-Georgian period, however, the clinical credibility of spa therapy –

always vulnerable due to its close bond with lay culture – was undermined by the decline of humoral theory and the rise of surgery. Reinforced by the authority of a specialist institution, Bath practitioners continued to assert that effective treatment required expert advice.[147] As localized pathology moved into the ascendency, however, their words had a hollow ring. Physicians and surgeons still accepted honorary positions at the Hospital; but with balneology translated to the margins of orthodox medicine, voluntary service brought fewer clinical returns. Therefore, doctors took up complementary posts at other charities in the city which were keeping pace with new developments in medical knowledge. The General Infirmary was becoming a backwater of local rather than national significance.

In this chapter, we have tried to unravel the motives which encouraged physicians and surgeons first to participate in and then to withdraw from the administration of the Georgian Bath Hospital. Throughout the period, a philanthropic portfolio was useful publicity for practitioners facing satire, competition and the stigma of trade. As Bath evolved into a residential town, however, the social capital afforded to medical staff was eroded by alternative cultural mechanisms, better at penetrating a settled community than an institution which barred the local sick poor. The emergence of these new forms of sociability broadly coincided with diminishing clinical status, as the Hospital's dedication to spa therapy demanded an ongoing commitment to the fading tradition of humoralism. Unlike surgeons at Bristol, therefore, doctors at the General Infirmary did not have to wield administrative power in order to thrust a new anti-phlogistic regime upon reluctant governors. It was this lack of a clinical rationale for participation, coupled with the falling social return, which underpinned the abdication of honorary physicians and surgeons from the management of the Bath Hospital. The rewards of service were no longer adequate to justify the costs of being an active governor.

Notes

1. Geoffrey Holmes, *Augustan England: Professions, State and Society 1680–1730* (London: George Allen and Unwin, 1982) p. 206.
2. See, for example, Juanita G.L. Burnby, *A Study of the English Apothecary from 1660 to 1760, Medical History* Supplement No. 3 (London: Wellcome Institute for the History of Medicine, 1983), pp. 27, 30; Corfield, *Power*, pp. 149–56; David Harley, '"Bred up in the study of that faculty": Licensed Physicians in North-West England, 1660–1760',

Medical History, 38 (1994), pp. 419–20; Wilfred Prest, 'Introduction: The Professions and Society in Early Modern England', in Wilfred Prest (ed.), *The Professions in Early Modern England* (Beckenham: Croom Helm, 1987), pp. 3–4.

3. Irvine Loudon, 'The Nature of Provincial Medical Practice in Eighteenth-Century England', *Medical History*, 29 (1985), pp. 2–3, 31–2.
4. Irvine Loudon, *Medical Care and the General Practitioner 1750–1850* (Oxford: Clarendon Press, 1986), pp. 24–6.
5. Holmes, *Augustan England*, pp. 183–4.
6. See also Loudon, *Medical Care*, pp. 27–8; Margaret Pelling, 'Medical Practice in Early Modern England: Trade or Profession?' in W. Prest (ed.), *The Professions in Early Modern England* (Beckenham: Croom Helm, 1987), p. 94.
7. Wood, *Bath*, p. 296. Minute Book, 1 May 1758; 1 May 1780; 1 May 1800; 1 May 1830. House Visitors Book 1, 6 September 1742.
8. Minute Book, 6 April 1774.
9. Woodward, *To Do the Sick No Harm*, pp. 28–9.
10. Minute Book, 27 February 1828.
11. Anning, *General Infirmary at Leeds*, pp. 44–5, 47; Brockbank, *Royal Infirmary, Manchester*, pp. 208–9; Eade, *Norfolk and Norwich Hospital*, pp. 219–20; Howie, 'Royal Salop Infirmary', pp. 45–6; Lawrence, *Charitable Knowledge*, p. 57.
12. Loudon, *Medical Care*, p. 19.
13. Wood, *Bath*, p. 296. See also Abel-Smith, *Hospitals*, pp. 6–7; Anning, *General Hospital at Leeds*, pp. 32–3; Brockbank, *Royal Infirmary, Manchester*, p. 208; Eade, *Norfolk and Norwich Hospital*, pp. 218; Shemilt, *Salisbury*, pp. 26–7.
14. See, for example, Minute Book, 27 January 1743; 28 November 1770; 28 May 1800; 28 October 1830.
15. Minute Book, 10 February 1830.
16. The bust commemorating John Harrison, for example, first surgeon of the London Hospital, proclaims him as the 'principal founder'; while at Worcester an early minute book not only thanked a group of local physicians 'for their useful assistance in promoting this good design' but also 'empowered [them] to forward and conduct all necessary measures for accomplishing the same'. See Owen, *English Philanthropy*, pp. 40–41; McMenemey, *Worcester Royal Infirmary*, p. 43. See also Frizelle and Martin, *Leicester Royal Infirmary*, p. 44; Leader, *Sheffield General Infirmary*, p. 7; McLoughlin, *Liverpool Infirmary*, pp. 13–14; O'Brien, *Charitable Infirmary*, pp. 2, 5; Pickstone, *Medicine and Industrial Society*, p. 11; Smith, *Bristol Royal Infirmary*, p. 7; Waddy, *Northampton General Hospital*, p. 4.
17. Porter, 'Gift Relation', p. 181.
18. Minute Book, 'Members of the Committee of Nov. 18 1728'; 21 September 1738; 5 October 1738; 25 January 1739. 12 Geo. II, p. 593.
19. Gibson, *Radcliffe Infirmary*, pp. 72–3; Rook, Carlton and Cannon, *Addenbrooke's Hospital*, p. 57.
20. Minute Book, 1 May 1740.
21. See also Lawrence, *Charitable Knowledge*, p. 58.
22. Minute Book, 17 May 1744; 1 May 1750.
23. In contrast, medical staffing at the eighteenth-century Middlesex

Hospital was more fluid with physicians staying an average of 5.9 years and surgeons 14.9 years. See Bronwyn Croxson, 'An Economic Analysis of a Voluntary Hospital: The Foundation and Institutional Structure of the Middlesex Hospital, 1745–1900' (unpublished doctoral thesis, University of Cambridge, 1994), p. 151.

24. Minute Book, 2 May 1748. Michael R. Neve, 'Natural Philosophy, Medicine and the Culture of Science in Provincial England: The Cases of Bristol 1796–1850 and Bath 1750–1820' (unpublished doctoral thesis, University of London, 1984), p. 100.
25. When the subscription scheme opened in 1741/42, the only holder of an honorary post to contribute was Dr William Oliver. In the sample year 1770/71, two of the physicians and all three surgeons were annual subscribers; in 1800/01, two physicians and two surgeons; and in 1830/31, one physician and two surgeons. See *Annual Reports*. This contrasts with the position reported in Berry's comparative study where the majority subscribed whilst filling hospital posts. See Berry, 'Patronage', p. 51.
26. See Appendix G.
27. Davies, *Deeds Not Words*, pp. 31–2; Lloyd, *United Hospital, Bath*, p. 11.
28. Clark-Kennedy, *The London*, p. 224; Turner, *Hampshire County Hospital*, p. 41.
29. Roy Porter, 'Laymen, Doctors and Medical Knowledge in the Eighteenth Century: The Evidence of the *Gentleman's Magazine*', in Roy Porter (ed.), *Patients and Practitioners: Lay Perceptions of Medicine in Pre-Industrial Society* (Cambridge: Cambridge University Press, 1985), p. 302; *Spectator*, 1, 24 March 1711, p. 88.
30. *The Diseases of Bath: A Satire* (London, 1737), p. 5.
31. Tobias Smollett, *The Adventures of Peregrine Pickle*, ed. James L. Clifford (Oxford: Oxford University Press, 1969), p. 375.
32. Christopher Anstey, *The New Bath Guide*, ed. Gavin Turner, first pub. 1766, repr. (Bristol: Broadcast Books, 1994), p. 57.
33. Smollett, *Peregrine Pickle*, pp. 372–3.
34. Granville, *Spas*, p. 402.
35. Peter Wagner, 'The Satire on Doctors in Hogarth's Graphic Works', in Marie Mulvey Roberts and Roy Porter (eds), *Literature and Medicine during the Eighteenth Century* (London: Routledge, 1993), pp. 216–17.
36. Corfield, *Power*, ch. 3. See also Anita Guerrini, '"A club of little villains": Rhetoric, Professional Identity and Medical Pamphlet Wars', in M.M. Roberts and R. Porter (eds), *Literature and Medicine during the Eighteenth Century* (London: Routledge, 1993), p. 231.
37. Benjamin Boyce, *The Benevolent Man: A Life of Ralph Allen of Bath* (Cambridge, MA: Harvard University Press, 1967), p. 77.
38. 'Hints to Young Practitioners, and Observations for the Benefit of Those Whom They May Concern', *Edinburgh Medical and Surgical Journal*, 5 (1809), p. 339.
39. James Ford, earning £42 a year in 1740, had an income of £495 three years later, after he had been appointed surgeon to the Bristol Infirmary. See Loudon, *Medical Care*, pp. 109–14. See also Porter, 'Gift Relation', p. 162; Dorothy Porter and Roy Porter, *Patient's Progress: Doctors and Doctoring in Eighteenth-Century England* (Cambridge: Polity Press, 1989), pp. 119–20.

40. Holmes, *Augustan England*, pp. 218, 221.
41. DNB, vol. 42, p. 154; Jerom Murch, *Biographical Sketches of Bath Celebrities, Ancient and Modern, with Some Fragments of Local History* (London: Isaac Pitman, 1893), pp. 137–8.
42. John Thomas, 'The Phillotts of Bath' (unpublished typescript, Bath Central Library, 1968), p. 1; Oliver Gray, 'The Rise of the Middling Sort and their Influence on Local Politics and the Economy of Seventeenth- and Eighteenth-Century Bath' (unpublished bachelor of science dissertation, University of Bath, 1985), p. 26.
43. Joan Lane, 'The Medical Practitioners of Provincial England in 1783', *Medical History*, 28 (1984), p. 359.
44. Barbara Brandon Schnorrenberg, 'Medical Men of Bath', *Studies in Eighteenth-Century Culture*, 13 (1984), p. 198.
45. G. Fletcher and G.I. Harris, 'Pharmacy in Bath during the Regency Period', *Pharmaceutical Historian*, 1 (1970), p. 2; Neve, 'Natural Philosophy', p. 79.
46. Ellen Wilson, 'A Shropshire Lady in Bath, 1794–1807', *Bath History*, 4 (1992), pp. 120–21.
47. Honorary positions at the General Hospital were included in the trade directory entries for later Georgian surgeons, along with their membership of the Royal College of Surgeons. See *Gye's Bath Directory* (Bath: H. Gye, 1819), p. 6.
48. Porter, 'Gift Relation', p. 162.
49. Loudon, 'Provincial Medical Practice', p. 31.
50. Mary Fissell, 'The Physic of Charity: Health and Welfare in the West Country 1690–1834', (unpublished doctoral dissertation, University of Pennsylvania, 1988), pp. 67–8.
51. *Annual Reports* contained this statement from 1747/48. For an *ad hoc* example, see [Bath General Infirmary], 'Short Account', in Bayly, *Sermon*, p. 31.
52. See, for example, Minute Book, 1 May 1773; 1 May 1800; 1 May 1830.
53. See, for example, Minute Book, 1 May 1761; 1 May 1781; 21 May 1806; 7 July 1830.
54. *Bath Journal*, 29 August 1757.
55. See, for example, Falconer, *Mineral Water Hospital*, p. 25; Murch, *Biographical Sketches*, pp. 136, 138, 148; Addison, *English Spas*, pp. 131–2; *Bath: Official Guide Book 1986* (Bath: Bath City Council, 1986), p. 14.
56. F.J. Poynton, 'An Address on the Occasion of the Unveiling of a Memorial Tablet at the Royal Literary Institution, Queen Square, to Dr William Oliver' (unpublished typescript, Bath Central Library, 1935), p. 3. See also R.A.L. Smith, *Bath*, 3rd edn (London: Batsford, 1948).
57. *Bath Journal*, 23 March 1752; 16 October 1786. *The Sixth Year's State of the Casualty Hospital in the City of Bath ... for the year 1793* (Bath: R. Cruttwell, 1794), p. 1; *The Bath Eye Infirmary 1811 to 1948* (no place of publication, publisher or date), p. 28; Murch, *Biographical Sketches*, pp 140–41.
58. See, for example, McLoughlin, *Liverpool Infirmary*, p. 36; McMenemey, *Worcester Royal Infirmary*, pp. 60–61, 80–81.
59. Boyce, *Benevolent Man*, pp. 87, 243.
60. *DNB*, vol. 25, pp. 67–8.

61. Sholem Glaser, *The Spirit of Enquiry: Caleb Hillier Parry, MD, FRS* (Stroud: Alan Sutton, 1995), pp. 23–6, 43–4, 57–9, 61–2, 84; T. Kirby, 'Royal Mineral Water Hospital, Bath: Catalogue of the Pictures' (unpublished manuscript, Bath Central Library, undated), p. 39; Mainwaring, *Annals*, pp. 234–5; W.J. Williams and D.M. Stoddart, *Bath – Some Encounters with Science* (Bath: Kingsmead, 1978), p. 13.
62. Glaser, *Caleb Hillier Parry*, pp. 53, 88, 96; Royal Mineral Water Hospital, 'Notes on the Pictures' (unpublished anthology of press cuttings, Bath Central Library, undated).
63. Roy Porter, 'Science, Provincial Culture and Public Opinion in Enlightenment England', in Peter Borsay (ed.), *The Eighteenth Century Town: A Reader in English Urban History 1688–1820* (London: Longman, 1990), pp. 243–67. See also Ian Inkster, 'Marginal Men: Aspects of the Social Role of the Medical Community in Sheffield, 1790–1850', in John Woodward and David Richards (eds), *Health Care and Popular Medicine in Nineteenth-Century England* (London: Croom Helm, 1977), pp. 128–63; Ian Inkster, 'Variations on a Theme by Thackray: Comments upon Provincial Science Culture, c. 1780–1850', *British Society for the History of Science Newsletter*, 8 (1982), pp. 15–18; Marland, *Medicine and Society*, pp. 336–7; Neve, 'Natural Philosophy', p. 108; Pickstone, *Medicine and Industrial Society*, p. 15; Arnold Thackray, 'Natural Knowledge in Cultural Context: The Manchester Model', *American Historical Review*, 79 (1974), pp. 672–709.
64. Hembry, *English Spa*, p. 152; Kirby, 'Mineral Water Hospital', p. 39; Jerom Murch, 'Bath in its Relation to Art, Science, Literature and Education', in J.W. Morris (ed.), *Handbook to Bath Prepared on the Occasion of the Visit of the British Association, 1888* (Bath: Isaac Pitman, 1888), pp. 110, 112, 123; Neve, 'Natural Philosophy', p. 80; Hugh Torrens, 'The Four Bath Philosophical Societies, 1779–1959', in R. Rolls, J. Guy and J.R. Guy (eds), *A Pox on the Provinces: Proceedings of the 12th Congress of the British Society for the History of Medicine* (Bath: Bath University Press, 1990), p. 181–5; Williams and Stoddart, *Bath*, pp. 72–3.
65. Philip Elliott, *The Sociology of the Professions* (London: Macmillan, 1972), p. 32.
66. Torrens, 'Four Bath Philosophical Societies', p. 185.
67. Jacqueline Jenkinson, 'The Role of Medical Societies in the Rise of the Scottish Medical Profession', *Social History of Medicine*, 4 (1991), pp. 253–4, 256–7.
68. Richard Fisher, *Edward Jenner 1749–1823* (London: André Deutsch, 1991), p. 20, 51–3, 61, 89, 225, 257, 289; William L. Proudfit, 'The Fleece Medical Society', *British Heart Journal*, 46 (1981), p. 589.
69. Rolls, *Hospital of the Nation*, p. 160. I am grateful to Emily Naish, Archivist of the British Medical Association, for supplying the date of foundation for the Bath branch.
70. Anning, *General Infirmary at Leeds*, p. 19; Philip Swan, 'A Brief Summary of the Role and Position of Medical Societies in the Early Nineteenth Century Medical Profession', *Journal of Local Studies*, 2 (1982), pp. 43–4.
71. Ivan Waddington, *The Medical Profession in the Industrial Revolution* (Dublin: Gill and Macmillan, 1984), p. 22.
72. John Bellers, 'An Essay Towards the Improvement of Physick', in George

Clarke (ed.), *John Bellers: His Life, Times and Writings* (London: Routledge and Kegan Paul, 1987), p. 184. See also Robert Nelson, *An Address to Persons of Quality and Estate* (London: 1715), pp. 210–11.

73. John Aikin, *Thoughts on Hospitals with a Letter to the Author by Thomas Percival* (London: Joseph Johnson, 1771), p. 76.
74. Othmar Keel, 'The Politics of Health and the Institutionalisation of Clinical Practices in Europe in the Second Half of the Eighteenth Century', in W.F. Bynum and Roy Porter (eds), *William Hunter and the Eighteenth-Century Medical World* (Cambridge: Cambridge University Press, 1985), pp. 207–56.
75. N.D. Jewson, 'The Disappearance of the Sick-Man from Medical Cosmology, 1770–1870', *Sociology*, 10 (1976), pp. 227–30; Ivan Waddington, 'The Role of the Hospital in the Development of Modern Medicine: A Sociological Analysis', *Sociology*, 7 (1973), pp. 211–12.
76. Dunthorne, *Enlightenment*, pp. 7, 9. See also Hankins, *Science*, p. 119.
77. Andrew Wear, 'Making Sense of Health and the Environment in Early Modern England', in Andrew Wear (ed.), *Medicine in Society: Historical Essays* (Cambridge: Cambridge University Press, 1992), p. 120.
78. N.D. Jewson, 'Medical Knowledge and the Patronage System in Eighteenth-Century England', *Sociology*, 8 (1974), pp. 371–2. See also Christopher Lawrence, *Medicine in the Making of Modern Britain 1700–1920* (London: Routledge, 1994), pp. 11–12; Lawrence, *Charitable Knowledge*, p. 232.
79. Roy Porter, 'Was there a Medical Enlightenment in Eighteenth-Century England?' *British Journal for Eighteenth Century Studies*, 5 (1982), pp. 52–3.
80. A proposal for a hospital in Exeter, reprinted in the *Bath Journal* on 14 January 1751, reported that the project would be 'as serviceable to the rich as to the poor, by furnishing the physicians and surgeons with more experience in one year, than they could have in ten without it'.
81. Minute Book, 16 February 1738, 'Plan and Elevation'.
82. Barrett, 'Spas', p. 69; Fawcett and Bird, *Bath*, p. 65.
83. Fawcett, 'Selling', p. 194.
84. Neve, 'Natural Philosophy', pp. 86–7.
85. Charles Lucas, *An Essay on Waters in Three Parts* (London: A. Millar, 1756), pp. 320, 323–5. See also Charles Lucas, *Cursory Remarks on the Methods of Investigating the Principles and Properties of Bath and Bristol Waters* (Bath: C. Pope, 1764).
86. William Baylies, *Practical Reflections on the Uses and Abuses of Bath Waters* (London: A. Millar, 1757), pp. 122–3, 131–2; William Baylies, *An Historical Account of the Rise, Progress and Management of the General Hospital or Infirmary in the City of Bath* (Bath: James Leake, 1758), pp. 126. 128.
87. G.S. Rousseau, 'Matt Bramble and the Sulphur Controversy in the Eighteenth Century', *Journal of the History of Ideas*, 27 (1967), pp. 585–6.
88. Neve, 'Natural Philosophy', pp. 87–9.
89. Jewson, 'Medical knowledge', p. 382.
90. *DNB*, vol. 34, pp. 231–4; E.A.B. Barnard, 'An Eighteenth-Century Worcestershire Doctor: William Baylies of Evesham, 1724–87', *Transactions of the Worcestershire Archaeological Society*, 4 (1945), pp. 36–8; Neve, 'Natural Philosophy', pp. 80–81, 84–92.

91. Lucas, *Essay*, p. xviii.
92. Neve, 'Natural Philosophy', p. 80.
93. Leyborne, *Charity Conducive*, p. 32.
94. Fawcett, 'Selling', pp. 201–3.
95. Hankins, *Science*, p. 84; Noel G. Coley, 'Physicians and the Chemical Analysis of Mineral Waters in Eighteenth-Century England', *Medical History*, 26 (1982), p. 133; Rousseau, 'Matt Bramble', pp. 585–6.
96. William Falconer, *A Practical Dissertation on the Medicinal Effects of the Bath Waters* (Bath: R. Cruttwell, 1790), p. xvii.
97. Daniel Lysons, *Practical Essays upon Continual and Intermitting Fevers, Dropsies, Diseases of the Liver, and the use of Bath Waters*, 2nd edn (Bath: S. Hazard, 1783), p. 135. See also William Oliver [the Elder], *A Practical Dissertation on Bath Waters*, 2nd edn (London: J.D. Varnam, 1716), pp. 14–15, 19; John Summers, *A Short Account of the Success of Warm Bathing in Paralytic Disorders*, 2nd edn (London: C. Hitch and L. Hawes, 1751), pp. 16–17; Charleton, *Three Tracts*, no. 2: 'An Enquiry into the Efficacy of Bath Water in Palsies', p. 96; Falconer, *Practical Dissertation*, pp. xvi–xxvii; Edward Barlow, *An Essay on the Medicinal Efficacy and Employment of the Bath Waters* (Bath: Longman, Hurst, Rees, Orme and Brown, 1822), p. 128.
98. James C. Riley, *The Eighteenth-Century Campaign to Avoid Disease* (London: Macmillan, 1987), pp. 1, 72.
99. Wood, *Bath*, p. 294.
100. See, for example, Alexander Sutherland, *An Attempt to Ascertain and Extend the Virtues of Bath and Bristol Waters*, 2nd edn (London: W. Frederick and S. Leake, 1764), p. 121.
101. Tobias Smollett, *An Essay on the External Use of Water*, ed. Claude E. Jones (Baltimore: John Hopkins Press, 1935), pp. 70–71.
102. Besides investigations of the spa, the honorary physicians conducted other medical research using patients of the General Hospital. Dr Edward Harington experimented with electrotherapy for paralytic conditions; while Dr William Falconer collaborated with John Haygarth – the Chester physician who retired to Bath – in an evaluation of 'metallic tractors' which, when applied to the skin, were supposed to relieve a raft of ailments. See Roger Rolls, 'From Balneology to Physiotherapy: The Development of Physical Treatment at Bath', in R. Rolls, J. Guy and J.R. Guy (eds), *A Pox on the Provinces: Proceedings of the 12th Congress of the British Society for the History of Medicine* (Bath: Bath University Press, 1990), p. 115; Rolls, *Hospital of the Nation*, p. 164.
103. *Cases of Persons Admitted into the Infirmary at Bath under the Care of Doctor Oliver* (Bath: Stephen Martin, 1760); Boyce, *Benevolent Man*, p. 243.
104. Sutherland, *Attempt*, p. 174.
105. John Summers, *Short Account*; *Narrative of the Efficacy of the Bath Waters, in Various Kinds of Paralytic Disorders Admitted into the Bath Hospital* (Bath: R. Cruttwell, 1787).
106. The eighteenth-century campaign for public health is discussed more fully in Chapter 5.
107. Ulrich Trohler, 'Quantification in British Medicine and Surgery 1750–1830, with Special Reference to its Introduction into Therapeutics' (unpublished doctoral thesis, University of London, 1978), pp. 62–4;

W.F. Bynum, *Science and the Practice of Medicine in the Nineteenth Century* (Cambridge: Cambridge University Press, 1994), pp. 42–3; Riley, *Eighteenth-Century Campaign*, pp. 4–7, 55. This use of medical records supports the conviction that political arithmetic did not disappear in the early eighteenth century and only re-emerge in the 1820s with the birth of 'the modern statistical age'. See Julian Hoppit, 'Political Arithmetic in Eighteenth-Century England', *Economic History Review*, **49** (1996), pp. 516–19.

108. Fawcett, 'Selling', p. 201.
109. Charleton, *Three Tracts*, no. 2, pp. 3, 12–14, 93–5.
110. William Falconer, *An Account of the Use, Application and Success of the Bath Waters in Rheumatic Cases* (Bath: W. Myler, 1795), pp. 50–63. See also William Falconer, *A Dissertation on Ischias; or the Disease of the Hip-Joint* (London: T. Cadell and W. Davies, 1805), pp. 29–35.
111. Eleven Georgian physicians had degrees from Oxford, five from Cambridge and five from Edinburgh, the latter all in post after 1780. See *DNB*; *Alumni Cantabrigienses: Part I to 1751*, 4 vols (Cambridge: Cambridge University Press, 1922–27); *Alumni Cantabrigienses: Part II 1752–1900*, 6 vols (Cambridge: Cambridge University Press, 1940–54); *Alumni Oxoniensis: The Members of the University of Oxford 1715–1886*, 4 vols (London: Joseph Foster, 1888); Falconer, *Mineral Water Hospital*; Loudon, *Medical Care*. I have been unable to confirm the educational backgrounds of two physicians.
112. Trohler, 'Quantification', pp. 182, 185–6.
113. Charleton, *Three Tracts*, no. 1: 'A Chemical Analysis of Bath Water', ch. 3; Falconer, *Practical Dissertation*, p. xvi; William Falconer, *An Essay on the Bath Waters* (London: T. Lowndes, 1770), p. 124.
114. Michel Foucault, *The Birth of the Clinic: An Archaeology of Medical Perception*, trans. A.M. Sheridan (London: Routledge, 1973), pp. 58.
115. Michael Neve, 'Orthodoxy and Fringe: Medicine in Late Georgian Bristol', in W.F. Bynum and Roy Porter (eds), *Medical Fringe and Medical Orthodoxy 1750–1850* (London: Croom Helm, 1987), p. 45.
116. Edward Jorden, *A Discourse on Naturall Bathes, and Mineral Waters, etc.* (London: 1631), p. 163.
117. Olive, *Particular Excellence*, p. 19.
118. Jewson, 'Medical Knowledge', pp. 373–6, 382–3; Waddington, 'Role', p. 213.
119. Fissell, 'Physic of Charity', pp. 254–5; Joan Lane, '"The doctor scolds me": The Diaries and Correspondence of Patients in Eighteenth Century England', in R. Porter (ed.), *Patients and Practioners: Lay Perceptions of Medicine in Pre-Industrial Society* (Cambridge: Cambridge University Press, 1985), p. 226; Loudon, *Medical Care*, pp. 101–3; Malcolm Nicolson, 'The Metastatic Theory of Pathogenesis and the Professional Interests of the Eighteenth-Century Physician', *Medical History*, **32** (1988), pp. 278, 283–5; Roy Porter, 'The Patient's View: Doing Medical History from Below', *Theory and Society*, **14** (1985), pp. 189–92; Porter, 'Laymen', pp. 283–314; Roy Porter and Dorothy Porter, *In Sickness and in Health: The British Experience 1650–1850* (London: Fourth Estate, 1988), p. 274; Porter and Porter, *Patient's Progress*, pp. 12–14, 27–9, 36, 69, 79–81, 85–90.
120. Porter and Porter, *Patient's Progress*, pp. 95, 208.

121. Minute Book, 16 February 1738, 'Plan and Elevation'.
122. Minute Book, 5 May 1743. See also Minute Book 10 October 1750; 7 May 1755.
123. Mary E. Fissell, 'The Disappearance of the Patient's Narrative and the Invention of Hospital Medicine,' in Roger French and Andrew Wear (eds), *British Medicine in an Age of Reform* (London: Routledge, 1991), pp. 92–4, 100–106. See also Loudon, *Medical Care*, pp. 73–5.
124. Berry, 'Patronage', p. 232.
125. Lawrence, *Charitable Knowledge*, pp. 21, 217.
126. See, for example, [William Oliver], *Cases*, p. 31; [Bath General Infirmary], *Narrative*, pp. 61, 85.
127. [Bath General Infirmary], *Narrative*, p 19. See also ibid., pp. 84–5.
128. Minute Book, 13 May 1795.
129. [Bath General Infirmary], *Narrative*, p. 46.
130. Minute Book, 11 November 1807.
131. Simon Schaffer, 'Natural Philosophy and Public Spectacle in the Eighteenth Century', *History of Science*, 21 (1983), p. 31. See also Frith, *Gloucester's Infirmary*, p. 11; Jacob, *Nottingham General Hospital*, p. 64; McMenemey, *Worcester Royal Infirmary*, p. 64; Waddy, *Northampton General Hospital*, p. 20.
132. Risse, *Hospital Life*, p. 217; Rolls, 'From Balneology', p. 115.
133. [Bath General Infirmary], *Narrative*, pp. 54–5. See also ibid., p. 59.
134. [William Oliver], *Cases*, pp. 31–5.
135. Ibid., p. 26.
136. [Bath General Infirmary], *Narrative*, pp. 32–3.
137. Minute Book, 10 February 1830.
138. [William Oliver], *Cases*, pp. 6, 8; [Bath General Infirmary], *Narrative*, p. 45.
139. [William Oliver], *Cases*, p. 39. See also ibid., p. 7; [Bath General Infirmary], *Narrative*, p. 48.
140. [William Oliver], *Cases*, pp. 30, 39; [Bath General Infirmary], *Narrative*, pp. 23, 51, 78.
141. [Bath General Infirmary], *Narrative*, p. 35.
142. Ibid., pp. 18, 20–21.
143. Barlow, *Essay*, pp. 108–14, 180.
144. Christopher Lawrence, 'Democratic, Divine and Heroic: The History and Historiography of Surgery', in Christopher Lawrence (ed.), *Medical Theory, Surgical Practice: Studies in the History of Surgery* (London: Routledge, 1992), pp. 20–23. See also Bynum, *Science*, pp. 32–3; Fissell, 'Physic of Charity', pp. 151–64.
145. Porter and Porter, *In Sickness*, p. 52; Wear, 'Making Sense', p. 120.
146. Barlow, *Essay*, p. 123.
147. George Smith Gibbes, *A Second Treatise on the Bath Waters* (Bath: W. Meyler, 1803), p. 11.

CHAPTER FIVE

The Limits of Autonomy

In Chapter 4, we examined the motives of physicians and surgeons who joined the staff of the General Infirmary, tracing their falling interest in its administrative affairs to the changing nature of social intercourse at Bath and the marginalization of spa therapy within medicine. Among the attractions which drew doctors to voluntary service in the first place was the opportunity to exercise clinical autonomy in a way that was impossible in private practice. Though the humoral framework of balneology preserved elements of the lay narrative, the Bath Hospital still provided a regulated environment for the implementation of medical orders. As well as a constituency of captive patients, however, clinical independence required freedom from the intervention of both lay governors and medical colleagues. Moreover, since the institution became embroiled in campaigns to police the application and evaluation of the spa waters, its influence over clinical discretion extended to medical practice in the city as a whole. The constraints imposed through the Infirmary were not uncontentious. In Chapter 5, therefore, we turn to the conflicts which they generated, focusing on the conspiratorial aspects of the sulphur controversy, the dismissal of the surgeon – Archibald Cleland – for sexual misconduct, the evolving relationship between doctors and governors, and the response to new ideas about institutional hygiene. The conclusion will weigh the limits of autonomy against the rewards of service in order to judge the role of the Bath Hospital in the development of the local medical profession.

The sulphur controversy: conspiracy and exclusion

Medical men in eighteenth-century Bath were a tightly knit community in which many physicians shared the experience of an Oxbridge education,[1] surgeons were bonded by the ties of apprenticeship, and practitioners of all kinds linked by family relationships. Recruitment to the General Hospital reinforced these networks. Although Edinburgh graduates were later appointed, most physicians in post before 1780 held qualifications from Oxford or Cambridge.[2] Kinship connections were also evident among the physicians. Henry Harington was the nephew of Edward Harington, Charles Parry the son of Caleb Parry,[3] and only a governor's fear that the Bath Hospital was becoming 'Oliver's hospital' allegedly prevented the election of William Oliver's son to a physician's post.[4] For surgeons it was apprenticeship which opened doors, with both Thomas Palmer and Joseph Phillott following their respective masters, Jeremiah Peirce and Henry Wright, to the Infirmary.[5] Family and occupational dynasties, and cries of nepotism, were a regular trait of Georgian voluntary hospitals,[6] but the extent to which they shut out 'outsiders' at Bath has been misrepresented. Just two physicians who obtained posts at the Georgian Bath Infirmary – John Ford Davis and Charles Parry – are known to have been born in the city;[7] and a number had previously practised elsewhere: David Hartley in Newark and Bury St Edmunds, Henry Harington in Wells, Daniel Lysons in Gloucester, William Falconer in Chester and Edward Barlow in Dublin.[8] These 'newcomers' integrated into the local medical community for two reasons. First, they were members of social élites: the Haringtons were 'an ancient and honourable family, who had long possessed considerable influence and property in the neighbourhood';[9] William Falconer's father was the Recorder of Chester;[10] Charles Parry and Edward Barlow were the sons of doctors;[11] and Sir George Smith Gibbes was the son of a Wiltshire rector.[12] But, equally important, these physicians were prepared to endorse the exceptional qualities of the waters and the conventional ways in which they were applied. What guaranteed exclusion was a critical attitude to the spa, perceived as disruptive to the future prosperity of the town and harmful to the vested interests of its medical practitioners.

When Charles Lucas and William Baylies ventured into the sulphur controversy, both these conditions were breached. Lucas came from a prodigal family and ran an apothecary's shop in Dublin before gaining an MD from Leyden in 1752.[13] Baylies was the son of a well-to-do Evesham apothecary who himself practised his father's trade prior to obtaining a medical degree from Aberdeen in 1748.[14] Lacking the social status to join the charmed circle of Bath physicians, Lucas and Baylies sought 'controversial visibility' in an attempt to destroy the 'closed shop'.[15] Lucas's attack did not confine itself to the chemical content of the waters; he also drew in the poor bathing facilities, condemning local politicians as well as doctors for their apathy and indifference.[16] The Bath Corporation, he argued, was rotten to the core because it had usurped ownership of the baths and denied the public their rightful free access.[17]

> For though ... [the citizens] be many, their best privileges, such as that of electing magistrates, common council and representatives in parliament ... are absorbed here, as in many other corporations, by the Few – a political epidemic distemper in Britain and Ireland, beyond the reach of physic, though seconded by Bath water.[18]

In short, the problems of the spa were symptomatic of a deep malaise which hinged on the exclusive, anti-democratic political system. The Bath élite was incensed by these medical and constitutional insults. Even before Lucas visited the city in the year after his *Essay* appeared, William Oliver was accused of 'exclaiming against him, and declaring, before he was asked, that he would hold no consultations with Dr Lucas'. Although an organized 'confederacy' was denied, Oliver – in correspondence which Lucas went on to publish – reaffirmed his unwillingness to co-operate: 'if I should ever hereafter hold any consultation, controversy, or conversation with the man, from whom I have received such usage, I should esteem myself to be really as great a scoundrel as he has represented me to be'. This refusal to interact lent substance to Lucas's claim that 'barely differing in opinion with Dr Oliver is a crime'. It helped to authenticate his view that, contrary to the public interest, there was 'an attempt to pervert a liberal profession into a sordid trade; to monopolize that trade, and to ingross the emoluments of a base craft, into the hands of a few'.[19]

William Oliver's role in this confrontation unavoidably associated it with the General Hospital, given his prominence as a physician and governor. After William Baylies entered the ring, however, the Infirmary was drawn more openly into the fray. For Lucas – described as the Wilkes of Ireland[20] – and for Baylies – who later stood as a Tory parliamentary candidate[21] – the sulphur controversy had radical connotations; it was a debate about exclusiveness in politics no less than medicine. But the dispute was also fired by commercial interest, and not just among the advocates of the spa. Lucas professed no intention of practising in the city,[22] but Baylies took up residence soon after graduating. For him, therefore, the discriminatory tactics of Oliver and his Hospital colleagues, Abel Moysey and Rice Charleton, were more serious, and ultimately led him to leave Bath for a career first in London and then abroad.[23] Baylies embellished Lucas's account of medical conspiracy with a direct attack upon the General Hospital, complaining of restrictive practices in the recruitment of staff. Objections focused on the number of honorary posts and the means used to fill them. In 1744, when the patient quota was 40, the governors had increased the complement of physicians and surgeons to six in each category; in 1750, with more beds occupied, the decision was taken to cut the number by half 'as soon as they shall be reduced ... by death or resignation'.[24] Baylies questioned the stimulus for this reversal, suggesting that 'a private and not public purpose' was at stake. There were, he insisted,

> others in Bath who are acquainted with hospital practice, with chemistry, pharmacy, and anatomy ... and the whole knowledge of physic has never yet been limited to the heads of any three

> individuals. Why, then, the patients of this Hospital should be prohibited the advantage, which the rest of the faculty may afford them, is to me inconceivable.[25]

As well as committing his thoughts to paper, Baylies campaigned for change by pursuing election to a Hospital post, the holding of which he regarded as a professional duty.[26] Even before his candidature, there had been breaches of the legal requirement to advertise vacancies a fortnight before the election;[27] Mr Philip Ditcher was appointed a surgeon in 1744 without prior public notice being given, while four years later Dr John Summers was unanimously voted a physician to replace Dr David Hartley at the very meeting at which the resignation was tabled.[28] The governors also failed to announce the post which Baylies sought in 1757 – at least until his letter of application prompted belated action. This letter, written because he did not have 'the honour to be personally aquainted with many of the governors', aired the case for greater openness. His own report of the ensuing general court tells of a lively debate about the merits of more medical staff. Baylies maintains, however, that the scales were tipped in favour of continued exclusiveness by the intervention of William Oliver who, from the chair, 'with the utmost heat and acrimony declared, if more than three physicians were elected, he, for his part, would be no longer concerned in the care of the charity, and that his colleague, Doctor Moysey, then absent, was fixed in the same resolution'. Two other physicians, to be candidates in a future election, let it be known that they were of the same persuasion. This threat of revolt scuppered any prospect of reform. Nor did William Baylies succeed in winning the position that was vacant. From his perspective, the effect was to monopolize 'most artfully ... all opportunities of improvement' that the Bath Hospital endowed.[29] But this improving discourse, no less than the conservatism of the medical élite, was a medium for economic self-interest as well as political idealism. Baylies ratified Lucas's critique of the spa and campaigned for an honorary post to advance his professional career; William Oliver and his supporters closed ranks against a censorious 'outsider' to defend their livelihoods.

The Cleland affair

The appropriation of the Infirmary to protect the local medical fraternity was also a theme in the earlier Cleland affair. In 1743 Archibald Cleland was first suspended and then dismissed from his surgeon's post on the grounds that he had committed 'indecent practices' against female patients.[30] Cleland was not a popular figure in Bath because he had found fault with the bathing facilities and recommended different ways of applying the waters. His proposals dated back to the 1730s when, after a visit to the city, he put forward a 'rational plan for rendering the Baths more safe and commodious'. Master of Ceremonies, Richard Nash, initially approved of the suggestion for a covered bagnio 'with proper conveniences for cupping, sweating, bathing, pumping, and fomentation', and presented the scheme to the Corporation at the instigation of the Prince of Wales. But enthusiasm waned. In his *Essay on the External Use of Water*, Smollett blamed lobbying on the part of local physicians for this loss of interest and reported that they had 'come to a resolution to exclude all surgeons from their consultations' on balneological improvements: 'an arrow directly levelled at ... [Cleland] (as it does not appear that any other of his profession has proposed any thing worthy of public notice)'.[31] Cleland himself also learned from George Cheyne of a plot to recall him to army service; and claimed that he was ostracized in Bath, being 'pointed at, both in public, and private, as a person not fit to be relied on, as not qualified in my profession'.[32] Yet despite this legacy, Archibald Cleland did succeed in becoming a surgeon to the General Infirmary, albeit amidst controversy.

Cleland's *Appeal to the Public*, published after his discharge, presented the Hospital's electoral procedures as highly informal. In 1742 the sole surgeon, Jeremiah Peirce, advised the governors that a second post was desirable and requested 'their interest, in favour of Mr Palmer, late his apprentice'. Other surgeons in the town soon heard of the opening through the grapevine and 'made their applications, with great assiduity, to all the governors'. Cleland, however, insisted that he was totally ignorant of the vacancy until the evening before the weekly committee gathered to receive applications and call an election. At this meeting, he was given 'leave to apply' after a governor had indicated his likely willingness to work for the charity. But, at the same time, Mr Peirce gained support for a motion which required a seven-year apprenticeship for surgeons. Archibald Cleland had impressive credentials; he had studied in London and Paris, and been employed by the South Sea Company, before becoming a surgeon to a 'regiment of horse' commanded by George Wade who was a Bath MP. However, his apprenticeship, under an eminent Edinburgh practitioner, had lasted only five years and, therefore, he was ineligible for the Hospital post.[33] In their *Short Vindication*, responding to Cleland's *Appeal*, the governors claimed that Mr Peirce's resolution 'was only intended to guard ... against persons unduly qualified for the office' and pointed to the subsequent amendment that 'any surgeon who has been regularly bred, and qualified in the opinion of the general court may be elected surgeon to this Hospital tho' he shall not have served seven years'.[34] Other accounts make Cleland the specific target. Ralph Allen's biographer argues that he was responsible for overturning the new rule, acting on the advice of the literary figure, Alexander Pope, who had been tackled by a grateful patient. Cleland himself thanked the Earl of Chesterfield for saving him from the crude manoeuvrings of an unscrupulous cartel.[35] But this skirmish was not the end of the affair. After appointment, Cleland was dogged by attempts to 'wound his character', even though he maintained that his Hospital attendance was diligent.[36] Moreover, when the sexual allegations came to light, they were handled with duplicity. Mr Cleland was informed of the complaints in the Pump Room by Dr Oliver. Next day he met with medical colleagues to justify his actions and since they seemed content with the explanation given, he assumed that the issue had been dropped. However, it seems that secret meetings – hotly denied – later took place, at which the Hospital apothecary, John Morris, drew up papers. These papers were then put before the weekly committee by a lay governor called Paul Bertrand to justify suspension pending a full 'trial' before the general court.[37] The long-standing animosity ensured that a 'guilty' verdict was almost inevitable.

Medical theory, surgical practice

The accusation of indecency stuck and discharge followed because Cleland's behaviour raised contentious questions about the relationship between physic and surgery, medicine and sexuality. The division of labour within medicine was a major source of conflict throughout the long eighteenth century. In voluntary hospitals, friction between the paid apothecary and visiting medical staff was not unknown,[38] but most antagonisms involved honorary practitioners. Both physicians and surgeons fought amongst themselves about the propriety of different treatments and their aptness for individual cases.[39] However, the interface between these two medical corporations was particularly troublesome. Physicians sought overall control of patient care, on the grounds that their knowledge of the body's internal constitution was required for the successful administration of external, surgical remedies.[40] Hospital regulations generally sanctioned these ambitions,[41] leaving surgeons resentful and belligerent for greater clinical autonomy.[42] The rules reproduced for the General Infirmary in John Wood's *Description of Bath* are less dogmatic: physicians and surgeons together admitted patients in rotation; the authorization of drugs was not explicitly tied to physicians; and although surgeons had to acquaint fellow practitioners of any forthcoming 'considerable operation' so that 'they may be present if they please', no formal consultation was directed.[43] The holistic assumptions of spa therapy made physicians its acknowledged superintendents and hence there was less need for the institutional reinforcement of occupational superiority.

The Cleland affair was not a straightforward dispute between the medical corporations. Although the apothecary may have taken his proactive stance because he feared the threat to his autonomy from a conscientious surgeon, it is more likely that he was an agent for leading governors, implementing enquiries and strategies which they had initiated. More significant was the way in which Jeremiah Peirce – the surgeon who had tried to obstruct Cleland's appointment – and two of the three honorary physicians combined with other governors – lay and medical – to expel a colleague who had broken the protocol which shaped interactions with patients as well as medical staff. The case did not revolve around the most serious accusation, namely that Cleland had – against her wishes – engaged in sexual intercourse with a patient called Sarah Appleby, who had subsequently died.[44] No doubt a charge of rape or assault would have been virtually impossible to prove, especially since the evidence came not from the woman herself but secondhand via one of the female patients who was also complaining of sexual abuse.[45] What the governors did was invoke the Hospital regulations to indict Mr Cleland on two other counts: first, he was accused of invading 'the province of the other physicians and surgeons, in treating their patients without their consent or knowledge';[46] and, secondly, in carrying out vaginal examinations, he was said to have undertaken a 'considerable operation' without giving notification.[47] Both complaints were of dubious validity. Since his activities had caused such offence, Cleland himself regretted that he had not acquainted the patients' doctors.[48] However, he correctly pointed out that whilst the orders of the Bath Infirmary allocated patients to the duty physician, they did not restrain surgeons from examining cases in general.[49] The designation of vaginal examinations as 'considerable' operations was equally exaggerated. In Cleland's words, 'every man of tolerable skill in surgery and midwifery' knew that they were 'of a kind very common, and often absolutely necessary to discover the true seat of several disorders incident to that sex. But because matters of this nature ... [were] rarely spoken of, and but very little known', the governors were able to present as exceptional a technique 'never yet deemed an operation, either by physicians or surgeons', much less an extraordinary one.[50] For his opponents, however, Cleland's interventions were not 'trivial'. On the contrary, 'very ill consequences would frequently attend ... subjecting the women patients to the vain curiosity, or vicious inclinations of every man of the profession belonging to the Hospital'.[51]

The reference to 'vain curiosity' in many respects holds the key to the dispute, suggesting that underneath the overt conflict were divergent views to the advance of medical knowledge and the exposure of women's bodies to the medical gaze. Discrepant attitudes to medical knowledge arose from Mr Cleland's practice of midwifery[52] and from more general developments of relevance to surgery. Cleland was one of the growing band of men-midwives who from the 1720s began to capture control of normal as well as complicated deliveries. Although this take-over has been closely linked to the availability of forceps, it was also assisted by fears of demographic decline at a time of population stagnation, and by social processes like cultural differentiation and an emphasis on companionate marriage; with or without the support of their husbands, wealthy 'ladies' began to break out of the 'collective culture' which in childbirth had united women of all ranks and so desert the traditional midwife for the fashionable male accoucheur who served as an emblem of superior status. Underlying this bid for politeness was the Enlightenment belief in science and progress. The man-midwife succeeded by boasting scientific expertise, in contrast to the primitive fumblings of his female rivals.[53] This was a self-interested ideology rather than an accurate reflection of lay competence, for as Ornella Moscucci has concluded, 'the onslaught on the female ceremony of childbirth must be read as an attempt to substitute women's customs for new medical rites masquerading as scientific practices founded on "objective" knowledge'. None the less, ideologies gain strength from resonating with practice.[54] Therefore, in consolidating his ambitions, and extending his practice outwards from obstetrics to gynaecology, the man-midwife resorted to the acquisition of medical knowledge via the 'scientific' paradigm. It is for these reasons that the women whom Cleland was accused of abusing were suffering from specifically female conditions: one was described as hysteric; the other he suspected (mistakenly) of being pregnant.[55] Given the transitional status of his specialism, researching these cases was likely to prove especially beneficial to his private work.

Complementing the influence of man-midwifery was the blossoming of anatomy and physiology. The humoral orthodoxy had been under challenge since the sixteenth century, when Vesalius (1514–64) published the first anatomical study based on dissections. From the 1740s, however, physiologists were beginning to query the mechanical concept of the body, derived from the Scientific Revolution; and in place of its accent on structure, advocate a focus on vital body functions.[56] The 'science of woman' was to be deeply affected. Anatomical dissection demonstrated that women had their own distinctive physical make-up that was geared to reproduction and thus overturned the Galenic position that the female genitalia were simply internal versions of the male. But nowhere were the limitations of mechanicalism clearer that in accounting for the generation of life.[57] These lesions in conventional knowledge, allied to the experimental ethos of Enlightenment science, set the stage for a more investigative approach to the study of medicine, which was to include the manual examination of women's bodies. In theory, the new anatomy and physiology were as pertinent to physicians as to surgeons. In practice, however, doctors of physic, educated classically in the texts of Galen, were more reluctant to spurn his authority.

This conservatism was reinforced by the long-standing elevation of mind over matter in Western value systems.[58] Malcolm Nicolson has attacked the stereotypical view that pre-modern diagnosis was almost without bodily contact. On the basis of Morgagni's *De Sedibus*,[59] published in 1761, he contends that physicians at Bologna and Padua frequently, if not routinely, applied techniques which involved touching patients and, with their consent, conducted rectal and vaginal examinations. In eighteenth-century Italy, however, 'close institutional and professional links' led physicians to mould 'forms of medical knowledge in which the perspectives of physic and surgery were, to some extent, combined'.[60] In Britain, there was no such osmosis to offset the stigma of handling the denigrated body. Rather, roles were polarized. Physicians, who had left autopsies to surgeons since the later seventeenth century,[61] concentrated on taking the patient history with little more than a cursory glance at appearance; surgeons conducted the hands-on diagnosis which was culturally constructed as 'dirty work', more appropriately dealt with by a labouring craftsman than by an 'ornate' professional gentleman.[62] There is a visual trace of this division of labour operating at the Bath Infirmary. In 1762 William Hoare, a local artist of national repute, presented the Hospital with a portrait of William Oliver and Jeremiah Peirce examining patients with paralysis, rheumatism and leprosy (Figure 5.1).[63] Painted in 1742, it offers an idealized interpretation of the Hospital in its first year.[64] Backed by the authority of the institution whose original 'Plan and Elevation' hangs behind them on the wall, the doctors are represented as caring co-operatively and benevolently for patients who are grateful and respectable. Yet even this unrealistic scene reveals clues to the medical hierarchy. Though there is no sign of detailed physical examination in the portrait, it is instructive that Mr Peirce, the surgeon, is holding the diseased hand in carrying out a diagnosis. Dr Oliver, conversely, holds the pen, his command confirmed by the mastery of the written record.

The physician's repudiation of bodily encounters enabled the surgeon to monopolize investigative medicine, using his grasp of anatomy and the knowledge gained by touching the patient to underwrite a bid for

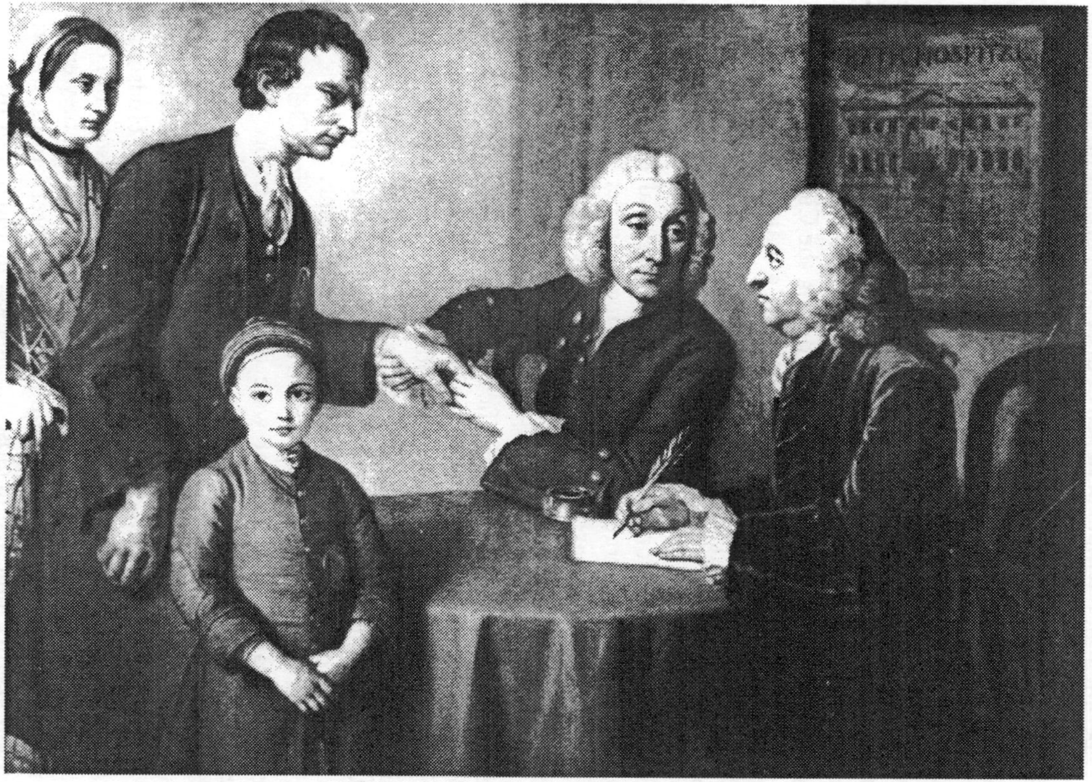

5.1 Mr Jeremiah Peirce and Dr William Oliver examining patients at the Bath Hospital

equal occupational status.[65] The role of the voluntary hospital in this campaign should not be overstated because post-mortems were also a feature of private surgical practice.[66] Moreover, for much of the eighteenth century, the infirmary's interest in anatomy was more pedagogic than experimental,[67] with experience of dissection becoming paramount for a growing number of surgical pupils. None the less, in the controlled environment of the hospital, surgeons did begin to research their captive patients, subjecting living bodies to physical examination and dead ones to autopsy. The Georgian Bath Infirmary was relatively unaffected by these changes. With no pupils attached to its own surgeons (or physicians), and no hospital-based medical training in the city until the 1820s, it managed to avoid the scramble for cadavers which disrupted other institutions.[68] Nor is there any suggestion that the honorary staff engaged regularly in post-mortems. Only during the Cleland dispute did the surgical investigation of patients emerge as a matter of controversy.

Mr Cleland's adversaries marshalled evidence drawn from a post-mortem, as well as his behaviour towards patients resident in the Hospital. The charge of indecent practices related to two particular women: Mary Hook and Mary Hudson each alleged that on several occasions, and without consent, the surgeon had 'put his finger up her body', causing pain and bleeding. Their stories were corroborated by two nurses.[69] Cleland not only denied that his interventions had been clumsy, but also claimed that the women had actively requested help after learning of his successful treatments. Of most significance, however, was the ready way in which he admitted performing the repeated vaginal examinations.[70] As a surgeon, Cleland did not eschew the bodily contact with patients which physicians avoided. In addition, he had experience of military medicine from where a number of eighteenth-century therapeutic initiatives emanated.[71] This occupational background was complemented by a keen personal interest in clinical innovation. During army service, Cleland had invented several instruments that were demonstrated before the Royal Society; and to these designs were later added 'a very ingenious apparatus ... for some complaints peculiar to the fair sex'.[72] On these grounds, Cleland was more inclined to see the Hospital as a site for medical 'trials'. Therefore, in defending the serial investigations of Mary Hudson, he stressed that his aim 'was to discover if the uterus was the seat and cause of ... her ... complaints, as it is in many hysteric cases'. This, he went on, was impossible 'without diligent inquiry, accurate observations, *frequent examinations* [my italics], and close attendance, in and out of fits; which may in time direct to a more rational method of relieving them'.[73] In short, Cleland was prepared to uphold clinical investigation as an experimental tool, to be deployed not simply to diagnose or treat the individual patient but to foster general rules of medical theory and practice.

The experimental use of the vaginal examination set Cleland apart from physicians and other surgeons at the General Hospital because even the arithmetic clinicians of the late eighteenth century assessed the spa waters through the indirect manipulation of routine statistics rather than the direct monitoring of patients' bodies. With the post-mortem, however, it was professional expertise which came under scrutiny. Cleland executed this post-mortem in the presence of Dr Oliver and Dr Rayner; four of the other Hospital surgeons; John Morris, the apothecary, and his journeyman; and one of the lay governors, Mr Paul Bertrand.[74] The patient was Sarah Appleby, who had made the allegation of rape. Admitted to the Infirmary with violent fits, she was treated both through bathing, and internal and external medicines. Examining her during a fit, Cleland had brought about the expulsion of what he judged to be a piece of retained placenta, and thereafter she was 'much relieved'. But the fits returned and Cleland therefore administered 'an injection' that was 'thrown into the uterus, upon her coming out of the bath, to procure further discharge'. He alleged that the governors had originally intended to charge him with Appleby's death, on the grounds that his management of the case was inept; but resorted to indecent practice after her physician, Dr Rayner, indicated his approval of the methods used and stated that the cause of death was venereal disease allied to a miscarriage.[75] The fact that the charge was dropped did not avert a heated exchange about the outcome of the post-mortem. In their *Short Vindication*, William Oliver and his colleagues rejected the diagnosis that Appleby had suffered from a retained placenta:

> it was the opinion of the gentlemen who examined it, that the womb could not have been the seat of the woman's disease: that the placenta, or any portion of it, had not remained in the uterus for so many months, as Mr Cleland supposed it to have done: that the substances which he brought away could not be parts of the placenta: that if matter was discharged from the vagina, it could not have proceeded from the womb; and that no injections could have entered the os tincae.[76]

In reply, Cleland acknowledged Oliver's 'superior knowledge of ... the natural way of all mankind', but devastated his reading of the post-mortem. First, Oliver was unable 'to distinguish between the state of the uterus of a virgin, and that of a woman, who not only has had a miscarriage, but the venereal disease'. Secondly, he asked 'Can the doctor know so little ... as to suppose that when the os tincae is once dilated, whether by a child, placenta ... or by the use of proper remedies ... [it] will never close again, or the uterus never appear clean, and regain its natural state?' Finally, Oliver's conclusion that a piece of placenta could not have been retained for so long was pronounced wrong, in view of the experience of those 'but moderately conversant in dissecting puerperous bodies, or even with the writings of those who have'. Cleland attributed the physicians' ignorance to their own deficiencies: 'I could not have believed that these two learned doctors ... could have been so little versed in these matters, if they had not in their *Vindication* thus publicly exposed themselves to the censure of every judicious reader'.[77] At the core of the physicians' confusion, however, was the structural division of medical knowledge, which grew out of the division of medical labour. Anatomy, requiring manual skill, was largely confined to the surgeon, leaving the profession of physic relatively untutored in the internal structure of the body. Therefore, disputed anatomical competence became a manifestation of the battle for preeminence between physicians and surgeons.

Women, medicine and morality

Archibald Cleland's position as a man-midwife placed him at the sharp end of controversy about the decency of physical contact as well as its epistemological utility. The Enlightenment has been celebrated as an age of sexual awakening, which saw the acceptance of sexuality as a natural and not a sinful activity, and the achievement of sexual gratification for women within more affectionate family relationships;[78] only romanticism, it was argued, together with the evangelical revival and a new breed of economic theory which stressed 'thrift, prudence and self-control' snuffed out the 'pleasure principle' later in the Georgian period.[79] Angus McLaren has challenged this thesis. From a reading of earlier moral and medical texts, he contends that marital sexuality was cherished in the puritan and humanist literature of the sixteenth century, and that doctors generally adopted 'an egalitarian model of procreation' in which male and female enjoyment was essential for conception. These ideas survived beyond 1700, especially in popular publications; but from the seventeenth century, this 'common culture' was undermined by 'a new "high culture" of scientific embryology ... [which] severed the traditional linking of pleasure and procreation'. The recognition that female satisfaction was unnecessary for conception, and the downgrading of the common culture to a 'low culture' – 'increasingly viewed by the educated and respectable as ... lewd and vulgar' – broadly coincided with a shift in the sexology literature. No longer elemental and unproblematic, the conjugal act was now envisaged as sordid and degrading.[80] The task of polite society was its refinement by, in Roy Porter's and Lesley Hall's words, 'stressing elevated sentiments, shunning licentious humours and gross anatomical discussion of organs and malfunctions, and indulging in lofty speculations about attraction and enticement, innocence and corruption, identity and ambivalence'.[81]

There are, of course, dangers in assuming that theological, scientific or sexological writings influenced sexual practice. But what they do suggest is that eighteenth-century attitudes to sexuality were variegated rather than uniformly liberated, particularly among the middling and upper orders. We must be wary about tracing a direct line from sexual to medical relationships because although both situations involve physical intimacy, the contexts are different.[82] Nevertheless, the experiences and practices of eighteenth-century medical men do accord with a society divided about sexuality. Early in the Georgian period, these anxieties came to a head in resistance to men-midwives who were blackened by accusations of debauchery and unmanliness.[83] William Hunter played a crucial part in relieving this antipathy by minimalizing clinical intervention in childbirth. If a response to the naturalism of the Enlightenment, however, the new social role for the man-midwife was also concordant with a concern for decency.[84] Sexual sensibilities were not confined to childbirth and private practice. Hospital patients, unable to enforce their own bodily taboos through the power of the purse, were likewise encompassed. Thus at the late eighteenth-century Edinburgh Infirmary, electric treatment in cases of amenorrhea was administered to the pelvic area through clothing to avoid 'shocking the delicacy of tender females', and certain surgical procedures on women were performed privately with no male spectators, rather than in the usual public amphitheatre, to prevent 'greater violence to female modesty than consists with decency'.[85] This commitment to decorum throws into sharp relief the audacity of Archibald Cleland in conducting vaginal examinations for research as well as clinical purposes. Yet only his methodology was forward-looking. Cleland's medical practice and his defence against dismissal upheld the conventional socio-cultural construction of women's role in Georgian society.

Eighteenth-century perceptions of women were underpinned by the dichotomized images of the sexes which Enlightenment thinking encouraged. Men were identified with 'culture' and hence with 'not just the progressive light of reason but also the corruption and exploitation of civil society'. Women were identified with 'nature' and hence were idealized as 'the carriers of a new morality through which the artificiality of civilization could be transcended'.[86] But if naturally 'good', women were also naturally 'emotional and passionate, needing constraint within social boundaries'.[87] The reproductive system was central to this process of control. The function of menstruation and the ovaries was little understood and so the woman's body was assumed to be in a constant state of readiness for conception.[88] It followed that the female was of 'a more amorous temper' than the male, a volatile creature whose unrestrained passions imperilled social stability.[89] Although the refinement of sexuality turned women into reluctant lovers whose feminine sensibilities had to be titillated, their weak-headedness, if not their instincts, left them prey to seduction by cunning suitors.[90] Therefore, from infancy girls were taught 'strong notions of honour', so that they hated 'a whore before they know what the word means' and grew up 'to find their worldly interest entirely depending upon the reputation of their chastity'.[91] Reinforcing the ethic of sexual purity was the social role derived from reproduction. Women were made 'only to conceive, to give suck, and to breed up children';[92] their greatest use to the community was in 'keep[ing] up a succession' and being of assistance to parents and husbands.[93] Man, conversely, 'acts with more firmness ... defends himself with more courage and presence of mind, reasons with more strength'; he turned to the female sex as 'playtoys' only after his 'more serious occupations' were over.[94] The image of early modern wives as fragile diversions for their husbands contradicts the essential if subservient economic role which even women of the middling sort played in urban and rural households.[95] But realism aside, the attempt to mould women into compliant angels – and condemn those who rebelled as deviant whores – retained an ideological potency. Moral and social virtue were thus fused through a hierarchical concept of marriage and the family which both negotiated or mediated the dissonance between sexual freedom and sexual inhibition, and sanctioned the recruitment of institutions besides marriage to rein in women's behaviour.

The Cleland affair illustrates how early Georgian medicine turned its hand to policing female virtue. Mary Hook provides the most obvious example of clinical practice articulating sexual morality. In justifying his management of the case, Cleland voiced a suspicion that the patient was pregnant, a judgement formed after his first external examination. The opportunity to probe further enabled him to ratify or reject this diagnosis. There was a therapeutic point to the exercise: if the patient was with child, then continuing the course of medicines and bathing would probably lead to miscarriage and 'a long train of illnesses, that might end in death'. Furthermore, medical practitioners at the Hospital might be upbraided 'for not having enquired into her case more minutely' before starting treatment. Above all, however, a positive confirmation would prevent the goodwill of benefactors 'from being imposed upon'.[96] In fact, Hook was not pregnant, but Cleland's argument is still revealing. Unlike other infirmaries,[97] Bath had no rules which excluded particular categories of patient. Nor were all Mary Hook's ailments associated with the suspected pregnancy; she also had leprosy and complained of 'a stoppage in her water'.[98] But even the lying-in hospitals, set up from mid-century,[99] catered largely for married women. Having crossed from respectability to disgrace, the single expectant mother was not a proper object of charity. It was the job of medicine to confirm her transgression and so guard the boundaries of propriety.

Moral policing also occurs in the cases of Mary Hudson and Sarah Appleby, both of whom were labelled hysteric. Hysteria was a common condition, embracing a broad spectrum of symptoms which ranged from sudden pain and physical convulsions to fits of laughing or weeping. Since the complaint was more prevalent among women than men, medical accounts focused on their anatomical and physiological differences. The most popular explanation was a malfunctioning of the uterus, but even where the cause was not peculiar to the female body – Thomas Sydenham's 'chemopathology of the spirits and nerves', for example – women's greater propensity to the disease was linked to their being the 'weaker vessel'.[100] Medicine did not stop at defining the female sex as biologically inferior to the male. Remedies for hysteria included social as well as clinical prescriptions. Since all women except married mothers were considered at risk, entering the conjugal state was advised. 'There still remains another highly natural, and efficacious method of cure', countenanced 'A Medical Dictionary' of 1743, 'which is, that to be expected from marriage. Reason, experience, and the authorities of the greatest physicians, concur in pronouncing matrimony highly beneficial in removing hysteric disorders'.[101] By blessing a social role with a clinical rationale, medicine became an agent of social control, adding its authority to the hierarchical marital relationship and pressuring women to conform to the angelic image.

Cleland's use of Hospital patients to explore the uterine origins of hysteria yoke him to what one sociologist has called 'probably the most dramatic and dynamic example of patriarchal medicine'.[102] Furthermore, his case against dismissal ruthlessly exploited the opposition between the virtuous and the fallen woman. These binary categories were most blatantly expressed in a robust retrospective pamphlet, published anonymously in 1748 by 'Britannicus'. '[H]ow unlikely it is', speculated the author, 'that Mr Cleland should have any taste for ravishing a nasty common prostitute, when he has so fine a woman for his wife, let the reasonable who know her judge.'[103] The evidence that Cleland himself arrayed to defend his character was also founded on dualistic assumptions about female virtue which he used to tarnish one of the governors, and Mary Hook and Mary Hudson. Among those present at the post-mortem of Sarah Appleby was Mr Paul Bertrand, a lay governor energetic in the surgeon's prosecution.[104] As the body was made ready for dissection, Mr Bertrand is said to have asked whether the patient 'was a maid, or not'. Replying that 'it was no affair of mine',

Cleland used the incident to infer a salacious interest on the part of the enquirer:

> It may here not improperly be asked, from what sort of principle this extraordinary curiosity of Mr Bertrand's did proceed? Since he had, or might have fully satisfied a more than modest degree of it, in his frequent examinations, or at least viewing of naked women, in the Academy of Painting ... of which ... he, and some other governors are members; and where one can scarcely think any modest maid, or woman, would expose herself.
>
> But, if it be supposed ... this same curiosity of his could possibly arise from a lewd and vicious inclination; it will not be difficult to account for the extraordinary part he has taken from the beginning; in charging me with acting from the same motives.[105]

This accusation of prurience recognized the 'sexual potential of medical anatomy'; the dissection – no less than representations of the female body – amounted to an 'undressing of the corpse'.[106] In deprecating the integrity of Bertrand, however, Cleland resorted to the very polarization of female sexuality upon which tales of his own lechery fed; nude modelling was an activity that no decent woman would contemplate.

Despite his avowed indifference to the virginal state of Sarah Appleby, Cleland used the sexual behaviour of Mary Hook and Mary Hudson to discredit their stories. Thus at the hearing, two witnesses – summoned from Mary Hook's home town of Cheltenham – described her as a 'common strumpet'; and one alleged that she had falsely accused a 'young gentleman' of rape, in order to extort money from him. Mary Hudson was not accused of prostitution; but the defendant informed the governors that 'he had several persons ready ... to prove that ... [she] was a cheat, an impostor, a great liar, [who] had miscarried by taking of medicines, and that no credit ought to be given to any thing she could say'.[107] The two house visitors on duty when the alleged indecencies took place endorsed these moral assassinations; they both denounced the accusations as 'false and scandalous' and went on to resign from the governing body, citing the 'hard treatment' of Mr Cleland as a reason.[108] Their suspicions may have been aroused because the charges were not uncovered during a routine tour of inspection.[109] Instead, the 'victims' were said to have 'complained to the nurses and patients ... not as informants to prosecute, but as poor creatures who had been injured, but were afraid to make higher appeal to justice'.[110] The failure to use official channels for a matter of such sensitivity is not surprising. However, was it fear of authority which led the women to confide in other women from a similar social background? Or were they members of a socio-cultural group whose attitudes to sexuality and physical touch were more relaxed than those of their élite and charitable patrons? In addition to Cleland's personal testimony, two former patients swore on oath that they had frequently heard Sarah Appleby say that Mary Hook and Mary Hudson 'had often teazed her' to ask Mr Cleland to examine them.[111] Consequently, we can speculate that Hook and Hudson did indeed agree to vaginal examination. What happened thereafter was that Cleland's enemies, hearing the gossip, saw the chance to trap him. The harassment to which witnesses were subjected after they had left the Hospital[112] suggests that pressure was applied to acquire the necessary evidence, with the governors and their paid officers extracting statements from patients and staff in a highly charged atmosphere. Under this scenario, the coercive circumstances rather than personal immorality explained any distortion of the truth which happened.

But if the charges were trumped up, why did the Hospital invest so much energy in securing a dismissal? Only four of the 11 governors present at the general court opposed the decision. In deciphering the motives of the majority who voted against him, Cleland made much of their connections: six, he claimed, were professionally or commercially dependent upon Ralph Allen who was himself 'an intimate acquaintance' of the Hospital's senior surgeon, Jeremiah Peirce.[113] However, the dispute was not simply a 'temporary disorder' between individuals but a structural conflict between interest groups,[114] which hinged primarily on the commercial welfare of the city and moral unease at the practice of controversial gynaecological techniques within the Infirmary. Cleland himself interpreted the incident wholly in economic terms: the local community was worried by his plans for the baths and jealous of his thriving private practice because he was 'likely ... to have prospered and fattened on their soil'.[115] His disapproval of the bathing facilities did not provoke universal retaliation from the four governors who, as members of the city Corporation, were managers of the baths; one, Mr Samuel Bush, supported a reprimand over dismissal.[116] Moreover, of the eight governors who were physicians, only a half attended the trial;[117] Dr Rayner was called away[118] and no vote was recorded for the surgeon, Jeremiah Peirce.[119] None the less, the two honorary physicians who were present did receive the backing of their professional colleagues who held no Hospital post, and at least two of the absentees were not greatly affected by criticism of the spa since they worked outside Bath. The foundation of early eighteenth-century medical ethics in 'manners' rather than professional competence[120] facilitated a conspiracy. Whereas Cleland's attack on William Oliver's anatomical ineptitude had little purchase, his own activities were perceived as highly dubious. An ambitious surgeon with new ideas, Archibald Cleland used methods which were tainted with midwifery and broke the conventions of bodily contact with patients. Therefore, after the charge of incompetence leading to the death of Sarah Appleby collapsed, what better ploy than a complaint that opened the hornet's nest of sexual morality?

Public opinion was a convenient means to that end. By the time Thomas Percival published his guide to medical ethics,[121] physicians and surgeons were beginning to recognize the advantages of settling their differences privately. Earlier in the century, however, conflicts were often adjudicated in the full glare of publicity.[122] With rumours that Cleland had debauched a female patient circulating, the governors faced an unenviable dilemma. Removing him put benefactions and subscriptions at risk. Lady Inchiquin, for example, in a trenchant letter of support to the surgeon, rejected reports that she had increased her contribution to the Hospital at the last collection and announced that she had 'not give[n] one sixpence; nor do I design it, 'till you have justice done your character'.[123] Yet, on the other hand, keeping Cleland in post would have offended not just the medical practitioners associated with the Hospital, but those visitors and residents upset by the allegations. The governors put on a brave face. To the public, they were adamant that the need to 'preserve all decency' justified their action and anticipated that when the 'passion and prejudice ... [had] subsided', true lovers of charity would double their benefactions to demonstrate approval for a decision which had been 'the duty of honest and impartial men'.[124] In private, however, they may have calculated that the dangers of retaining Mr Cleland surpassed those of sacking him. If Georgian society as a whole was torn between eroticism and prudity, that disquiet was all the more acute in Bath where, according to the satirists, the rich and famous came to indulge their libidinous appetites.[125] As the city's premier charity, the General Hospital played a central part in counterbalancing this negative image; and, therefore, any inkling of sexual waywardness was damaging in the extreme. However creditable from a clinical perspective, Cleland's vaginal examinations were an affront to élite notions of decency; even the Earl of Chesterfield, who had actively canvassed for his appointment, observed that 'To suppose him innocent one must suppose him uncommonly curious ... to a degree of incredulity, into the state of his female patients'.[126] Medical colleagues capitalized astutely on this breach of respectability, commandeering the bodies of women patients in an attempt to wreck the career of a commercial rival. Caught in the middle, the lay governors put the reputation of the Hospital first; whatever their attitudes to Cleland's behaviour, sexual impropriety was an insinuation that no charity could afford to ignore.

Clinical autonomy: the doctor–governor relationship

With the Cleland affair and the sulphur controversy, there were efforts to limit clinical autonomy outside the General Infirmary, as a coterie of medical governors seized the institution to exclude from local practice those who challenged the conventional methods of spa therapy. However, the dismissal of Archibald Cleland also suggests that professional discretion over patients within the Hospital was not absolute but conditional upon the approval of both fellow medical staff and lay governors. Whereas other voluntary infirmaries began to exclude physicians and surgeons from governor status,[127] at Bath they retained throughout the long eighteenth century the representation that had enabled such full participation in the Cleland and Baylies affairs. But though doctors were involved in running the Infirmary,[128] and requests for medical equipment were granted,[129] their professional activities were overseen by a governing body in which the majority of members were laymen. Thus if Dr Hartley and Dr Harington escaped censure for the irregular attendance of which William Baylies claimed they were guilty,[130] the honorary surgeons were on two occasions in the 1740s reprimanded for their lax attendance and subjected to the scrutiny of lay house visitors.[131] More importantly, the admission and discharge of patients remained in the realm of lay as well as medical judgement.

Although benefactors and subscribers did not obtain the right to sponsor patients at the Bath Infirmary, the physicians and surgeons were still hamstrung by recruitment policy. Since residents of the city were barred in favour of the more distant sick poor unable to visit the spa, aspiring patients did not usually present themselves for clinical examination. Instead, the 1739 Act required that the details of each case be drawn up by 'some physician or person of skill in the neighbourhood' and forwarded to the Hospital, together with a statement of the individual's 'poverty or circumstances ... attested by the minister and church-wardens ... or other creditable persons'. Commanding officers were to vouch for regular soldiers and militia men.[132] The register then sent in turn for those minuted for admission when vacancies arose. The Casebook of letters recommending patients, which survives for 1750 to 1758, shows that at times the honorary staff did propose admissions. Some of these applicants were relatively local, often inhabiting the outer Bath parishes;[133] others were temporarily lodged in the city, whether as servants or self-funding visitors.[134] Whatever their grounds for qualifying, this group allowed the physicians and surgeons direct access to prospective patients. Thus Thomas Deluke, deaf and without speech after smallpox, had 'been examined by the gentlemen of this Hospital and thought a very proper object of it', when he was put forward by the honorary surgeon, Philip Ditcher, in 1758.[135] However, these local patients were the exception; diagnosis from afar was the norm. The Hospital made strenuous efforts to ensure a flow of suitable cases. In 1741, 12 000 copies of the admission conditions were printed and sent to diocesan bishops in an attempt to penetrate as many parishes as possible.[136] Until the later Georgian period, advertisements were placed in the *Bath Journal*;[137] after 1747/48, details were included in the *Annual Reports*; and local histories and guidebooks also held the information.[138] Despite these endeavours, the Casebook contains copies of letters which were vague and of little clinical value. 'Alice Murdain, of the parish of Walford ... has, for some time, had nervous complaints of various kinds' ran one unsigned entry in 1756.[139] Henry Steele of Northampton even recommended himself, concluding – after a lengthy account of 'growing weakness' from a fall downstairs – that 'unless I shall be so happy as to meet with any success at Bath, I must expect soon to be totally incapacitated for any business'.[140] The Infirmary deplored such defective medical reports:

> Another great grievance this Hospital has to complain of is, that many of the lower class of the Faculty of Physic, who are applied to by the parishes to draw up the cases of paupers, do it in so short and general a manner, that scarce any judgement can be formed about them by the gentlemen here ... Others omit such circumstances, which if known, would at once show the patients improper to be admitted ... [141]

Yet these reproaches were not followed by a specification of the clinical conditions most appropriate for spa treatment. Of greater concern were procedural breaches of the regulations, which led to the arrival of the sick poor without prior permission and exposed them to prosecution under the vagrancy laws.[142]

The priority given to the non-medical characteristics of patients was reflected in their selection. Lack of formal sponsorship rights did not prevent lay governors from exercising patronage. In 1755, for example, Benjamin Bathurst, one of the treasurers, recommended the widow of a Paris miniature-portrait painter who had 'been seized a few days ago with a hemiplegia which has in some degree affected her brain and her speech. She appear[ed] to be a proper object of charity'.[143] More restrictive was the routine involvement of lay governors in the admissions process. All applications were considered by the weekly committee at which medical staff were expected to be present, but differences of opinion were resolved by majority voting and the physicians and surgeons enjoyed no special privileges.[144] The discharge of patients was likewise a shared responsibility. In September 1742, Mr Paul Bertrand and the Hospital apothecary, John Morris, whilst serving as house visitors, 'queried of the physicians if George Cotton should not be discharged as incurable'. Earlier in the same year, the weekly committee had thought it 'proper to continue John Lewis a little longer',[145] seemingly overturning a recommendation from the medical faculty. The lay supervision of dismissal was quickly absorbed into the administrative structure. In the Autumn of 1743, a monthly meeting of the governors was set up 'to view the patients', so that those who had 'been here long enough may be discharged'. Four years later a time limit was imposed; all inmates resident for six calendar months were to be dismissed automatically, unless benefit had been received and their physician or surgeon believed that further improvement was possible. This respect for clinical opinion did not extend to procedural lapses; for in 1768 the physicians were asked 'to be more cautious of discharging patients without their appearance at the committee'.[146] Towards the end of the century, however, a shift in the balance of power is discernible. From the mid-1780s, *Annual Reports* began to voice regret each year about the 'very imperfect description of cases' which had previously been expressed only at intervals. Simultaneously, fevers, abscesses and external ulcers were singled out as unfit for treatment at the Hospital. 'Patients with coughs attended with pain in the chest, or spitting of blood' were added to the exclusions in 1825/26,[147] and at the turn of the decade, the admission conditions were thoroughly overhauled to include a list of suitable ailments:

> For the information of applicants respecting the diseases capable of being benefited by Bath waters, it may be stated that these are palsy, gout, rheumatism; certain nervous derangements, in which the brain is not materially affected, amongst which chorea sancti viti may be particularly noticed; diseases of the skin, palsy from lead, poisonous effect of mercury or other minerals, injuries sustained through exposure to cold; pain, weakness, or contraction of limbs from any cause; dyspeptic complaints, biliary and visceral obstructions ... but even these cases are deemed improper where there is pain of chest, cough, spitting of blood, palpitation or other disturbances of the heart, evidence of too great a determination of blood to the head, acute inflammation in any part, or general fever; absess, suppuration of the joints, or ulcer of any kind. If epileptic fits have occurred, the case is always deemed improper.[148]

If this comprehensive catalogue 'extolled [the spa] for too many virtues',[149] it none the less represented an erosion of the lay perspective that had been a thorn in the flesh of Georgian medical practitioners across the voluntary hospital sector.[150] By the early nineteenth century, the Bath Infirmary was no longer at the coal-face of medical knowledge, but its physicians and surgeons, like colleagues elsewhere,[151] were engaged in the medicalization of their institution, subordinating charitable motives to clinical ones.

Public health and hospital hygiene

The campaign to improve the physical environment of the General Hospital also implies an acceleration in medical power as, contrary to the growing movement for institutional hygiene, the physicians and surgeons managed to block plans for new premises in the 1790s. This dispute between governors and honorary staff has to be explicated within the context of changing attitudes to health and the environment. Throughout the early modern period, this relationship was interpreted through a neo-classical model of the non-naturals; whereas the intrinsic, 'natural' humours were seen as shaping the bodily constitution, the overall health of the individual depended upon his or her interaction with a set of external factors: air, diet, exercise, climate and weather.[152] Until the mid-seventeenth century, doctors believed that these outside agents were responsible for releasing 'the seeds of disease or pain ... within the body' and tried to control them by prescribing 'appropriate health regimens, purges, diaphoresis, and sometimes bleeding'. With the Scientific Revolution of the 1660s, however, an alternative to this 'humoural pathology' emerged in which the non-naturals alone were considered capable of generating sickness. Although the pathogens in the environment which produced disease were unknown, a mechanical conception of the atmosphere as 'composed of and holding in suspension minute particles' identified a plausible instrument for causation and transference which made air 'the primary agent of disease'. Furthermore, the extension of the term 'miasma' to cover not just these particles but also 'vaporous exhalations' enabled the new 'environmental pathology' to accommodate the 'principal element' of earlier contagion theory. As James Riley has extrapolated, 'Not only emanations from earth but also emanations from diseased people, corpses, rotting vegetable matter, and other sources might add to the atmospheric constitution the properties and qualities necessary to provoke an epidemic'. Thus the environment became a 'remote cause' as well as the mechanism for transmission. It was from the combination of these ideas with the improvement ethos of the Enlightenment that a concept of public health or social medicine was born. Therapy was no longer confined to the individual and quarantine was no longer the main means of prevention. Epidemics indicated that man was improperly adjusted to his habitat and this symptom of disorder demanded a collective medicine that treated the environment as a whole.[153]

Epidemic fevers were critical in bringing about this transformation. Although 'symptomatic' fevers distinguished by local inflammation and 'intermittent' fevers like ague were familiar to early modern physicians and surgeons, 'continuous' fevers were less common before 1700.

Associated with headaches, delirium and small red spots, they were most prevalent amongst the growing institutional population in prisons, military establishments and hospitals, and generated a wave of medical texts from the second quarter of the eighteenth century. By 1750, innovative military doctors like John Pringle and James Lind were correlating continuous fevers with vitiated air.[154] The most famous application of this discourse to hospitals was John Howard's *Account of the Principal Lazarettos in Europe*, published in 1789.[155] Howard – a Bedfordshire landowner with an influential survey of prisons already under his belt – was not the only source of advice; a number of medical men – John Aikin, Thomas Percival, William Blizard[156] – also went into print. Their didactic texts reveal a basic consensus about the aetiology of continuous fevers and the means to prevent them. Quality of air was the cause. As Aikin observed, when the visitor

> walks through the long wards of a crowded hospital, and surveys the languid countenances of the patients, when he feels the peculiarly noisome effluvia so unfriendly to every vigorous principle of life, and compares their transient effect upon him, with that to be expected by those who are constantly breathing them and imbibing them at every pore, he will be apt to look upon a hospital as a dismal prison, where the sick are shut up from the rest of mankind to perish by mutual contagion.

The solution to this 'inbred pestilence of crowded receptacles for the sick' lay in ventilation, drainage and cleanliness. Ventilating machines to freshen the air were not ruled out, especially in confined spaces; but the careful location and design of hospitals was the chosen course of action. 'The situation of the building', wrote Blizard, 'should be a little elevated: out of a town: the soil gravelly, or, at least, dry ... [the] ground to be possessed to an extent that will always be a security against detriment to the air by buildings, [and] obnoxious manufactories'. Just as important was the construction of the infirmary. Circular, quadrangular, and trilateral structures with parallel sides were all condemned for impeding the circulation of air, and plans with wings which diverged were recommended in their place. Also advocated was the accommodation of patients preferably on one floor, and not more than two; wards that were no less than 15 feet high; passages that were a minimum of six feet wide; and windows that had mechanisms to prevent them from being shut at the wrong times. In addition to design, the wards were to be treated regulary with white lime; nearby nuisances removed; offensive sanitation improved; and iron bedsteads and straw mattresses promoted over wood and flock because they were less likely to harbour bugs and retain infectious exhalations. Finally, overcrowding was to be avoided.

The policy of admitting patients only when there were vacancies protected the Bath Infirmary from over-occupancy. However, commitment to the non-naturals had long fostered an awareness of the virtues of fresh, dry air and in his *Description of Bath*, the Infirmary's architect, John Wood, emphasized that the building stood on a well-drained 'fine gravel' facing the northern perimeter of the city, with a large garden to the west. Moreover, he went on to regret the Corporation's decision to permit the construction of a house in front of the Hospital, thus threatening 'all the advantages of a free and open situation' required by 'poor diseased objects ... while they are trying the effects of the hot waters'.[157] The management of smallpox likewise reflected traditional attitudes. Although a number of Georgian hospitals specifically excluded contagious diseases,[158] there was no such explicit ban at Bath. Nevertheless, the rules printed by Wood specified 'That all patients who, after their admission, shall be found to have an infectious distemper, shall be ordered into a particular ward, appropriated for that purpose'.[159] In 1747, the register was asked to advise when he sent for patients that if they contracted smallpox whilst resident, the cost of treatment would be deducted from their caution money,[160] and this information was added to the *Annual Report* in 1751, where it remained until the early nineteenth century. In 1752 several patients discharged themselves prematurely 'for fear of the smallpox'.[161] Their anxieties were not unfounded. In November the Prince's Ward was earmarked for patients with smallpox or any other infectious disease, as was the Duke's Ward three years later.[162] Furthermore, at the beginning of 1757, a subcommittee was set up to investigate the possibility of a separate house for smallpox patients.[163] No such accommodation was acquired, but in the 1790s patients who fell victim to smallpox were being transferred to private dwellings. Their personal prognoses were poor; for according to one report, three out of five subsequently died.[164] But the strategy of isolating these cases demonstrates that an imperfect aetiology did not preclude an effective reaction to infectious diseases.

The Bath Hospital was also responsive to some of the more novel aspects of social medicine. In 1743 a model of the ventilating machine, devised by Dr Stephen Hales, was installed 'in the most commodious place in the House'.[165] A more ambitious scheme was afoot in 1780 when a 'report respecting ventilators ... [was] referred to the physicians and surgeons', the implementation of which may account for the high cost of Hospital expenses in 1780/81.[166] The windows had received attention at an earlier stage. In 1756 John Wood and Philip Allen, on duty as house visitors, recommended for consideration by the weekly committee that the lower sashes become fixed and the upper sashes movable 'as a means to render the wards warmer and more easy to be ventilated'. It is not clear whether this particular proposal was acted upon; but in 1778 sliding upper sashes were ordered for the front of the Infirmary.[167] White-liming[168] and the treatment of bugs[169] appear in the Minute Books only during the early 1750s when the publications of Sir John Pringle – a governor of the General Infirmary – gave hospital hygiene a high profile. Throughout the long eighteenth century, however, sanitation prompted a series of alterations 'to remove offensive smells and stench' from the 'necessary houses'[170] or the sewers.[171] These piecemeal measures may have helped to avert outbreaks of hospital fever,[172] but the Bath Hospital was constrained by its premises. During the early stages of construction, the size of the wards was increased in line with 'a new plan brought this day by Mr Wood and the physicians, apprehending that large wards will be conducive to the health of the patients'.[173] Nevertheless, the overall designs which Wood prepared did not anticipate the prescriptions of the later institutional reformers. In 1727, when plans for a 60–bed Infirmary were drawn up, he offered the trustees the choice of a circular or quadrangular form. After the projected capacity of the institution was increased, the layout was revised and a U-shaped mansion block for just over 100 patients was produced, with the potential for expansion to the south.[174] When John Howard paid an inspection visit in May 1788, he found the site congested. Several windows were open and the Infirmary was 'cleaner and fresher than at my visit last year', but ventilation problems persisted; in particular, many upper sashes in the wards, passages and staircases did not 'let down', which was 'the more necessary in such close and confined spaces'.[175] Yet despite these negative observations, subsequent plans to relocate the institution were scuppered.

In May 1791, the weekly committee, asked 'to enquire into the expediency of building a new Hospital', commissioned a feasibility study from the physicians and surgeons. When their report expressed unanimous opposition to a move, it was agreed to enlarge the existing premises and the offer of plans from Mr Thomas Baldwin was accepted.[176] But not all the governors concurred with this decision and the presentation of financial estimates for the extension enabled these dissidents to reopen the question of an alternative site.[177] Furthermore, convinced that the issue had 'not ... received that ample and candid discussion which its importance certainly deserves', they published an *Address* detailing the protracted handling of the affair, reproducing the text of the medical report and taking apart the objections of the physicians and surgeons.[178] The authors of this pamphlet were not ignorant of the issues involved, ten of the 14 being members of a subcommittee set up to consider the options after the costings for the enlargement became available.[179] Their starting-point was the Hospital's continuing dereliction of its duty 'to supply the public demand for assistance': the waiting list was too long, with the result that subscribers were deterred; and many prospective patients died, became more difficult – if not impossible – to cure, or found relief from other local charities.[180] Infused throughout the dispute, however, were public health principles.

In commencing their report, the honorary physicians and surgeons had maintained that although the density of occupation was high, there was 'no account of any putrid or contagious distemper, such as frequently occur in other hospitals, having ever made their appearance in this'. The rebel governors were sceptical, contending that the disease profile of Bath patients meant that they were rarely vulnerable to infection and that if they were, the regular bathing gave protection. The case against the proposed location was similarly dismissed. The physicians and surgeons objected to the site for the new building – in the vicinity of the Hot Bath and the Pump Room – on the grounds that it was lower than the current one 'and not many feet above the level of the river in rainy seasons'. The effects of this dampness, 'though scarcely manifest when mankind inhabit separately, and are spread over a large space ... are materially to be apprehended when a large number of persons are enclosed in the same building, and many of these obliged to sleep in the same ward'. The problem was compounded by the daily warm bathing of patients, which prevented 'the admission of air, by opening windows'. In reply, the *Address* conceded that the soil on which the Hospital stood was dry, and acknowledged that the new location was lower. But it denied the adverse conditions during wet seasons and cleverly turned the ventilation argument on its head; if bathing inhibited the safe influx of 'outward air' through doors and windows, the only remedy was a new building 'in which a proper quantity and degree of internal circulation of air may be provided for, by lofty ceilings, spacious wards, and prudently placed ventilators'. The debate extended beyond the Hospital's structure to its immediate setting. The medical staff maintained that the current situation was convenient for patients, who could 'be easily carried into the fields for the benefit of the air'. Their protagonists, however, observed that this opportunity – a disappearing asset as the growing city encroached upon the countryside – was seldom taken, even in the summer months; and had to be set against the 'painful and tedious' journey of patients to the Hot Bath, carried by chairmen, the cost of whom inflated annual expenditure. The location suggested for the new Hospital was much nearer to the bath and hence more economical for transport. Furthermore, it stood to gain from a general improvement programme for the area, which comprised two broad new streets, a wide paved passage for foot passengers and chairs, and a sanitation system in which the sewers would be cleansed daily by waste water from the bath.[181]

For the authors of the *Address*, the logic of a move was irresistible. Only a new infirmary could offer a more healthy external environment and neither plan for enlarging the premises – an extra storey or two additional wards to the south – could 'remedy that essential defect now existing, from the lowness of the wards, of the passages, and appertenances, and from want of a free circulation of air'.[182] But this 'progressive' case for a relocated hospital failed and contrary to the strictures of institutional hygiene, the governors decided to add an attic storey,[183] thus increasing the density of occupation and accommodating patients on three levels rather than the recommended one. The reasons for this outcome are complex. We cannot ignore the position of the influential Dr Henry Harington, honorary physician but also an Improvement Commissioner[184] whose vested interest in upgrading the precincts of the proposed site may have been threatened by an institution for the sick poor. However, his ability to carry his medical colleagues with him points to the contested nature of the late eighteenth-century public health debate. 'Modern' ideas about social medicine first affected the Bath Hospital through the clinical research of Rice Charleton and William Falconer, whose statistical techniques owed much to the medical and social reformers. Charleton held an Oxford MD and his work predated the most vigorous phase of the public health movement. The younger Falconer, on the other hand, had been educated at the advanced Edinburgh medical school where William Cullen and his followers were by the 1780s teaching that if poor nutrition and anxiety predisposed the constitution to continuous fever, breathing exhausted air was a principal exciting cause. A contemporary of Thomas Percival and John Haygarth, he had subsequently held an honorary post at Chester Infirmary where Haygarth had carried out a series of hygienic improvements; and he moved to Bath at the suggestion of the Quaker physician, John Fothergill, who was a leading figure among London reformers.[185] However, these close connections with the dissenting medical community did not stop William Falconer from joining forces with his Oxford colleagues, Dr Harington and Daniel Lysons, and the honorary surgeons, to condemn the removal of the Bath Infirmary to a new site.

This reaction was underpinned by a number of factors. Armed with a scientific knowledge of the 'atmospheric economy', medical practitioners were able to broaden their area of expertise to include habitats as well as patients and so assert the right to police sickness in society as a whole.[186] But environmental pathology held little appeal for élite spa doctors who made their money by peddling personalized therapies and had no wish to threaten their exclusivity by meddling too much with the masses. Religion and politics were also central to the public health discourse. Since dissenters were excluded from Oxbridge and barred from legal and political office, a medical education north of the border offered the prospect of a respectable career in public service. The puritanical values which they brought to medicine fortified its commitment to progress, and the contemporary revival of political radicalism offered a vehicle for reform. Not every dissenter was a Whig, but the party's critique of electoral and administrative deficiencies both reinforced, and was reinforced by, the accounts of social and institutional malaise made public by the movement for social medicine.[187] It is unfortunate that we cannot trace the political and religious affiliations of all those on both sides of the Bath dispute. It is unlikely, however, that the honorary medical staff were in any way radical; indeed, Henry Harington was renowned for the firm stand which he took against political protest during his period as mayor of the city in 1793/94.[188] Conversely, amongst those campaigning for new premises was Baron Dimsdale, a retired physician, banker and politician from a Quaker family who had written a treatise on inoculation for smallpox and set up an 'inoculating house' in Hertford.[189] No details survive of how the 34 governors who gathered to adjudicate between the two camps cast their votes, but it would seem that a die-hard medical establishment exerted its authority to hold the line against a corps of more progressive governors. Whereas in Manchester the radical, dissenting community was sufficiently wealthy and powerful to force through a series of public health reforms (including a dedicated fever block),[190] in Bath conservatism prevailed.

From the early nineteenth century, the medical context of hospital improvement began to alter, as localized pathology was applied to epidemic disease and a concomitant regime of bleeding adopted. But if local inflammation was now a more popular explanation for continuous fever than constitutional debility, overcrowding was still seen as a causative effect and, therefore, environmental strategies complemented phlebotomy.[191] At the Bath Infirmary, where spa therapy circumscribed venesection, the rooftop extension did not extinguish calls to expand and upgrade the premises. In 1806, a subcommittee was appointed to discuss once again 'the propriety and eligibility' of rebuilding; but the ground offered to the Hospital was too small and the scheme was dropped.[192] Twelve years later, another elevation of the Infirmary roof was explored to make 'an extra ward with proper conveniences', but this project was abandoned after the governors concluded that the lower offices would be 'considerably darkened', access to the Princess Ward restricted and the chairmen fatigued by carrying patients upstairs.[193] Only in 1828 was a major refurbishment finally inaugurated. The public health imprint was clear in the raising of ceilings for passages on the second (attic) floor and in the 'regulated introduction of warm and cold air for the purposes of completely warming and ventilating the whole House'.[194] Moreover, just before the work was completed in 1829, the subcommittee for repairs was asked 'how far it might be advisable or eligible to adopt iron lathes with straw mattresses for the bedsteads in the future; as preferable, in many respects to the sacking at present in use'.[195]

A proud report in the *Bath Journal*, celebrating the benign usage of machines at a time when they were becoming metaphors for antipathy to industrialization,[196] emphasized that the steam boiler was employed for cooking, washing and drying as well as extracting 'all the air which is not proper for respiration'. The interior was now 'more complete than that of any Hospital, perhaps, in or out of London'.[197] The annual statement, prepared for the general court in May 1830, was also complimentary, claiming that the new arrangements had not only 'given great satisfaction' to all those visiting the Infirmary but also benefited the patients' health; even during the severe winter weather, they had 'suffered very little from coughs and colds, which may fairly be attributed to the regular temperature of the wards and passages'. What the bitter cold had affected was access to the Hot Bath. The construction of baths within the Hospital, already in the hands of a subcommittee as an outgrowth of the refurbishment programme, was put forward as a response to this problem.[198] Simultaneously, however, the Hot Bath itself was undergoing reconstruction with the addition of a new reservoir and a tepid swimming-pool.[199] These enhanced amenities were designed to increase the attractiveness of the spa. Therefore, given the respectability of the early nineteenth-century city, patient use may have now been regarded as inappropriate.

The procedural haggling which accompanied the improvement scheme at the Bath Hospital hints that the changes may have been more controversial than the anodyne reports suggest. However, it was now lay governors who were balking at modernization;[200] the physicians and surgeons had become receptive to public health ideas, giving higher priority to internal ventilation and discarding earlier objections to baths within the Hospital on the grounds that damp air spread infection.[201] The honorary staff in the late 1820s included the radical physician, Edward Barlow – a leading figure in the national campaign to reform the medical profession – and William Tudor, a surgeon who with Barlow later participated in the local activities of the British Medical Association.[202] But environmental pathology was an orthodoxy even by 1800 and its obsession with miasmas was later to become an impediment to innovation.[203] Therefore, the belated endorsement of a public health discourse at the Bath Infirmary echoed the medical traditionalism of its balneology. Yet despite the substantial refurbishment eventually sanctioned, concern about atmospheric quality persisted. Within months of the project being finished, two governors were asked to inspect the Princess Ward and the nurses' bedrooms in the King's and Queen's Wards in order to 'better' their ventilation,[204] and when an appeal was launched for the Hospital extension, which opened in 1861, the building was described as poorly aerated as well as too small and lacking in recent 'conveniences'.[205] Therefore, the problem of institutional hygiene, identified by Georgian reformers, was inherited by the Victorians. Not until 1865 was the first major hospital built according to Nightingale principles, developing the concept of pavilions which had first appeared at the Royal Naval Hospital in Plymouth a century before.[206]

In this chapter, we have assessed the extent to which the Bath Infirmary facilitated clinical autonomy. Within the institution, the exercise of professional discretion was qualified in two main ways: first, the superior position of the physician, prolonged by spa therapy, constrained the honorary surgeons; and, secondly, freedom of action depended upon the condonation, if not the active approval, of institutional colleagues. An inability to obtain such tacit support enabled Archibald Cleland's enemies to hang his discharge upon a breach of the conventions governing bodily contact with female patients. Underlying this prosecution, however, was Cleland's attack on the spa facilities. The Hospital was harnessed to drive out other critics of the medical establishment, notably William Baylies who was forced to leave the city after questioning the content of the waters. The penumbra of the Bath Infirmary thus spread to the local medical community as a whole, the threat of exclusion limiting the autonomy of any physician or surgeon who wished to dispute the sulphur orthodoxy. Such unwillingness to engage in a critical debate, confirmed by the traditional character of research within the Hospital, sits uneasily with concepts of professional status which stress the accumulation of a systematic core of theory and practice. Furthermore, though voluntary service at the Bath General Infirmary was losing its socio-cultural rationale by the late eighteenth century, the rise of localized pathology marginalized balneology, undermined its clinical credibility and weakened claims to technical competence. But defining professionalization in terms of a static list of traits is less useful than seeing it as a dynamic process of 'occupational control ... [which] structures the relationship between experts, patrons and clients'.[207] The General Hospital may have limited the autonomy of its surgeons and expert outsiders who found fault with the spa. From its foundation, however, honorary staff were provided with a regulated environment in which 'clients' were subjected to medical directives. By the later Georgian period, lay governors or 'patrons' too were conceding power as, despite withdrawing from routine administration, doctors dictated the pace of hygienic reform and tightened the clinical criteria for admission. Like other voluntary hospitals, therefore, the Bath Infirmary did further the prestige of its doctors and hence the development of their profession.

Notes

1. Lane, 'Medical practitioners', p. 368.
2. See Chapter 4, footnote 111.
3. Kirby, 'Mineral Water Hospital', p. 37; Royal Mineral Water Hospital, 'Notes on the Pictures'; Minute Book, 20 October 1816.
4. Baylies, *Historical Account*, pp. 121–2.
5. *An Appeal to the Public ... Relating to the Proceedings of a Party of the Governors of the New General Hospital at Bath Against Mr Archibald Cleland* (London and Bath: A. Dodd and W. Frederick, 1743), p. 1; Thomas, 'Phillotts of Bath', p. 2.
6. See, for example, Cherry, 'Voluntary General Hospitals', p. 141; Frizelle and Martin, *Leicester Royal Infirmary*, pp. 51, 54; Holmes, *Augustan England*, p. 217; Jacob, *General Hospital*, p. 105; Lane, 'Medical practitioners', pp. 367–8; Loudon, *Medical Care*, p. 34; Rook, Carlton and Cannon, *Addenbrooke's Hospital*, p. 67; Turner, *Hampshire County Hospital*, pp. 48–9.
7. *DNB*, vol. 14, p. 168; vol. 43, p. 372.
8. *DNB*, vol. 25, p. 67; vol. 24, p. 384; vol. 34, p. 360; vol. 18, p. 165; Loudon, *Medical Care*, p. 311.
9. Mainwaring, *Annals*, p. 162.
10. Francis M. Lobo, 'John Haygarth, Smallpox and Religious Dissent in Eighteenth-Century England', in Andrew Cunningham and Roger French (eds), *The Medical Enlightenment of the Eighteenth Century* (Cambridge: Cambridge University Press, 1990), p. 223.
11. Minute Book, 20 October 1816; Loudon, *Medical Care*, p. 310.
12. Kirby, 'Mineral Water Hospital', p. 91.
13. *DNB*, vol. 34, pp. 231–4.
14. Barnard, 'William Baylies', pp. 37–8.
15. Neve, 'Natural Philosophy', p. 88.
16. Lucas, *Essay*, pp. 346–7; Boyce, *Benevolent Man*, p. 234.
17. Neve, 'Natural Philosophy', p. 86.
18. Lucas, *Essay*, p. 244.
19. *Letters of Doctor Lucas and Doctor Oliver Occasioned by a Physical Confederacy Discovered in Bath* (Bath: James Leake, 1757), pp. iii, 2, 10, 18.
20. *DNB*, vol. 34, p. 234.
21. Barnard, 'William Baylies', p. 41.
22. *Letters of Doctor Lucas and Doctor Oliver*, p. 21.
23. Barnard, 'William Baylies', pp. 38, 40; *DNB*, vol. 3, p. 447; David Harley, 'Honour and Property: The Structure of Professional Disputes in Eighteenth-Century English Medicine', in A. Cunningham and R. French

(eds), *The Medical Enlightenment of the Eighteenth Century* (Cambridge: Cambridge University Press, 1990), pp. 150–51.

24. Minute Book, 15 May 1744; 15 August 1744; 1 May 1750.
25. Baylies, *Historical Account*, pp. 49, 62–71, 85–6, 88–9; William Baylies, *A Narrative of Facts Demonstrating the Actual Existence and True Cause of that Physical Confederacy in Bath made Known to the Public in the Printed Letters of Dr Lucas and Dr Oliver* (London: A. Millar, 1757), pp. 34–5; Baylies, *Reflections*, pp. 124–30.
26. Baylies, *Historical Account*, p. 82.
27. 12 Geo. II, p. 584.
28. Baylies, *Historical Account*, pp. 65, 69–70. See also Minute Book, 15 August 1744; 2 November 1848.
29. Baylies, *Historical Account*, pp. 65, 69–70, 82, 90, 99–106, 111, 114, 117–18, 120. Baylies, *Reflections*, p. 124. Minute Book, 18 May 1757; 2 June 1757.
30. Minute Book, 7 September 1743; 21 September 1743; 19 October 1743.
31. Smollett, *Essay*, pp. 71–2, 74–7, 79–81.
32. Manuscript letter, quoted in Neve, 'Natural Philosophy', p. 82.
33. *Appeal*, pp. 1–3; Minute Book, 3 June 1742.
34. *A Short Vindication of the Proceedings of the Governors of the General Hospital at Bath in Relation to Mr Archbald Cleland* (Bath and London: J. Leake and A. Dodd, 1744), p. 4.
35. *Short Vindication*, p. 4; Boyce, *Benevolent Man*, p. 151; *Appeal*, pp. 2–3. See also Letter Book, F. Fauquier to Earl of Chesterfield, 29 October 1743.
36. *Appeal*, p. 4.
37. *Appeal*, pp. 4–8; *Short Vindication*, p. 16; Archibald Cleland, *A Full Vindication of Mr Cleland's Appeal to the Public* (Bath and London: W. Frederick and A. Dodd, 1744), pp. 30–32.
38. See, for example, Gibson, *Radcliffe Infirmary*, p. 250.
39. See, for example, Humble and Hansell, *Westminster Hospital*, p. 18; Smith, *Bristol Royal Infirmary*, p. 76; Philip K. Wilson, '"Sacred sanctuaries for the sick:" surgery at St Thomas's Hospital, 1725–26', *London Journal*, 17 (1992), p. 48.
40. Nicolson, 'Metastatic Theory', pp. 285–6.
41. See, for example, Anning, *General Infirmary at Leeds*, pp. 32–3; Brockbank, *Royal Infirmary, Manchester*, p. 208; Eade, *Norfolk and Norwich Hospital*, pp. 218–19; Frizelle and Martin, *Leicester Royal Infirmary*, p. 52; Jacob, *General Hospital*, pp. 338–9; McLoughlin, *Liverpool Infirmary*, pp. 75–6.
42. See, for example, Clark-Kennedy, *The London*, pp. 85–7; Hume, *Newcastle Infirmary*, p. 23; McMenemey, *Worcester Royal Infirmary*, pp. 123–4, 162–72; Smith, *Bristol Royal Infirmary*, pp. 109–10, 117; Waddy, *Northampton General Hospital*, p. 18.
43. Wood, *Bath*, pp. 296–7.
44. *Short Vindication*, p. 6.
45. Mary E. Fissell, 'Innocent and Honourable Bribes: Medical Manners in Eighteenth-Century Britain', in Robert Baker, Dorothy Porter and Roy Porter (eds), *The Codification of Medical Morality: Historical and Philosophical Studies of the Formalization of Western Medical Morality in the Eighteenth and Nineteenth Centuries*, 2 vols (Dordrecht, Nether-

lands: Kluwer Academic, 1993), vol. 1: *Medical Ethics and Etiquette in the Eighteenth Century*, pp. 27–8.
46. *A Letter to Mr Archibald Cleland Occasioned by his Full Vindication of his Appeal to the Public against the Proceedings of the Bath Hospital* (London: J. Roberts, 1744), p. 2. See also Minute Book, 19 October 1743.
47. *Short Vindication*, pp. 28–9.
48. *Appeal*, p. 37.
49. Cleland, *Full Vindication*, p. 25; *Short Vindication*, pp. 27–8.
50. Cleland, *Full Vindication*, p. 26.
51. *Short Vindication*, p. 29.
52. Cleland, *Full Vindication*, p. 28–9.
53. Adrian Wilson, *The Making of Man-Midwifery: Childbirth in England 1660–1770* (Cambridge, MA: Harvard University Press, 1995), pp. 1–6, 185–92. See also Adrian Wilson, 'William Hunter and the Varieties of Man-Midwifery', in W.F. Bynum and Roy Porter (eds), *William Hunter and the Eighteenth-Century Medical World* (Cambridge: Cambridge University Press, 1985), pp. 343, 346; David Harley, 'Provincial Midwives in England: Lancashire and Cheshire, 1660–1760', in Hilary Marland (ed.), *The Art of Midwifery: Early Modern Midwives in Europe* (London: Routledge, 1993), pp. 39–40, 42–4; Ornella Moscucci, *The Science of Women: Gynaecology and Gender in England 1800–1929* (Cambridge: Cambridge University Press, 1990), pp. 10–12, 46–7.
54. Moscucci *Science of Woman*, pp. 50–51. See also Harley, 'Provincial Midwives', pp. 28–9.
55. *Appeal*, pp. 21, 23.
56. W.F. Bynum, 'Health, Disease and Medical Care', in G.S. Rousseau and Roy Porter (eds), *The Ferment of Knowledge: Studies in the Historiography of Eighteenth-Century Science* (Cambridge: Cambridge University Press, 1980), pp. 218–20; Hankins, *Science*, pp. 119–20, 123–4; Bryan S. Turner, *Medical Power and Social Knowledge* (London: Sage, 1987), pp. 31–3.
57. Hankins, *Science*, p. 130; Angus McLaren, 'The Pleasures of Procreation: Traditional and Biomedical Theories of Conception', in W.F. Bynum and R. Porter (eds), *William Hunter and the Eighteenth-Century Medical World* (Cambridge: Cambridge University Press, 1985), p. 327; Roy Porter, 'Bodies of Thought: Thoughts about the Body in Eighteenth-Century England', in Joan H. Pittock and Andrew Wear (eds), *Interpretation and Cultural History* (London: Macmillan, 1991), pp. 96–7.
58. Roy Porter, 'History of the Body', in Peter Burke (ed.), *New Perspectives on Historical Writing* (Cambridge: Polity Press, 1991), pp. 206, 212–13.
59. The full title of this text was *De Sedibus et Causis Morborum per Anatomen Indagatis*, which in translation means *The Seats and Causes of Diseases as Revealed by Anatomy*.
60. Malcolm Nicolson, 'Giovanni Battista Morgagni and Eighteenth-Century Physical examination', in C. Lawrence (ed.), *Medical Theory, Surgical Practice: Studies in the History of Surgery* (London: Routledge, 1992), pp. 101–27.
61. David Harley, 'Political Post-Mortems and Morbid Anatomy in Seventeenth-Century England', *Social History of Medicine*, 7 (1994), pp. 21–3.

62. Roy Porter, 'The Rise of Physical Examination', in W.F. Bynum and R. Porter (eds), *Medicine and the Five Senses* (Cambridge: Cambridge University Press, 1993), pp. 182–5; Risse, *Hospital Life*, p. 281; Christopher Lawrence, 'Ornate Physicians and Learned Artisans: Edinburgh Medical Men, 1726–1776', in W.F. Bynum and R. Porter (eds), *William Hunter and the Eighteenth-Century Medical World* (Cambridge: Cambridge University Press, 1985), p. 153.
63. *DNB*, vol. 27, p. 28–9; Minute Book, 28 July 1762.
64. Peter Burke, 'Overture: The New History, its Past and its Future', in P. Burke (ed.), *New Perspectives on Historical Writing* (Cambridge: Polity Press, 1991), pp. 13–14; Ludmilla Jordanova, 'The Representation of the Family in the Eighteenth Century: A Challenge for Cultural History', in J.H. Pittock and A. Wear (eds), *Interpretation and Cultural History* (London: Macmillan, 1991), pp. 114–16; Wagner, 'Satire', pp. 200–201.
65. Fissell, 'Physic of Charity', p. 158; Pickstone, *Medicine and Industrial Society*, p. 12.
66. Glaser, *Caleb Hillier Parry*, p. 35; Joan Lane, 'Eighteenth-Century Medical Practice: A Case Study of Bradford Wilmer, Surgeon of Coventry, 1737–1813', *Social History of Medicine*, 3 (1990), pp. 375, 376, 379–80; Robert Martensen, 'The Transformation of Eve: Women's Bodies, Medicine and Culture in Early Modern England', in Roy Porter and Mikulas Teich (eds), *Sexual Knowledge, Sexual Science: The History of Attitudes to Sexuality* (Cambridge: Cambridge University Press, 1994), pp. 118–19.
67. Bynum, 'Health', p. 236; Langford, *Polite and Commercial People*, pp. 138–9; Ruth Richardson, *Death, Dissection and the Destitute* (Harmondsworth: Penguin, 1988), pp. 47–8.
68. Bath United Hospital Minute Book, 20 December 1830; Clark-Kennedy, *The London*, pp. 107–9; Fissell, 'Physic of Charity', pp. 159–62, 267–8; Pickstone, *Medicine and Industrial Society*, p. 48.
69. Minute Book, 19 October 1743; *Short Vindication*, pp. 3–8, 11–12.
70. *Appeal*, pp. 18–23.
71. N.A.M. Rodger, *The Wooden World: An Anatomy of the Georgian Navy* (London: Fontana, 1986), pp. 98–112.
72. Roger Rolls, 'Archibald Cleland: c. 1700–71', *British Medical Journal*, 288 (14 April 1984), p. 1134; Smollett, *Essay*, p. 71.
73. *Appeal*, p. 23; Minute Book, 19 October 1743.
74. Cleland, *Full Vindication*, pp. 37–8.
75. *Appeal*, pp. 17–18, 24–5.
76. *Short Vindication*, pp. 17–18.
77. Cleland, *Full Vindication*, pp. 41–2.
78. For a subtle statement and evaluation of this position, Roy Porter, 'Mixed Feelings: The Enlightenment and Sexuality in Eighteenth-Century Britain', in Paul-Gabriel Boucé (ed.), *Sexuality in Eighteenth-Century Britain* (Manchester: Manchester University Press, 1982), pp. 1–21.
79. McLaren, 'Pleasures of Procreation', p. 324, 339.
80. McLaren, 'Pleasures of Procreation', pp. 324–40. See also Patricia Crawford, 'Sexual Knowledge in England, 1500–1750', in R. Porter and M. Teich (eds), *Sexual Knowledge, Sexual Science: The History of Attitudes to Sexuality* (Cambridge: Cambridge University Press, 1994), pp. 84, 86–7.

81. Roy Porter and Lesley Hall, *The Facts of Life: The Creation of Sexual Knowledge in Britain 1650–1950* (New Haven and London: Yale University Press, 1995), pp. 68–9, 82.
82. Talcott Parsons, *The Social System* (London: Routledge and Kegan Paul, 1951), p. 451. See also Ludmilla Jordanova, *Sexual Visions: Images of Gender in Science and Medicine between the Eighteenth and Twentieth Centuries* (London: Harvester Wheatsheaf, 1989), p. 138; Waddington, 'Role of the Hospital', p. 214.
83. Porter and Porter, *Patient's Progress*, pp. 182–3; Loudon, *Medical Care*, pp. 90–91.
84. Wilson, 'William Hunter', p. 362.
85. Risse, *Hospital Life*, pp. 65, 216.
86. Ludmilla Jordanova, 'Natural Facts: A Historical Perspective on Science and Sexuality', in Carol P. MacCormack and Marilyn Strathern (eds), *Nature, Culture and Gender* (Cambridge: Cambridge University Press, 1980), p. 43.
87. Carol P. MacCormack, 'Nature, Culture and Gender: A Critique', in C.P. MacCormack and M. Strathern (eds), *Nature, Culture and Gender* (Cambridge: Cambridge University Press, 1980), p. 6.
88. Crawford, 'Sexual Knowledge', p. 95; Vivien Jones (ed.), *Women in the Eighteenth Century: Constructions of Femininity* (London: Routledge, 1990), p. 58.
89. 'Philogamus', from *The Present State of Matrimony ...* , 1739, in V. Jones (ed.), *Women in the Eighteenth Century: Constructions of Femininity* (London: Routledge, 1990), p. 77. See also Anne Laurence, *Women in England: A Social History 1500–1760* (London: Weidenfeld and Nicolson, 1994), p. 67; Turner, *Medical Power*, p. 85.
90. A.D. Harvey, *Sex in Georgian England: Attitudes and Prejudices from the 1720s to the 1820s* (London: Duckworth, 1994), chs 2 and 3.
91. 'Colonel Harry Mordaunt' [Bernard Mandeville], from *A Modest Defence of Public Stews ...* , 1724; 1740 edn, in V. Jones (ed.), *Women in the Eighteenth Century: Constructions of Femininity* (London: Routledge, 1990), p. 65.
92. 'A Physician' from *The Pleasures of Conjugal Love Explained ...* , [1740], in V. Jones (ed.), *Women in the Eighteenth Century: Constructions of Femininity* (London: Routledge, 1990), p. 82.
93. [Daniel Defoe], from *Some Considerations Upon Street-Walkers ...* , [1726], in V. Jones (ed.), *Women in the Eighteenth Century: Constructions of Femininity* (London: Routledge, 1990), p.69. See also Martensen, 'Transformation', p. 109.
94. 'A Physician' p. 82.
95. Bridget Hill, *Women, Work and Sexual Politics in Eighteenth-Century England* (Oxford: Basil Blackwell, 1989), ch. 3; Mary Prior, 'Women and the Urban Economy: Oxford, 1500–1800', in Mary Prior (ed.), *Women in English Society 1500–1800* (London: Routledge, 1985).
96. *Appeal*, p. 21.
97. Anning, *General Infirmary at Leeds*, p. 81; Brockbank, *Royal Infirmary, Manchester*, p. 207; Eade, *Norfolk and Norwich Hospital*, pp. 217–18; McLoughlin, *Liverpool Infirmary*, pp. 73–4.
98. *Appeal*, p. 20; Minute Book, 19 October 1743.
99. Owen, *English Philanthropy*, pp. 50–51; Rhodes, *Dr John Leake's Hos-*

pital, p. 20; Lindsay Granshaw, 'The Rise of the Modern Hospital in Britain', in Andrew Wear (ed.), *Medicine in Society: Historical Essays* (Cambridge: Cambridge University Press, 1992), p. 205.

100. Roy Porter, *Mind-Forg'd Manacles: A History of Madness in England from the Restoration to the Regency* (Harmondsworth: Penguin, 1987), pp. 48–9. See also Audrey Eccles, *Obstetrics and Gynaecology in Tudor and Stuart England* (London: Croom Helm, 1982), pp. 78–9; Turner, *Medical Power*, p. 89.
101. R. James MD, from *A Medicinal Dictionary*, 1743, in V. Jones (ed.), *Women in the Eighteenth Century: Constructions of Femininity* (London: Routledge, 1990), p. 86. See also Crawford, 'Sexual Knowledge', p. 91.
102. Turner, *Medical Power*, p. 88.
103. 'Britannicus', *Remarks on an Appeal to the Public by Mr Cleland* (London: J. Woon, W. Owen, E. Amey and W. Frederick, 1748), pp. 14–15.
104. *Appeal*, pp. 7, 11, 14.
105. Cleland, *Full Vindication*, pp. 37–8.
106. Jordanova, 'Natural Facts', pp. 54, 57.
107. *Appeal*, pp. 27–8, 33–4.
108. *Appeal*, pp. 38–9; 'Short Narrative', p. 18; Cleland, *Full Vindication*, pp. 48, 50.
109. *Appeal*, pp. 11–13.
110. *Short Vindication*, p. 10.
111. Cleland, *Full Vindication*, p. 51.
112. Cleland, *Full Vindication*, pp. 51–4.
113. 'Short Narrative', p. 18; Cleland, *Full Vindication*, pp. 13–14.
114. Harley, 'Honour and Property', p. 140.
115. *Appeal*, pp. 39–40; Cleland, *Full Vindication*, pp. 45–6; *Remarks*, p. 48.
116. 'Short Narrative', p. 18; Bath Corporation Minute Book, 6 September 1743.
117. 12 Geo. II, p. 573; 'Short Narrative', p. 18.
118. *Appeal*, p. 39.
119. Despite this failure to vote, the attendance list does include Mr Peirce. See Minute Book, 21 September 1743.
120. See Fissell, 'Innocent and Honorable Bribes', pp. 19–20.
121. Chauncey D. Leake, *Percival's Medical Ethics*, first pub. 1803 (New York: Robert E. Krieger, 1975).
122. Fissell, 'Physic of Charity', p. 289; Harley, 'Honour and Property', pp. 156–7; Risse, *Hospital Life,* p. 186; Ivan Waddington, 'The Development of Medical Ethics: A Sociological Analysis', *Medical History*, 19 (1975), pp. 37, 39.
123. Cleland, *Full Vindication*, p. 56.
124. Letter Book, 19 October 1743, E. Brett to M. Steward.
125. Peter Borsay, 'Image and Counter Image in Georgian Bath', *British Journal for Eighteenth-Century Studies*, 17 (1994), pp. 172–3.
126. Letter Book, 1 November 1743, Earl of Chesterfield to F. Fauquier.
127. Clark-Kennedy, *The London*, p. 224; Turner, *Hampshire County Hospital*, p. 41; Davies, *Deeds Not Words*, pp. 31–2; Lloyd, *United Hospital, Bath*, p. 11.
128. Minute Book, 20 March 1754; 1 May 1754; 28 January 1795; 24 May 1797; 25 June 1828.

129. Minute Book, 31 July 1745; 15 November 1749; 15 December 1819.
130. Baylies, *Historical Account*, p. 124.
131. Minute Book, 2 May 1743; 30 January 1745. The attendance of medical staff also posed problems at other institutions. See Cherry 'Voluntary General Hospitals', p. 147; Perry, *Medical Institutions*, p. 3; Rhodes, *Dr John Leake's Hospital*, p. 83; Rook, Carlton and Cannon, *Addenbrooke's Hospital*, p. 83; Waddy, *Northampton General Hospital*, p. 11.
132. Minute Book, 16 February 1738, 'Plan and Elevation'; 12 Geo. II, pp. 575–6; Minute Book, 1 May 1746; 6 February 1760.
133. Casebook, admitted 27 January 1752; 21 October 1752; 27 April 1754.
134. Casebook, admitted 15 May 1754; 2 March 1758.
135. Casebook, admitted 25 March 1758. See also Casebook, admitted 27 January 1752; 21 October 1752; 27 April 1754; 6 July 1754; 15 August 1754.
136. Minute Book, 4 March 1742; 11 March 1742; 15 June 1743.
137. In 1747, for example, notices were published on 8 June, 15 June and 22 June; in 1757 on 14 February, 2 May, 1 August and 7 November; and in 1786 on 30 January, 27 February, 10 April, 1 May, 29 May, 24 July, 28 August, 25 September, 27 November and 18 December.
138. See, for example, *Bath and Bristol Guide*, pp. 18–19; *Improved Bath Guide*, pp. 48–9; *The Original Bath Guide* (Bath: Meyler and Sons, 1840), pp. 101–2; Wood, *Bath*, pp. 300–301.
139. Casebook, admitted 5 October 1756.
140. Casebook, admitted 13 April 1756.
141. [Bath General Infirmary], 'Short Account', in Bayly, *Sermon,* p. 25. See also [Bath General Infirmary], 'Short Account', in Dalton, *Religious Uses*, p. 22.
142. *Bath Journal*, 3 June 1745; 18 May 1747.
143. Casebook, 27 December 1755; 26 February 1755.
144. 12 Geo. II, p. 575; Minute Book, 7 December 1738.
145. House Visitors Book 1, 4 September 1742; Minute Book, 24 March 1743.
146. Minute Book, 26 October 1743; 11 February 1747; 13 April 1768.
147. *Annual Report*, 1785/86; 1825/26.
148. *Annual Report*, 1830/31.
149. Smith Gibbes, *Second Treatise*, p. 14.
150. See, for example, Clark-Kennedy, *The London*, pp. 109, 170, 222–3; Fissell, *Patients*, pp. 136–7.
151. Fissell, *Patients*, p. 147.
152. Porter and Porter, *In Sickness*, pp. 30–31; Ginnie Smith, 'Prescribing the Rules of Health: Self-Help and Advice in the Late Eighteenth Century', in R. Porter (ed.), *Patients and Practitioners: Lay Perceptions of Medicine in Pre-Industrial Society* (Cambridge: Cambridge University Press, 1985), pp. 256–62; Wear, 'Making Sense', pp. 131–2.
153. Riley, *Eighteenth-Century Campaign*, pp. Introduction, ch. 1, pp. 89–90, 145. See also John Pickstone, 'Dearth, Dirt and Fever Epidemics: Rewriting the History of British "Public Health", 1780–1850', in Terence Ranger and Paul Slack (eds), *Epidemics and Ideas: Essays on the Historical Perception of Pestilence* (Cambridge: Cambridge University Press, 1992), pp. 128–9.
154. Christopher Lawrence, 'Priestley in Tahiti: The Medical Interests of a

Dissenting Chemist', in R.G.W. Anderson and Christopher Lawrence (eds), *Science, Medicine and Dissent: Joseph Priestley (1733–1804)* (London: Wellcome Trust/Science Museum, 1987), pp. 5–6.

155. John Howard, *An Account of the Principal Lazarettos in Europe* (Warrington, 1789), especially pp. 136, 141–2.
156. Aikin, *Thoughts*, especially pp. 8–10, 14–16, 18–19; William Blizard, *Suggestions for the Improvement of Hospitals and Other Charitable Institutions* (London: C. Dilly, 1796), especially pp. 34–9, 41–2, 46; Thomas Percival, 'A Letter from Thomas Percival MD FRS', in J. Aikin, *Thoughts on Hospitals with a Letter to the Author by Thomas Percival* (London: Joseph Johnson, 1771), especially pp. 88–91.
157. Wood, *Bath*, p. 292. See also Anning, *General Infirmary at Leeds*, p. 7; Brockbank, *Royal Infirmary, Manchester*, pp. 18–19; Leader, *Sheffield General Infirmary*, p. 10; McLoughlin, *Liverpool Infirmary*, pp. 19–21.
158. See, for example, Anning, *General Infirmary at Leeds*, p. 81; Brockbank, *Royal Infirmary, Manchester*, p. 207; Davies, *Deeds Not Words*, p. 38; Eade, *Norfolk and Norwich Hospital*, p. 218; McLoughlin, *Liverpool Infirmary*, p. 74.
159. Wood, *Bath*, p. 297.
160. Minute Book, 20 July 1747.
161. Minute Book, 6 May 1752; 20 May 1752; 17 June 1752; 8 November 1752; 22 November 1752.
162. Minute Book, 29 November 1752; 30 July 1755. The ordering of a prayer book for the 'foul' ward in August 1752 suggests that infectious patients may have occupied more than one ward. See Minute Book, 26 August 1752.
163. Minute Book, 26 January 1757.
164. *Address*, p. 17.
165. Minute Book, 17 August 1743. With John Pringle, Dr Hales was responsible for the ventilators used at Newgate following the infection of the Old Bailey by prisoners on trial in 1750. See Michael Ignatieff, *A Just Measure of Pain: The Penitentiary in the Industrial Revolution* (Harmondsworth: Penguin Books, 1978), pp. 44–5.
166. Minute Book, 19 April 1780; *Annual Report*, 1780/81.
167. House Visitors Book 2, 24 May 1756; Minute Book, 28 January 1778.
168. Minute Book, 25 July 1750; 28 August 1751; 4 July 1753; 21 August 1754.
169. Minute Book, 1 May 1751; 8 May 1754.
170. Minute Book, 7 February 1753. See also House Visitors Book 1, 1 February 1743; Minute Book, 9 November 1763; 13 January 1796; 20 September 1826.
171. Minute Book, 3 February 1796.
172. *Address*, p. 17.
173. Minute Book, 25 August 1738.
174. Wood, *Bath*, pp. 284–5. For a discussion of the 'courtyard' and 'block' plans adopted for British voluntary hospitals, see John D. Thompson and Grace Goldin, *The Hospital: A Social and Architectural History* (New Haven: Yale University Press, 1975), pp. 83–96.
175. Howard, *Account*, p. 190. The Casualty Hospital did not open until 1 January 1788 and the Pauper Charity was not extended to become the Bath City Infirmary and Dispensary until 1792. Therefore, given the

reference to a visit in 1787, Howard's entry for the 'Bath Infirmary' in all probability refers to the General Hospital.

176. Minute Book, 2 May 1791; 4 May 1791; 18 May 1791; 27 July 1791.
177. Minute Book, 25 January 1792; 1 February 1792; 21 March 1792. Subcommittee Book, 26 January 1792.
178. *Address*, p. 5. The medical report was also entered in the Minute Book on 18 May 1791.
179. Minute Book, 25 January 1792; *Address*, p. 33.
180. *Address*, pp. 6–7, 28.
181. *Address*, pp. 17–21, 29.
182. *Address*, pp. 23–5.
183. Minute Book, 1 May 1792; 2 January 1793; 6 March 1793. See also Subcommittee Book, 15 June 1792; 6 July 1792; 27 July 1792; 27 July 1792; 1 November 1792; 22 November 1792; 10 January 1793.
184. Neale, *Bath*, p. 256.
185. Lawrence, 'Priestley in Tahiti', pp. 5–6; Pickstone, 'Dearth', p. 130; *DNB*, vol. 18, p. 164; Lobo, 'John Haygarth', pp. 220, 222–3, 229.
186. Lawrence, 'Ornate Physicians', p. 171. See also Schaffer, 'Natural Philosophy', pp. 22–8.
187. Lawrence, 'Priestley in Tahiti', pp. 1, 3; Ignatieff, *Just Measure*, pp. 60–68. See also Robert Kilpatrick, '"Living in the light": Dispensaries, Philanthropy and Medical Reform in Late-Eighteenth-Century London', in A. Cunningham and R. French (eds), *Medical Enlightenment in the Eighteenth Century* (Cambridge: Cambridge University Press, 1990), pp. 254–80.
188. Steve Poole, 'Radicalism, Loyalism and the "Reign of Terror" in Bath, 1792–1804', *Bath History*, 3 (1990), pp. 114–15.
189. Lewis Namier and John Brooke, *The House of Commons*, 3 vols (London: HMSO, 1964), vol. 2: *Members A–J*, pp. 325–6.
190. Pickstone, *Medicine and Industrial Society*, pp. 18–20. See also J.V. Pickstone and S.V.F. Butler, 'The Politics of Medicine in Manchester, 1788–1792: Hospital Reform and Public Health Services in the Early Industrial City', *Medical History*, 28 (1984).
191. Pickstone, 'Dearth', pp. 138–42.
192. Subcommittee Book, 13 May 1806; Minute Book, 14 May 1806.
193. Minute Book, 1 May 1818; 28 October 1818. Subcommittee Book, 2 June 1818; 4 July 1818.
194. Minute Book, 29 October 1828; 1 May 1829.
195. Minute Book, 27 May 1829.
196. 'Men are grown mechanical in head and in heart, as well as in hand' bemoaned Thomas Carlyle, also in 1829. See 'The Signs of the Times', in *Thomas Carlyle: Selected Writings*, ed. by Alan Shelston, repr. (Harmondsworth: Penguin Books, 1986), p. 67.
197. *Bath Journal*, 10 August 1829.
198. Minute Book, 1 May 1830.
199. Phyllis Hembry, *British Spas from 1815 to the Present: A Social History*, eds Leonard W. Cowie and Evelyn E. Cowie (London: Athlone, 1997), p. 58.
200. Minute Book, 18 February 1829; 25 February 1829; 18 March 1829; 15 April 1829; 29 April 1829; 1 May 1829.
201. *Address*, p. 20. The baths came into use in January 1831 after permis-

sion had been obtained from Bath Corporation to draw water from their springs, and an Act of Parliament passed to allow the introduction of mineral water into the Hospital and the sinking of pipes to convey it from the King's Bath. See Falconer, *Mineral Water Hospital*, pp. 56–7; 11 Geo. IV.

202. Loudon, *Medical Care*, pp. 147–51. When the Bath branch merged with Bristol in 1842, Barlow became its first secretary with William Tudor, probably the former Hospital surgeon, as president. I am grateful to Emily Naish, Archivist of the British Medical Association, for providing this information.

203. Riley, *Eighteenth-Century Campaign*, pp. xv, 139.

204. Minute Book, 7 July 1830.

205. Bath Chronicle, *The Bath General or Hot Water Hospital* (Bath: H.E. Carrington, 1857), p. 3. See also G.D. Kersley and John Cosh, 'The Royal National Hospital for Rheumatic Diseases, Bath', *The Practitioner*, **195** (1965), p. 816.

206. This was the Herbert Military Hospital in Woolwich. See Jeremy Taylor, *Hospital and Asylum Architecture in England 1840–1914: Building for Care* (London: Mansell, 1991), pp. 56–7, 82; Thompson and Goldin, *Hospital,* pp. 142–3, 146, 155–69; Harriet Richardson, *English Hospitals 1660–1948: A Survey of their Architecture and Design* (Swindon: Royal Commission on the Historical Monuments of England, 1998), pp. 5–7, 27–31, 90–94.

207. Turner, *Medical Power*, pp. 133–5. See also Paul Wilding, *Professional Power and Social Welfare* (London: Routledge and Kegan Paul, 1982), pp. 2–7.

PART FOUR

The Moral Economy

CHAPTER SIX

The Obligations of Paternalism

In Parts Two and Three of this book, we looked at the management and finance of the Bath Infirmary and at its contribution to the development of the medical profession during the long eighteenth century. Although only a minority of governors actively engaged in hospital administration, the structures and procedures which they put into practice enabled the institution both to personify civic virtue and to achieve financial solvency, despite the volatility of the Georgian economy and a dependence upon casual benefactions rather than a more stable diet of annual subscriptions and investment income. For the physicians and surgeons who served the Infirmary in a voluntary capacity, there were opportunities to police the activities of commercial rivals and to wield clinical power over patients and increasingly lay governors as well. These advances by a key Georgian profession benefited the prestige of professional groups in general, and since they 'shared many social and political assumptions with their commercial and manufacturing peers', the position of the middling orders as a whole was strengthened.[1] Among the areas of common concern was charity. The honorary medical staff wanted specifically occupational spin-offs for their benevolence, but they also joined with non-medical patrons in seeking economic and moral, social and political returns. Parts Four and Five address these issues. In Part Five, medical philanthropy is explored with reference to social status, the integration of the political élite, and the education of the lower orders. But first we turn to the moral economy of Georgian medicine as it was worked through at the Bath Infirmary. Chapter 6 asks for how long paternalist obligations survived the impact of commerce and prosperity, focusing on the underlying partnership between medicine and providence, changing attitudes towards luxury, and the resulting movement away from a tributary towards a proprietary relationship between rich and poor. Chapter 7 will then examine the shift from mercantilism to *laissez-faire* in economic thought, and assess the consequences of the eclipse of paternalism for the operation of medical philanthropy.

Property, charity and moral discourse

At the moral centre of charity in early modern England was the concept of paternalism, which construed society as a hierarchical but organic whole held together by reciprocal responsibilities. Of medieval origin, paternalism was rooted in the relations between lord and vassal, and reinforced by the church and royal government. The decline of the feudal system prompted a redefinition in terms of Renaissance civic humanism; backed up by a strong central state, the independent property owner, whose dedication to the public good also protected against corruption, was expected to be benevolent towards his social inferiors who now worked for a wage.[2] For R.H. Tawney, this market orientation, aggravated by the rapid post-Restoration growth in trade and industry, opened up a 'chasm' in English society which, aided and abetted by Puritan religion, destroyed the moral authority of the established Church over economic relations; material rewards, argued Tawney, were bracketed with divine providence and poverty regarded as the just desert for idleness, improvidence and vice.[3] His analysis was fundamentally flawed. Though humanism, and a decline in traditional hospitality, had brought greater discrimination to almsgiving, the Protestant belief in justification by faith alone did not invalidate the charity which under Catholicism had been a route to salvation. Quite the opposite, acts of philanthropy, appropriately exercised via institutional mechanisms, were both an outward and visible sign that the Protestant had been saved by grace and a defence against the Catholic charge that reformed theology exonerated men from behaving with social responsibility. Puritanism shared this commitment to community obligation. Therefore, paternalism was not snuffed out because, as Puritans themselves recognized, blaming the undeserving poor for their poverty was wholly consistent with a commitment to selective good works.[4]

Of more significance than capitalism or religion was the political environment which paternalism encountered in the aftermath of the English Revolution. With the constitutional settlement of 1688 came a firm rejection of absolutist administration, parliamentary sovereignty going hand in hand with local autonomy. Simultaneously, the granting of toleration to Dissenters both encouraged the theological latitude for which early eighteenth-century Anglicanism was renowned and potentially undermined the authority of the Established Church, previously weakened by the Civil War and the Interregnum. Compounding these politico-ecclesiastical developments was the emergence of a new political philosophy. Inspired by Enlightenment science, mechanical models of the natural world provided an intellectual basis for mechanical models of the state, in which traditional reciprocal obligations were supplanted by a social contract between governors and governed. The individualism of political theorists like Hobbes and Locke provoked a backlash from Tory traditionalists like Bolingbroke who, fearing the collapse of the old deferential order, reasserted the values of paternalism and equated the body politic with the patriarchal family, hierarchical but united by a common interest. Bolingbroke concentrated on the obligations of property rather than the needs of the poor. However, the Anglican Church, increasingly under the influence of latitudinarianism, preserved the charitable imperative as a feature of its reasonable and rational doctrine which, in John Gascoigne's words, sought 'theological breadth rather than depth and an emphasis on the few essentials which could unite English protestants rather than the inessentials which divided them'.[5] Therefore, if no longer a social ideal reinforced by an all-powerful church and state, paternalism remained a familiar part of the intellectual furniture of Hanoverian England.

The theological rationale for paternalism was debated through two moral discourses which jostled for position during the long eighteenth century. Following Donna Andrew's characterization, the first discourse was based on a providential view of poverty in which charity was regarded as 'the rent annexed to the use of property' and almsgiving as 'merely the workings of justice'.[6] Under such a tributary relationship, the rich man was obliged to be generous in his support of the disadvantaged because he was 'no more than God's steward and the poor man's treasurer'. The poor man had corresponding responsibilities for, being free from the temptations of mammon and hence nearer to God, he was obliged to intercede on behalf of the rich with his prayers.[7] A classic statement of early eighteenth-century paternalism belongs to the Quaker, John Bellers: 'it's as much the duty of the poor to labour when they are able, as it is for the rich to help them when they are sick'.[8] But the tributary relationship was also endorsed by Established churchmen. In the words of Knightly Chetwood, speaking before the assembled governors of the London chartered hospitals in 1708, 'We are apt to take it for granted that our Estates ... are entirely at our own Disposal, legal debts being discharg'd; but this is a great Mistake, Charity is a principal Branch of Justice ... we are but Stewards, not Proprietors, even when Estates are gotten by the most justifiable Means'.[9]

Coexisting with this tributary discourse – where paternalist obligations were exercised through Christian stewardship – was an alternative moral relationship in which justice became 'detached from the duty to charity and attached to the promulgation of private property'.[10] The new ethic attempted to tailor civic humanism to the circumstances of affluence in the same way that the institutions of commercial society were reinforced against villainy. Political economy provided the means for this adaptation. The eighteenth century is commonly identified with a transition from mercantilism to *laissez-faire*, as the free-market principles of Adam Smith dislodged 'the belief that the economic welfare of the state ... [could] only be secured by government regulation of a nationalist character'.[11] In reality, the passing of mercantilism was more complex; for protectionism outlived the Georgian age in overseas if not domestic economic policy,[12] and *laissez-faire* ideas penetrated economic thought long before *The Wealth of Nations* was published in 1776.[13] Yet though practice and theory defy easy classification, mercantilism was their 'central tendency' from the late sixteenth- to the mid-eighteenth century[14] and, therefore, national prosperity was associated with a favourable balance of payments. For *laissez-faire* thinkers, the outcome was a 'zero-sum game' which falsely assumed that 'there was a fixed quantum of gain from trade, and that what one country gained another must lose'.[15] Coming to maturity in Adam Smith was a different conception of material progress which emphasized the scope for greater productivity through an ever more sophisticated division of labour. Stressing the economic benefits of increasing demand opened the door to a moral justification for the escalating consumption of non-essential goods which under mercantilism had been denigrated as a source of financial and social disaster.[16] Furthermore, the 'invisible hand' of the free market necessary to release this economic potential would convert the personal interest of individuals into the public good of society as a whole;[17] as the *Wealth of Nations* explained, 'It is not from the benevolence of the butcher, the brewer or the baker, that we expect our dinner, but from their regard to their own interest'.[18] Under this economic individualism, moral responsibility became 'a private question of choice'. However, Smith – full of the optimism of the Enlightenment – was confident that commercial society would not degenerate into a jungle of self-interest. Rather, he believed that the 'mutual dependence' of the market would create a 'bond of sympathy and imagination' which fear of social disapproval would translate into a compassionate code of ethics. Morality was private, but 'a matter of social interaction'.[19]

The challenge to paternalist obligation extended beyond political economy to culture and sociability. As Adam Smith himself recognized, 'The whole industry of human life is employed not in procuring the supply of our three humble necessities, food, cloaths, and lodging, but in procuring the conveniences of it according to the nicety and delicacy of our taste'.[20] Although Bernard Mandeville's satirical defence of luxury in *The Fable of the Bees* was greeted with antagonism when first published in 1714,[21] a cultural accommodation of civic humanism to prosperity had been in progress since the late seventeenth century. Not only was the simplicity and frugality of the classical aesthetic superseded by a set of 'polite manners', which were 'sociable, conversible, urbane, decorous' and hence less disinterested and severe, but 'the softer virtues of universal benevolence', before regarded as unselfish but private, were also incorporated into a broader definition of public spirit. Through the authorship of his *Characteristics*, the third Earl of Shaftesbury became a leading figure in this campaign, but the endeavour to moralize polite society was broadly based and transcended the political boundaries between commerce and land, court and country.[22] By the 1760s, these efforts were shaping into the 'sentimental revolution' which was to exert such a formative influence on art and literature, architecture and landscape later in the eighteenth century. Excessive indulgence in gambling and ostentatious display continued to elicit moral condemnation and so this 'birth of sensibility' was no licence to sin.[23] Celebrating the emotions of the individual, however, did shore up the view that morality was the preserve of personal conscience and not public prescription. Applied to charity, where the tributary relationship was polarized between rich and poor,[24] these individualist perspectives construed the act of giving as an optional badge of civility and not a paternalist obligation ordained by rank and property. This was the proprietary discourse. Charity remained 'the very expression of Christian devotion', argued Bishop Thomas Sherlock as early as mid-century. But 'Property is established ... by the positive law of God', who did not 'force us to part with our estates to the Poor, or give the Poor *any Right* to serve themselves out of the Abundance and Superfluity of others'. Rather, they were to be supported 'by the *free and voluntary* Gift of such as can spare from their own subsistence some Part of what they enjoy'.[25]

The proprietary relationship had special appeal for middling men because its economic and cultural individualism enabled them to carve a philanthropic identity that was refined but not dependent upon lineage and land ownership. By the late 1780s, 'the foundations of what was to become a middle-class social and political sensibility had been laid' and moral virtue 'no longer rested on ... acknowledged reciprocities between rich and poor'.[26] Since paternalism died no sudden death, however, we cannot assume a straightforward, linear movement from the tributary relationship based on civic virtue to a proprietary relationship based on social virtue. At Bath, the changing moral relations of poverty and plenty were explicitly articulated in the charity sermons preached on behalf of the General Infirmary to raise funds. Though services were organized biannually, the published texts of only seven clerics have been located. Just one sermon has been traced for the later Georgian period: a discourse on *The Ameliorated Condition of the Poor*, delivered by the Reverend Joseph Hunter at his local Presbyterian chapel in 1810. The remaining preachers in print were all Anglicans addressing congregations in Bath Abbey before 1760: William Warburton, Bishop of Gloucester from 1759 (October 1742); John

Dalton, Fellow of the Queen's College in Oxford (December 1745); Edward Bayly, Rector of Kilkeel in Ireland (April 1749); John Brown, MA (April 1750); Robert Leyborne, DD (April 1753);[27] and R. Olive, Vicar of Burnham (April 1759). In the remainder of this chapter, these sermons – along with complementary evidence from hospital records, diaries, legislation and local newspapers – are used to excavate the transition from a tributary to a proprietary relationship. First, the discursive twists and turns are charted with reference to the partnering of providence, the embarrassment of riches, and the rise of sensibility. Secondly, the ethics of medical charity in Bath are related to the development of the city, and this chronology is associated with the socio-economic profile of residents and visitors.

Partnering providence

The charity sermons for the early Georgian Bath Infirmary were dominated by paternalism. Thus, echoing Knightly Chetwood, William Warburton argued in the Anglican paternalist mould that: 'Charity should incline us, but strict justice will oblige us, to aid our needy and distempered brethren, in their partaking, with the best convenience, of a common blessing'[28] – namely the spring waters. Other preachers referred directly to the tributary relationship, identifying both sides of the equation. First, the barriers to salvation erected by wealth were acknowledged and the intercessionary powers of the poor affirmed. Riches were not 'in themselves criminal, but' counselled Mr Bayly, 'it is so extremely difficult for those that possess them in any great degree, to keep themselves unspotted from the world'. In comparison, the poor were spiritually privileged because poverty allowed them to sleep 'undisturbed either by the pangs of guilt, or fumes of luxury'.[29] Consequently, they were able to intervene, their prayers lengthening the lives of those who follow 'after righteousness and mercy'.[30] As Mr Olive advised, 'the thankful poor ... [will] continually send up their prayers for you to the throne of grace; and He who sitteth thereon, and heareth the supplications of the poor and needy, shall pour down upon your heads the abundance of his blessings'.[31] Far greater exposure was given to the second strand of the tributary relationship: to the function of the rich as 'stewards and agents for the poor'. Every man was 'accountable to God for every worldly blessing he enjoyed'[32] and those with 'superfluities' providence had entrusted to relieve and comfort 'our indigent brethren'.[33] But the needy were not alone in gaining from good works, for by 'the proper application of ... [his] external advantages', the benefactor was also able 'to purchase for himself more permanent, and more excellent possessions in a future state'.[34]

The interface between medicine, health and providence prepared fertile soil in which to sell these paternalist obligations. The early modern period saw a gradual waning of providential accounts of the human condition, as the empiricism of the Scientific Revolution displaced the *a priori* reasoning of formal logic. God remained the supreme architect of the universe, but its day-to-day operation was determined by a set of natural laws which manifest his will. There was thus no tension between providence and science because, as Newton put it, God's purpose was revealed 'by the light of Nature'.[35] Religious explanations of illness declined as doctors and laity adjusted accordingly.[36] This development was facilitated by the latitudinarian thrust of Anglican theology which supported natural rather than revealed religion; the physical world bore witness to the game plan of its creator and hence study of 'the human frame as one of the noblest achievements of the divine handiwork' helped to confirm the essentials of Christian revelation.[37] Water therapy at Bath reflected the evolving partnership between medicine and providence. Doctors used science rather than religion to validate the healing qualities of the spa[38] and to distance themselves from the lay culture of balneology.[39] Simultaneously, however, they cherished the collaboration with God which their professional skills enabled. So William Baylies, disputant in the sulphur controversy, finished his *Reflections* with a flourish which paid homage to the religious dimensions of treatment.

> As the waters ... are a medicine, prepared and delivered to us by the hand of the omnipotent; it is the duty of all who are benefited by them, in gratitude to their bountiful CREATOR, and in charity to their fellow-creatures, to make known to the world the good they have received from these healing fountains; that their brethren, who in like manner are visited with sickness, may share in the blessing, *take up their beds and walk*; while with thankfulness unfeigned, and voices raised, all join in the praises of the great AUTHOR of their HEALTH, and with inraptured seraphs sing,
> GLORY BE TO GOD ON HIGH!
> ON EARTH PEACE!
> GOOD-WILL TOWARDS MEN![40]

For Bath doctors, medicine and theology were not in conflict; rather, secular expertise was applied within a providential framework which honoured the divine origins of the waters and recognized the religious responsibilities that a cure imposed.

The Anglican clerics who preached for the General Infirmary during the 1740s and 1750s were equally committed to co-operation between God and medicine. Again, the divine source of the spa was hammered home. '[N]ature, or providence, or ... God himself, had, for ages, by the peculiar blessing of these copious and salutary springs, marked out this spot for a Bethesda, or House of Mercy, for the distempered poor.'[41] However, it was in justifying the Hospital as a legitimate cause for benevolent concern that the direction of medicine to God's purposes was most forcefully expounded. '[It] cannot, it should not be concealed ... that the most excellent, the most necessary and the most laudable kind of charity is that which provides for the spiritual good and eternal happiness of others.' But continued Mr Olive:

> this, tho' the brightest part, is very far from being the whole of charity. That extends itself to all our wants as well as of the body as of the soul. Else, where would be the force of that reason which the Son of Man shall give for the blessedness of those who shall stand at his right-hand in the Day of Judgement? *I was an hungered, shall he say, and ye gave me meat, I was thirsty and ye gave me drink, I was a stranger and ye took me in ...*

Bath congregations were alerted to the unique opportunity which the General Infirmary offered to patronize this type of corporeal philanthropy: physicians had at their disposal a one-off remedy in the form of the spa waters and, therefore, the traveller who passed indifferently by was unable to 'compensate for former omissions' by giving to another hospital.[42] But over and above this special facility, there were the advantages shared with other medical charities: the centrality of health, 'without which no other worldly thing can give us pleasure', and the 'very distant ... yet an evident and pleasing likeness' to the earthly work of Christ, who 'tho' the great physician of our souls ... condescended ... to cure the bodily diseases and infirmities of men. For', concluded Olive, 'when *the multitude brought their sick unto Jesus, He healed them all*'.[43] Like doctors, Anglican clergy at Bath preached a symbiotic relationship between medicine and theology, physicians and surgeons doing God's will within a divine scaffolding.

Yet despite the reconciliation of orthodox religion and medical science, the idea of a providential God did not entirely die out, even among the élite, and hence illness remained a 'direct hit', warning the victim to moderate earthly pleasures with spiritual awareness or punishing 'some particular sin, crime, or evil'.[44] The didactic function of sickness was colourfully rendered by Mr Dalton who, berating 'the inordinate desires of the sensualist' and 'the proud aspirations of the ambitious', cautioned that when the 'frantic race is over', death would ultimately show 'these restless and repining animals ... their just and proper dimensions'. Because 'man's state of trial ... [was] confined to this life only', however, God in his mercy had 'not left it to death alone, to convince him of so fatal an error'; he had also provided 'for the timely instruction of his mortal creatures ... another, and ... a sufficient teacher ... sickness. By whom, when others, more gentle, are not listened to, he often speaks home to the consciences of mighty and impertinent sinners'.[45] Nor was divine retribution ruled out. If love and gratitude for health and wealth were not enough to instill a sense of obligation towards the lower orders, argued Mr Leyborne, 'Then let fear of punishment teach us better':

> Is the health, lately gained, so firmly established, that we no longer want the favour of God, and dare now provoke his anger? ... Can we promise ourselves, that in the moment we go hence, we shall not want that relief ourselves, which God now asks us to give? Or that the hand which we shall stretch forth, like Jeroboam, in disbelief of the divine threatening, may not, like the king's, be dried up, that we cannot pull it in again unto us? Tho' these springs, in such cases, sometimes can work miracles, as effectually as did the prophet's prayers, and we may think the remedy at hand; will any be entitled to such a miracle, who hath no hand open to the poor?[46]

Running throughout these educative and punitive constructions of divine intervention was an astute critique of polite society and its 'embarrassment of riches'.[47] Therefore, the rich Company remained receptive to providential explanations of personal misfortune which preached the obligations of paternalism by stressing the sins of affluence.

The embarrassment of riches

This religious attack on prosperity mined a deep-seated seam of ambivalence in early Georgian society. The Societies for the Reformation of Manners had begun their campaign against vice, debauchery and profaneness in the 1690s, and though the Anglican establishment was deserting them for charity schools and workhouses by the early eighteenth century, the conviction that wealth induced moral degeneration became more widespread. Like the absorption of polite values, the 'embarrassment of riches' cut across political factions: Henry Fielding, a staunch supporter of the Whig supremacy, rehearsed the 'country' argument that luxury caused crime; Samuel Johnson, opponent of the Whigs, disagreed.[48] Legislation in the 1730s and 1740s to curtail gin consumption, gaming, horse-racing and playhouses was indicative of this cross-party concern for the moral fibre of the nation. The fact that these restrictions were applied more rigorously to popular participation suggests that élite morality was judged less fragile.[49] The impact of luxury was socially selective, declared Fielding in 1751. The wealthy invested their assets in projects which were a tribute to the age; only the morally feeble lower orders were corrupted, squandering their money on gambling, alcohol and trivial amusements.[50] None the less, wealth remained an acute worry for the prosperous members of polite society and one that was compounded by the Evangelical Revival sweeping through all the Protestant churches from the 1730s. Far from being an exuberant reaction to religious rationalism, the Revival was a product of the same Enlightenment thinking that underpinned trust in the material progress of mankind. At its core was a revivification of justification by faith alone, which inevitably relegated acts of charity to second place behind redemption. But whereas orthodox Protestantism taught the uncertainty of salvation, 'the Evangelicals believed it to be general, normally given at conversion and the result of simple acceptance of the gift of God'. For these enthusiasts, 'the quest for assurance' no longer sapped spiritual energy and detracted from good works. The person certain of a seat in eternity was free to cast aside nervous introspection and use philanthropy as well as the Gospel to disseminate the good news with confidence.[51]

Being a fashionable resort, Bath especially felt the 'Fatal effects of luxury and ease!'[52] and its notoriety for opulence and decadence enticed Evangelical reformers. Both the Wesley brothers pronounced the city to be 'Satan's throne', and John preached there on no fewer than 150 occasions.[53] His presence was not without controversy and during a public confrontation in 1739, Richard Nash – high priest of Bath sociability – attempted to challenge his authority to teach the Gospel by imputing sedition.[54] None the less, the Wesleys maintained that their congregations were not drawn solely from the underprivileged and they enjoyed a friendly relationship with the Countess of Huntingdon, who was a member of the Methodist Society and financed them generously during the 1740s. When her exclusive chapel opened in Bath in 1765, with its mission of moral rescue for the rich Company, both John and Charles participated in services.[55] Furthermore, contact with the élite may have included hospitality from Ralph Allen because an entry in John Wesley's *Journal* for 1755 indicates that he was invited to Prior Park, Allen's home outside the city: 'I dined with some serious persons in a large stately house standing on the brow of a delightful hill. In this paradise they live in ease, in honour and in elegant abundance. And this they call retiring from the world!'[56]

The hilltop mansion offered more frequent shelter to less stern critics of luxury, not all of whom shared Allen's Whig politics; Pope as well as Fielding was entertained, despite his association with Bolingbroke and the 'country' cause.[57] Charity played an important part in allaying this broadly based moral concern and early Georgian Bath was fiercely proud of its philanthropic record. There were, wrote John Wood, no fewer than six institutions for 'aged, infirm, sick, impotent and otherwise helpless poor people ... the chief of which is that lately built under the name of the General Hospital or Infirmary'.[58] The Infirmary itself was closely (though not exclusively) connected with the moral crusade. The first president – Thomas Carew MP – carried legislation to prohibit 'a certain pernicious game called roulet or roly-poly', and followed this anti-gaming legislation with a bill to prevent cursing and swearing by imposing a scale of fines.[59] Lady Elizabeth Hastings, a pioneer of the initial scheme, had strong Evangelical sympathies, being both an aunt of the Countess of Huntingdon and a personal friend of the Puritan protagonist of hospitals, Robert Nelson.[60] Moreover, one of her collaborators, Master of the Rolls, Sir Joseph Jekyll, was active in the parliamentary battle against playhouses.[61] A set of *Proposals for a National Reformation of Manners*, published anonomously in 1694, had proclaimed that playhouses fostered 'delight in idleness, excessive vanity, revellings, luxury, wantonness, lasciviousness, [and] whoredoms'.[62] The General Hospital stood on the site of the old Bath theatre.[63] What better antidote to corruption in a spa town than a charitable hospital which made the medicinal waters available to poor strangers? A den of iniquity had been demolished; a place of moral virtue erected in its stead.

The charity sermons for the General Infirmary amplified this symbolic stand against the 'embarrassment of riches' into an outspoken castigation of the moral deficiencies which affluence bred. For Mr Dalton, 'civil society ... [possessed] scarce any character of vice more detestable, than that of the selfish voluptuary; whose God is his belly, to the gratification of which, he sacrifices every creature upon the earth, without once remembering its heavenly creator'. John Brown reserved his most virulent criticism for immoderate gaming, rife in Bath and practiced in defiance of the law:

> Here we may often see a numerous assembly of both sexes, chained down by the magic of the fatal circle; the sorcerer seated triumphant in the midst, with his instruments of deceit before him: At length the spell begins to work, and the engine of falsehood is put in motion: The enchanted crowd stand fixed with anxious eyes and beating hearts, 'till, in the end, fate proclaims the magician victorious; who, by secret and unsuspected arts, hath conveyed the wealth of his followers into his own pocket; leaving them nothing in return but the just reward of grief and vexation, indignation and remorse ... [64]

No doubt the deployment of a supernatural metaphor was designed to shock the polite Company for whom Enlightenment rationalism was a hallowed cultural value. But reason was not the only virtue in jeopardy, and gambling was not the only threat to personal peace of mind and public morality. '[A] variety of principles ... [had] been found to predominate in human nature ... In one age, a sense of religion and duty ... In another, the prospect of future glory: In a third, the contracted views of interest and cunning: In a fourth, the dissolute maxims of luxury and pleasure.' According to Brown, and his fellow preachers for the Bath Infirmary, there was no disputing that early Georgian Britain fell into the fourth category. 'We are cunning, indeed, and laborious to heap up; but we only heap up, that we may squander. Immediate gratification is the great object of pursuit; and futurity is lost, amidst our rage for present enjoyment.'[65]

Preachers intent upon teaching careful stewardship confronted church congregations with the ethical ambiguities of this 'rage for present enjoyment', exploiting the psychological tensions of affluence through a manipulation of guilt and anxiety. Since paternalism decreed that charity was not a voluntary option but a mandatory duty stemming from the ownership of property,[66] any failure to meet the legitimate needs of the sick poor was a moral offence of which their negligent masters were guilty. Mr Dalton adopted this reasoning. Pointing out that beds at the Bath Infirmary were closed due to financial insufficiency, he reminded his audience that the patients who sought admission had fulfilled their part of the tributary relationship:

> before we shut the doors of mercy against these humble petitioners, let us consider, who they are that desire admittance. Is it not the faithful servant, the painful labourer, the diligent artificer, or the gallant soldier; those, who have attended our pleasures in health, and our distresses in sickness; have cultivated our lands, augmented our commerce, or bravely defended the rights, the liberties, the religion of our country?[67]

But the worthy poor were not only entitled to assistance because a paternalist obligation had been fulfilled; gratitude also demanded action because their labour, which enabled the rich to have ease, was not infrequently responsible for the ill health with which they were afflicted.[68] William Warburton pushed furthest this thesis that the advance of civilization was responsible for the progress of disease.[69] '[T]o the poor ... it is', he argued, that 'we are immediately, and almost solely, indebted for every advantage of ease and pleasure, which improved and refined society affords ... it being by their incessant toil and labour that these elegancies are procured for us'. The health risks which this work presented were many:

> For toiling, in pursuit of the commodities of life, some are confined to the pestilential damp of mines; while others are exposed to all the rage of elementary and solar fires: These subject to every various inclemency of distempered air; and those to the rotten humidity of fens, or the corrosive vapours of salt waters. Here, a too sedentary occupation viciates the torpid fluids; and there, a too violent destroys the overstretched tone of the solids. In some of the baleful materials, employed or worked upon, strike with acute distempers;

> in others, the very manner of working brings on chronical: So that the shop of the artificer may be truly styled the warehouse of death.

These 'maladies' – 'chiefly contracted in our service, in an incessant application of all their faculties to the supplial of our imaginery, and ... endless wants and conveniences' – were contrasted with the medical 'mischiefs' which the 'distempered rich' brought upon themselves 'by their own follies and vices' and 'licentious appetites'.[70] The different ramifications of illness aggravated this injustice. As Edward Bayly observed, 'the far greater part of mankind must rise early, and eat the bread of carefulness; they must work out their maintenance in this world, as well as their salvation in the next, with pains and labour'. For these men and women 'not born to fortunes ready-made', health was 'the source of all ... happiness' and sickness deprived them of their livelihoods. Therefore, whereas the culpable rich had the resources to buy treatment for their self-inflicted ailments, the innocent poor did not. By highlighting this inequity, Mr Bayly encouraged the privileged to become conscious of, and even chastened by, their easy circumstances:

> If all the assistance that human art can afford; if downy pillows, and obsequious attendants cannot ease their pains, or cause the temples of their heads to take any rest, they must thence judge the misery which those poor wretches necessarily endure; who, like their suffering Saviour, have not a place to lay their heads; who have no cordial draughts to cheer their spirits; who have no means, no lenitives to soften the rigour of disease.[71]

How dreadful then it was that the General Hospital still lacked the funds to treat those who 'want and continually solicit an admission'. Above all, 'how unpardonable our guilt, (if we are able to grant their request) in refusing it!'[72]

In addition to stoking the fires of guilt, charity sermons for the Bath Infirmary inflamed and appeased anxiety by expounding the temporal and eternal fate of man and the protections which charity afforded. Present good fortune was precarious, warned Mr Brown. '[W]hatever prosperous conditions you may now enjoy, yet as age and infirmities steal on, the evil days will come, when you shall say, you have no pleasure in them ... when neither wealth, palaces, attendance, titles, or distinction, can yield you comfort.'[73] According to Mr Leyborne, the very act of indulging in the Bath's social whirl put well-being at risk: ''Tis often questioned, whether the waters in this place, do more promote the health of the body, than some of the customs and diversions do endanger not only health, but your substance also; perhaps the welfare of your souls; perhaps your happiness, both here and hereafter.'

For the 'truly virtuous' who heeded these threats and decided to 'lay up alms in ... [the] store-house' of charity, the return on their investment was both material and spiritual.[74] Leyborne explicitly linked the city's increasing prosperity to its philanthropic endeavours.

> [M]ay we not remember, that with your care of the poor in this city, the rich Company ever has increased? With your charity school were the beginnings of your prosperity; and with the building of this Hospital, how many more buildings arose? ... and how greatly has the trade and substance of the inhabitants since multiplied, together with their numbers?

Further benefits might follow.

> [W]ho knows but, when this good design shall be accomplished, and your Hospital in its full extent completed, God may put it into the hearts of the worthy members of this Corporation, to proceed to those improvements in the baths, which the physicians have represented as necessary, and most men long wished for and wanted.[75]

Complementing this naked material bribery was the assurance of an untroubled conscience.[76] Mr Bayly stressed the comforts of such 'a self-approving mind' during 'the last closing scenes of life ... [when] all else, that the wealth of empires could purchase for you, will be lost and useless'.

> Believe me! At that hour, the smallest bounty bestowed upon these, your distressed brethren, will more avail, than millions employed in the best-concerted worldly schemes: For, They shall perish and wax old, as doth a garment, but this shall endure; works of charity will not deceive you; or, like false friends, desert you, in the time of trial. On the contrary, they will support thee on thy bed of languishing, they will attend thee to thy grave ...

Moreover, philanthropy conferred eternal as well as earthly tranquility. Even after death:

> where all things are forgotten; when all the pageant glories of this world shall be buried in one common undistinguished mass of ruin; when the everlasting mountains shall melt, like wax, before the Sun; and even the heavens and earth shall pass away. –
>
> Yet then, even then, shall works of charity remain; they shall be had in everlasting remembrance.
>
> They shall rise up as a memorial before God.
>
> They shall stand recorded in that book, where all our deeds are written; and according to which, we shall, one day, be finally judged.

This spiritual consolation was most dramatically portrayed by the use of two contrasting vignettes: one of those who employed the 'valuable gifts of heaven ... worthily and wisely'; the other of those who abused or misapplied them. Members of the former group were entitled 'to consider themselves as the favourites and substitutes of heaven; as the agents of providence; the dispensers of God's bounty to his creatures; the channels which convey the plenteous streams of His diffusive goodness, as chosen guardians of the distressed, and protectors of the helpless'. In opposition was the 'sordid miser or lavish libertine', tormented by his future fate: 'what shall I do, when my Lord calleth for an account of my stewardship? ... those precious trusts I have either tied up in a napkin, or wasted on my sins: How then shall I stand the inquisition of my injured master?'[77] For the charitable good steward of God's gifts came deliverance from such eternal perils.

The overblown language of the charity sermons when fulminating against vice makes it tempting to dismiss them as empty pieces of theatre, designed to entertain a visiting Company in holiday mood. The extent to which preachers seriously wished to liberate polite society from false pleasure is open to question. Nor did fashionable visitors who listened to the 'ceremonial polemics against wealth'[78] from the pulpit forsake the forbidden fruits. In the playground of early Georgian England, however, charity sermons were able to capitalize on the psychological dissonances of affluence. If no transformation of behaviour ensued, verbal flagellation did prompt the symbolic dispensation of charity; the rich Company laundered their wealth with philanthropy, experiencing a temporary catharsis which purged the soul whilst leaving the lifestyle essentially intact. For this service of moral cleansing, they were willing to pay. Therefore, cash was forthcoming to salve the consciences of Bath's opulent clientele.

The rise of sensibility

The florid use of guilt and anxiety to exhort church congregations to the paternalist obligations of the tributary relationship exposed the degree to which early Georgian Bath society was racked by the 'embarrassment of riches'. Cohabiting with this civic definition of virtue, however, was the more benign moral sensibility of polite society – later to develop into the proprietary relationship – that emphasized the common predicament of humanity and the pleasure of showing compassion.[79] The 'Plan and Elevation' of 1738, for example, argued that allowing the poor access to the curative waters 'would be so sincere a pleasure to all good minds, that they must think it cheaply purchased by a generous contribution towards so good a work'.[80] The Infirmary likewise traded in moral sensibility when, as a result of financial crisis during the 1780s, Christopher Anstey was commissioned to pen a poetic advertisement. Anstey, author of the satirical *New Bath Guide*, had settled in the city and become a governor of the Hospital.[81] Though closing with a reference to the physical and spiritual rewards of giving, he chose to milk the compassionate nature of his readers.

Oh pause a while, whoe'er thou art
  That drinks this healing stream,
If e'er compassion o'er thy heart
  Diffused its heavenly beam.

Think on the wretch whose distant lot
  This friendly aid denies;
Think how in some poor lowly cot
  He unregarded lies.

Hither the helpless stranger bring,
  Relieve his heartfelt woe,
And let thy bounty like this spring
  In genial currents flow.

So may thy years from grief and pain,
  And pining want be free,
And thou from heaven that mercy gain
  The poor receive from thee.[82]

The governors were delighted with the 'very just and elegant manner' in which their wishes had been fulfilled, and decided to hang the inscription in the Pump Rooms as well as print 1 000 copies for distribution to well-wishers.[83] Moreover, when the New Pump Room opened in the 1790s, the 'beautiful effusion' was attached to the wall of the pumping enclosure in gilt letters.[84] Presumably, the verses were judged an effective money-spinner because they pulsated with the moral tempo of the times.

The social virtue harnessed in printed publicity was also displayed at cultural events and charity services. Georgian culture acted as a moral barometer for Georgian society, its moving arm tracking the changing conditions. In art, the falling popularity of Hogarth's 'secular sermons in print' reflected a greater tolerance of luxury from mid-century,[85] while in music the London flop of Handel's *Messiah* until its 1750 performance in the Foundling Hospital chapel demonstrated the ambivalence towards the theatre; playhouses were too full of sin and immorality to host a sacred 'Act of Religion'.[86] In addition to measuring morality, cultural activities – John Brewer's 'pleasures of the imagination stimulated by the arts'[87] – were regarded as educative or reforming, given the right content and context.[88] The approval of charity as an uplifting pursuit created the opportunity for partnership with the new polite pastimes, anxious to enhance their image. At Bath, wealthy visitors donated to the General Infirmary in lieu of bells to announce their arrival, as well as paying over bets and gambling fines and making contributions via social events and venues. In seeking the moralizing effects of philanthropy, these 'suspect' activities used their fund-raising occasions to promote the sensitivity of polite society. In December 1751, for example, two plays were staged at Mr Brown's Bath theatre in aid of the General Infirmary, one a tragedy of the *Orphan* and the other a pantomime called *Harlequin Restored*. The prologue to this mix of serious and light entertainment, spoken by the proprietor himself, relied on the carrot rather than the stick to extract donations:

> To raise the tender passions and impart
> The softest anguish to the hardest heart,
> For this the tragic muse, melodious Queen!
> Tunes her soft lays, or swells the lofty scene.
> But need we now the personated woe,
> The studied pang, the tear that's taught to flow,
> The feigned distress, though drawn from nature's pen,
> To rouse the soul, and tell you, you are men?
> When every breast with generous pity glows,
> For more, alas! than visionary woes?
> For real wants, misfortunes baleful train,
> The smart of anguish, and the rack of pain?
> Such are the woes with which the afflicted grieve,
> Such are the woes your bounteous hearts relieve.
> Vain were the talk, a glorious deed to raise,
> With all the soft impertinence of praise;
> Nobly you act in virtue's heavenly cause,
> And your own conscience is the best applause.
> To praise such merit, though our forces fail,
> At least our gentle wishes shall prevail.
> If you who take the wretched to your care,
> Some little strokes of human anguish share,
> Oh! may you feel (like those you aid) no more
> Your former pangs, or be what you deplore;
> May joys returning wave their gladsome wing,
> And health flow largely from this vital spring.[89]

This piece obliquely mentions the relief of 'former pangs' but, essentially, theatre-goers were being complimented for their sensibility. The negative critique of luxury was therefore opposed. Culture might be a vehicle for moral elevation, but the artificial stimulus of drama was unnecessary to prod a polite audience into good works because they were naturally 'soft' and caring.

Whilst we might expect cultural venues to become mouthpieces for social virtue, its presence in religious discourse is more suggestive of moral change. The theological nucleus of moral sensibility was the directive: 'Thou shalt love thy neighbour as thyself'[90] – a fundamental duty to God which believers aspired to by imitating the earthly example of Jesus.[91] Charity sermons for the General Infirmary insisted that this Christian love demonstrated the superiority of 'our holy Religion, and the numerous defects of all other forms of wisdom and Godliness'.[92] Glorious former ages possessed impressive architectural structures, claimed Mr Bayly, overlooking the medicinal role that pagan temples had played;[93] but until the arrival of Christ and his apostles, there were no hospitals for the relief of the poor and helpless.[94] Yet despite being a Christian obligation, love for fellow man was only released through human agency and at Bath this had been sadly delayed. In creating 'these copious and salutary springs ... Heaven had long done its part'. The rich, however, 'those faithless or careless stewards of its bounty', had neglected their contribution ''till the anger or spirit of charity also descended to move the hearts of some among us, with a just, generous, and wise compassion for the numerous distressed inconveniences, here suffered by their sick and needy brethren'. As Mr Dalton elaborated:

> They had seen with tender concern many of these unhappy objects, after having despaired of all relief at home, and every other place, that charity had established for their assistance, and, with incredible pain and difficulty, arrived at the very brink of what they fondly hoped would again restore them to their greatest happiness on earth; they had often seen them, from the sole want of that necessary shelter, care, and attendance ...meet their ruin here, where alone they expected relief.[95]

To awaken such 'tender concern' in others, charity sermons evoked the empathy and pleasure deployed in secular publicity for the General Infirmary. 'We stand here in the presence of God', observed Mr Brown, 'before whom the greatest of us are but dust and ashes; in whose eyes no distinction can take place, but that of virtue and vice, the righteous and the sinner.' Those in the rich Company who were ill, and those who had been restored by the waters, were urged to 'Let the sense and feeling of your own infirmities teach you to pity those of others'.[96] For visitors without personal experience of ill health, who came 'purely for amusement, to pass the fleeting hours in gaiety and delight', it was the sight of the sick poor that was spiritually instructive.

> [T]hey can scarce avoid reflecting ... that they were made by the same God, and formed of the same materials; that they are, or at least were, capable of the same enjoyments, which they now glory in; that they themselves are likewise liable to the same miseries, which now render them the objects of compassion.[97]

The genuine satisfaction of charitable giving was most heralded by John Brown, its rewards being heightened by comparison with the superficial gains from self-indulgent vices and pastimes.[98] Despite any initial attractions, debauchery and intemperance destroyed 'the health of the body, and all the powers of the mind'; luxury and prodigality were 'no less fatal to our fortunes', and every breech of social duty was 'attended with some embittering or ruinous circumstance', so that arbitrary, oppressive or uncharitable behaviour would always evince 'a just and public ignominy'. Voicing the hope that none of his congregation were 'declared and determined enemies of virtue', Mr Brown went on to alert them to 'the folly of expecting true and permanent pleasure' from innocent diversions or amusements which squeezed out opportunities for benevolence. These activities constantly or immoderately followed grew tedious and tiresome; and, if relinquished, gave pain rather than pleasure in reflection.

> We toil, like children in pursuit of rainbows, after these chimeral and air-painted objects of delight: When we come upon the spot, we find, that what at a distance appeared so gay, had but a false splendour, which is vanished on a nearer approach. Yet still, as new objects rise before us, we renew our pursuit, find ourselves again deceived, and thus pass our time between expectation and disappointment.

Even 'the temperate pursuit of a single amusement', which left room for 'pursuits of a higher nature', endangered true pleasure because 'when the soul becomes totally immersed in trifling or idle gratifications, the superior faculties of the mind lie dormant and neglected', enabling 'the latent seeds of corruption ... to spring up in tares and thistles'.[99]

It is unfortunate that these early Georgian murmurings of compassion and pleasure cannot be followed through in religious discourse for the later eighteenth century. In 1810, however, the Presbyterian minister, Joseph Hunter, preached a charity sermon on *The Ameliorated Condition of the Poor* which has survived. In common with his mid-century clerical predecessors, Hunter stressed the providential nature of the waters, which allowed benevolence to avail 'itself of one of the richest presents from the great Giver of all good'. Eternal reward was also promised for 'assisting especially those who ... cannot be expected to make you any return, under the expectation that ... yet you shall be recompensed at the resurrection of the just'. But gone was the engineering of guilt and anxiety to propel sinful man in the direction of charity. Instead, all the emphasis fell on 'the Christian precepts of gentleness and love; the effects of that *new* commandment given by our Lord, that men should love one another'. Whereas earlier sermons had alluded to the moral shortcomings of past times, Mr Hunter constructed his entire sermon around 'a noble contrast' between the benevolence of opulent but Christian Bath and 'the barbarous conduct of the falsely-called liberal and enlightened Romans!' Turning to advantage the recent abolition of the British slave trade, he argued that despite their reputation for civility and refinement, the citizens of antiquity behaved abominably towards their slaves. '[E]steeeming them born only to minister to their luxury, they treated them as if they belonged to some inferior order of animated existences.' Therefore, though the 'venerable remains' of classical civilization 'astonish ... by their vastness, and delight by their extraordinary beauty and exquisite proportions ... we do not find among them one which was devoted to the reception of the man by whose labour they were erected, when sickness had enervated his limbs, or age weighed down his head'. To 'the ears of a Christian audience', this oppression was shocking because they mistook 'for the native dictates of the human heart the suggestions of a mind with its moral sensibilities formed by the precepts and genius of a heaven-descended religion'. 'Where there was no love', however, 'no fellow-feeling, no sense of a common origin, no prospect of being hereafter brought to the same level, it could not be expected that there should be any consideration respecting ... [the lower stations in life], but how they might be made to minister to the emolument or pleasure of their masters'.[100]

Hunter's reasoning overturned the moral status of the labouring classes by no longer representing them as the victims of an affluent but insensitive élite. Thanks to Christianity, 'the practice of depressing the lower orders to a state of slavery' had been outlawed by so 'humanizing the manners and softening the heart' that those blessed with wealth were willing to communicate their 'abundance to the necessities of ... poorer brethren'. Therefore, when the labouring man saw 'the numberless structures erected in every part of this happy island by the benevolence of the rich, out of the most disinterested wish to relieve him from a portion of his burden, he has reason to bless his God that he became poor in a Christian country'. This argument for a common humanity was anachronistic because sensibility had been 'finally wrecked by the storms over the French Revolution', its rejection of 'indiscriminate benevolence' evident in the exclusionary charitable practices that took hold from the late eighteenth century.[101] But if Hunter's attitude to the poor was outdated and idealistic, his ethics of giving were contemporary and consistent with the economic and cultural individualism which underpinned polite society. Despite hailing benefactors as 'good stewards of the manifest grace of God', the relationship which he described was more a proprietary than a tributary one. '[T]he rich had *voluntarily* [my italics] made a legal surrender to the poor of a right to a certain portion of all their possessions ... nor satisfied with this, they have provided *other extraordinary means of relief* [my italics] for cases of distress which make larger claims upon the community than ordinary instances of poverty'.[102] In short, rich and poor no longer inhabited a world of mutual obligation; statutory and charitable assistance was now an optional concession, not a duty of paternalism.

The changing ethics of charity

Joseph Hunter's consecration of sensibility sets him apart from the fiery clerical critics of early Georgian Bath, but we must be cautious about drawing general conclusions from a single sermon, particularly one delivered by a Dissenter. In the first place, Hunter was addressing a different audience, more middling and residential than the élite visitors who had earlier populated the Abbey. Furthermore, since Nonconformity favoured religious and political pluralism, he would have lacked the commitment to paternalist obligation which Anglicans absorbed from the integration of church and state. He himself acknowledged a longstanding Presbyterian commitment to moral sensibility by prefacing the published version of his text with lengthy extracts from William Robertson's address to the Society in Scotland for Promoting Christian Knowledge.[103] '[T]he genius of the gospel ... civiliz[ed] the fiercest and most barbarous nations', preached Dr Robertson in 1755; and 'not only sanctifi[ed] our souls, but refine[d] our manners'.[104] Identification with this tradition of politeness may have blinded Hunter to the ambivalence that leisure and luxury continued to stir up in Bath. Although the later Georgian city acquired an increasingly respectable image, moral reproof was still voiced. In an 1810 journal entry, for example, the American ship owner, Louis Simond, was reminiscent of the early Hanoverians in insinuating sexual as well as material intemperance:

> Bath is a sort of great monastery, inhabited by single people, particularly superannuated females. No trade, no manufactures, no occupations of any sort, except that of killing time, the most laborious of all. Half of the inhabitants do nothing, the other half supplies them with nothings:- Multitude of splendid shops, full of all that wealth and luxury can desire, arranged with all the arts of seduction.[105]

For the Evangelical reformer, Hannah More, the city was a 'foolish, frivolous place',[106] from which she sought protection in prayer: 'O Lord! fit me for the duties and keep me from all the temptations of it. I thank thee that the vain and unprofitable company with which this place abounds, is a burden to me.'[107] Katherine Plymley was more gentle in her reproach, but still considered that the 'great business' of Bath was 'pleasure'. Returning home to Shropshire after a stay in 1794, she wrote in her diary of life being

> seen through a false medium. Of the numbers that resort to it [the city], the greater part come with a wish to see and be seen ... to leave all care behind ... and though the fixed inhabitants of Bath are now more numerous, yet they must be influenced by the gay shifting scene around them.[108]

The development of the city as a residential centre helps to explain why the Lower Assembly Rooms were not rebuilt after a catastrophic fire in 1820; not only was the location now inconvenient for the most fashionable lodgings, but in a more permanent community sociability was increasingly conducted not in the public arena but privately behind closed doors. However, the construction of a Literary and Scientific Institution on the site of the former Rooms also served to appease the ongoing 'embarrassment of riches' which haunted the city. Symbolizing a 'change from the indulgent pleasures of the eighteenth century to the more earnest activity of the nineteenth', the Institution enabled a revision of the reputation for superficiality.[109] 'It is well known', admitted Roland Mainwaring in 1838,

> that when the Institution was first projected, there were many who imagined that the literary character of Bath was not sustained by the existing race of inhabitants, and regarded as hopeless any attempt to interest a sufficient number of persons in the completion of a design which was chiefly destined for scientific and literary purposes.

But these fears had proved 'groundless'; Bath stood 'redeemed from the imputation of being a city devoted only to pleasure and dissipation'.[110] Equally redemptive was the impressive array of charitable enterprises in existence by the early nineteenth century. 'Amply furnished as Bath is with edifices devoted to the glory and worship of God', proclaimed *The Improved Bath Guide* of 1812:

> it is not less accommodated with institutions dedicated to the service and comfort of men. Not withstanding the most fascinating amusements are ever open to occupy the attention, and drain the purses of our visitors and inhabitants, yet the softer calls of charity and benevolence are still heard amidst the gaiety of dissipation and the frivolities of fashion; and no place in the kingdom exhibits any more asyla for disease and wretchedness, for the support of the poor, the relief of the sick, and the instruction of the ignorant than Bath.[111]

This trilogy of religion, philanthropy and sociability was no accident. Although the values of polite society which the city epitomized had come to dominate the later Georgians' moral frame of reference, the pleasures of affluence provoked a residual unease. This anxiety was intensified by the early nineteenth-century Evangelical Revival which from the 1820s swept 'enthusiastic' ministers into local churches and chapels.[112] Therefore, marketing 'the softer calls of charity and benevolence' helped to lance the boil of prosperity by drawing on the sensibility with which politeness was associated.

The moral discourse which surrounds the Georgian Bath Infirmary suggests that philanthropy embodied a hybrid of civic and social virtue. On the one hand, charity sermons sought compliance with the obligations of paternalism by exploiting the guilt and anxiety manufactured by luxury.[113] On the other hand, they vaunted the civilizing influence of Christian love, urging the wealthy to picture the plight of the sick poor and enjoy the satisfaction of responding to their needs with compassion. Far from diminishing their credibility, this explosive combination of contradictory elements is indicative of a society in the process of adapting to change. However, the experience of Bath does challenge the universality of Donna Andrew's conclusion for London philanthropy that a proprietary interpretation of property relations was overtaking the older tributary relationship between 1670 and 1740. Unfortunately, sermons elsewhere by the preachers most animated in their advocacy of paternalism – notably Edward Bayly – were apparently never printed or have not survived and, therefore, we cannot be sure that the discrepancy is not due to variations in clerical opinion rather than a differentiated reaction to the particular circumstances of Bath. Yet even in the moderate John Dalton, there are signs that the performance was geared to the local audience. Addressing the governors of the Middlesex Hospital in 1751, he maintained that despite the loss of many virtues to luxury, wantonness, licentiousness and profanity, 'the guardian angel of charity has not yet relinquished his charge' and so the sick poor still excited compassion; 'open acts of beneficience ... [would] not only be seen but felt by the rich as well as the poor, and may kindle in the coldest and most insensible hearts a noble and useful emulation'.[114] While these words share with Dalton's sermon for the General Infirmary a belief in the educative role of sickness, their gentle hope of moral improvement departs markedly from the savage attack on sensuality which he rained down on his Bath congregation.[115]

But if there are grounds for thinking that traditional paternalism was more resilient in Bath, what are the reasons for this difference? The disintegration of established authority structures partially accounts for the early rejection of the tributary relationship in London. So, too, do the socio-economic characteristics of benefactors. Whereas Bath's visiting Company was drawn extensively from the aristocracy and gentry who were more closely wedded to paternalism, metropolitan patrons were more heterogeneous and included a larger bourgeois faction more sympathetic to the capitalist concept of welfare.[116] Reinforcing this economic logic, however, were the values of polite society which, by defining the élite in terms of refined sociability rather than land ownership, struck a chord with London's middling orders. The resulting interpretation of charity as an optional emblem of civility underpins the 'free and voluntary' character of the proprietary relationship which was quick to find favour in the capital. From the 1760s, the ethical values embodied within this relationship became increasingly influential outside the mercantile community of London. Bath was not unaffected. Although sentiment had coexisted with obligation in early Georgian discourses focusing on the city, the 'exhortary aspect'[117] had privileged paternalism. Local ambivalence towards leisure and luxury did not entirely evaporate, but in the second half of the eighteenth century the balance began to tip in favour of sensibility. Therefore, though Joseph Hunter's 1810 sermon on behalf of the General Hospital exaggerated humanity towards the poor, it was essentially in tune with moral attitudes to giving; an abrasive purgative was no longer required, but charity as a manifestation of refinement became a prerequisite for ethical and social approval. It follows that his suggestion of a proprietary relationship beween rich and poor is also convincing. Philanthropy exercised as a paternalist duty in the name of civic virtue was obligatory and hence tributary; philanthropy exercised as a personal expression of social virtue was voluntary and hence proprietary.

In this chapter, we have charted the decline of paternalism during the Georgian period. Though Donna Andrew's study of London philanthropy dated the rise of the proprietary relationship from the early decades of the eighteenth century, charity sermons on behalf of the Bath Infirmary upheld a tributary relationship for longer, exposing the ethical ambivalences of affluence and luxury in an attempt to enforce paternalist duties. From 1760, however, the moral sensibilities of politeness accelerated in influence, encouraged especially by the growing prosperity of the middling orders and their search for a gentility that was acquired not ascribed. The one charity sermon which survives for the late Georgian Bath Hospital is an eloquent testimony to the new ethics of benevolence because refinement, rather than hell-fire and damnation, was used to inspire voluntary gifts rather than to extract compulsory stewardship. In tandem with this apparent sensibility, however, was a hardening attitude towards poverty which not only reduced the labouring classes to economic chattels but also increasingly banished them to the realms of moral degeneracy. In Chapter 7, we search for the origins of this change in economic thought, pondering how medical charity was affected by the transition from mercantilism to *laissez-faire*.

Notes

1. Corfield, *Power*, p. 237.
2. David Roberts, *Paternalism in Early Victorian England* (New Brunswick, NJ: Rutgers University Press, 1979), pp. 1–15. See also Maxine Berg, *The Age of Manufactures: Industry, Innovation and Work in Britain 1700–1820* (London: Fontana Press, 1985), pp. 26–30; David Levine, 'Industrialization and the Proletarian Family in England', *Past and Present*, 107 (1985), pp. 169, 171–2; Rule, *Vital Century*, pp. 16–18; E.P. Thompson, 'Patrician Society, Plebeian Culture', *Journal of Social History*, 7 (1974), pp. 382–7.
3. R.H. Tawney, *Religion and the Rise of Capitalism: A Historical Study* (New York: Harcourt, Brace and Co., 1926), p. 13.
4. Baugh, 'Poverty', pp. 66–75; A.L. Beier, *The Problem of the Poor in Tudor and Early Stuart England*, (London: Methuen, 1983), pp. 14–16; Felicity Heal, *Hospitality in Early Modern England* (Oxford: Clarendon Press, 1990), pp. 122–5; Slack, *Poverty*, pp. 9–10; Slack, *English Poor Law*, pp. 14–15.
5. Gerald R. Cragg, *The Church and the Age of Reason 1648–1789*, repr. (Harmondsworth: Penguin Books, 1990), pp. 71–3, 157–9; John Gascoigne, 'Anglican Latitudinarianism and Political Radicalism in the Late Eighteenth Century', *History*, 71 (1986), p. 23; A.D. Gilbert, *Religion and Society in Industrial England: Church, Chapel and Social Change 1740–1914* (London: Longman, 1976), pp. 3–12; Gertrude Himmelfarb, *The Idea of Poverty: England in the Early Industrial Age*, (London: Faber and Faber, 1984), pp. 23–4; Roberts, *Paternalism*, pp. 16–19.
6. Andrew, *Philanthropy and Police*, p. 17.
7. Slack, *Poverty*, pp. 18–19.
8. Bellers, 'Essay', p. 181.
9. Andrew, *Philanthropy and Police*, p. 14.
10. Ibid., p. 17.
11. This definition, taken from the Unesco *Dictionary of the Social Sciences*, is cited in Rule, *Vital Century*, p. 315.
12. Sydney Checkland, *British Public Policy 1776–1939: An Economic, Social and Political Perspective* (Cambridge: Cambridge University Press, 1983), pp. 16–19; Langford, *Polite and Commercial People*, pp. 174–82; Rule, *Vital Century*, pp. 315–16.
13. Terence Hutchison, *Before Adam Smith: The Emergence of Political Economy, 1662–1776* (Oxford: Basil Blackwell, 1988), pp. 4–5, 115–26.
14. Mark Blaug, *Economic Theory in Retrospect*, 3rd edn (Cambridge: Cambridge University Press, 1978), p. 10.
15. Checkland, *British Public Policy*, p. 16.
16. Andrew, *Philanthropy and Police*, p. 94; Christopher J. Berry, *The Idea of Luxury: A Conceptual and Historical Investigation* (Cambridge: Cambridge University Press, 1994), pp. 103, 123; Neil McKendrick, 'The Consumer Revolution in Eighteenth-Century England', in Neil McKendrick, John Brewer and J.H. Plumb, *The Birth of a Consumer Society: The Commercialization of Eighteenth-Century England* (London: Hutchinson, 1982), pp. 13–15.

17. William J. Barber, *A History of Economic Thought* (Harmondsworth: Penguin Books, 1967), p. 27; D.D. Raphael, *Adam Smith* (Oxford: Oxford University Press, 1985), pp. 46–51. See also Hutchison, *Before Adam Smith*, pp. 229–30, 362; Roberts, *Paternalism*, p. 17.
18. Adam Smith, *An Inquiry into the Nature and Causes of the Wealth of Nations*, ed. J.R. McCulloch, 4th edn (Edinburgh: Adam and Charles Black, 1855), p. 7.
19. Berry, *Idea of Luxury*, pp. 160–68.
20. Adam Smith, *Lectures in Jurisprudence*, quoted in C.J. Berry, *The Idea of Luxury: A Conceptual and Historical Investigation* (Cambridge: Cambridge University Press, 1994), p. 166.
21. Andrew, *Philanthropy and Police*, pp. 32–5; Hutchison, *Before Adam Smith*, pp. 115–20; McKendrick, 'Consumer Revolution', pp. 16–18.
22. John Barrell, *The Political Theory of Painting from Reynolds to Hazlitt* (New Haven: Yale University Press, 1986), pp. 45–6, 54–5, 58. See also Lawrence Klein, 'Liberty, Manners and Politeness in Early Eighteenth-Century England', *Historical Journal*, **32** (1989), pp. 586–7, 593, 603.
23. Langford, *Polite and Commercial People*, chs 10 and 12.
24. Colin Jones, 'Some Recent Trends in the History of Charity', in Martin Daunton (ed.), *Charity, Self-Interest and Welfare in the English Past* (London: UCL Press, 1996), pp. 57–8.
25. Andrew, *Philanthropy and Police*, p. 17.
26. Nicholas Rogers, 'The Middling Sort in Eighteenth-Century Politics', in Jonathan Barry and Christopher Brooks (eds), *The Middling Sort of People: Culture, Society and Politics in England 1550–1800* (London: Macmillan, 1994), p. 178.
27. This sermon was repeated at St James' Church, Bath in May 1754.
28. William Warburton, *A Sermon Preached at the Abbey-Church at Bath* (London: J. Leake, 1742), p. 20.
29. Bayly, *Sermon*, pp. 10, 16.
30. Leyborne, *Charity Conducive*, p. 34.
31. Olive, *Particular Excellence*, pp. 26–7.
32. Bayly, *Sermon*, pp. 7, 15.
33. J. Dalton, *The Religious Use of the Visitation of Sickness* (Bath: Thomas Boddely, 1746), p. 14.
34. Bayly, *Sermon*, p. 7.
35. Hankins, *Science*, pp. 3, 6; Speck, *Stability and Strife*, pp. 87–8.
36. Wear, 'Making Sense', pp. 121–2.
37. Roy Porter, 'Medicine and Religion in Eighteenth-Century England: A Case of Conflict?' *Ideas and Production*, 7 (1987), pp. 4–5, 9, 11. See also Gascoigne, 'Anglican Latitudinarianism', p. 23.
38. Christopher Hamlin, 'Chemistry, Medicine, and the Legitimization of English Spas, 1740–1840', in R. Porter (ed.), *The Medical History of Waters and Spas, Medical History*, Supplement No. 10 (London: Wellcome Institute for the History of Medicine, 1990), p. 68.
39. Neve, 'Orthodoxy and Fringe', p. 45.
40. Baylies, *Reflections*, pp. 253–4. See also Henry William Freeman, *The Thermal Baths of Bath: Their History, Literature, Medical and Surgical Uses and Effects* (London: Hamilton, Adams and Co., and Bath: Charles Hallett, 1888), p. 245; John Kent Spender, *The Bath Thermal Baths: Historical, Social and Medical* (London and Bath: W. Lewis, 1877), p. 19.

41. Dalton, *Religious Use*, p. 16. See also Bayly, *Sermon*, p. 14; Olive *Particular Excellence*, p. 16; Warburton, *Sermon* [1742], pp. 17–20.
42. Leyborne, *Charity Conducive*, pp. 20–1.
43. Olive, *Particular Excellence*, pp. 8, 10–11, 14. See also Dalton, *Religious Use*, p. 20; Andrew Wear, 'Religious Beliefs and Medicine in Early Modern England', in Hilary Marland and Margaret Pelling (eds), *The Task of Healing: Medicine, Religion and Gender in England and the Netherlands 1450–1800* (Rotterdam: Erasmus, 1996), p. 162.
44. Porter, 'Medicine and Religion', pp. 6, 8. See also Jonathan Barry, 'Piety and the Patient: Medicine and Religion in Eighteenth-Century Bristol', in R. Porter (ed.), *Patients and Practioners: Lay Perceptions of Medicine in Pre-Industrial Society* (Cambridge: Cambridge University Press, 1985), p. 172; Porter and Porter, *In Sickness*, pp. 170–75; J.A. Sharpe, *Early Modern England: A Social History 1550–1760* (London: Edward Arnold, 1987), p. 252.
45. Dalton, *Religious Use*, pp. 5–7. See also 'Of Sickness and its Uses', *Bath Journal*, 15 January 1753.
46. Leyborne, *Charity Conducive*, pp. 29–30.
47. Simon Schama, *The Embarrassment of Riches: An Interpretation of Dutch Culture in the Golden Age* (London: Fontana, 1987), pp. 289–371.
48. Andrew, *Philanthropy and Police*, pp. 92–5; Jeremy Black, *The English Press in the Eighteenth Century* (London: Croom Helm, 1987), pp. 267–8; Frank McLynn, *Crime and Punishment in Eighteenth Century England* (Oxford: Oxford University Press, 1989), p. 243; Robert B. Shoemaker, 'Reforming the City: The Reformation of Manners Campaign in London, 1690–1738', in Lee Davison, Tim Hitchcock, Tim Keirn and Robert B. Shoemaker (eds), *Stilling the Grumbling Hive: The Response to Social and Economic Problems in England 1689–1750* (Stroud: Alan Sutton, 1992), pp. 100–101, 109–10, 114–15; Speck, *Stability and Strife*, pp. 86–7.
49. Borsay, *English Urban Renaissance*, pp. 303–5; Hembry, *English Spa*, pp. 136–7; Langford, *Polite and Commercial People*, pp. 48–9, 127; McIntyre, 'Bath', p. 238; Neale, *Bath*, p. 28.
50. McLynn, *Crime*, pp. 244–6. See also Langford, *Public Life*, pp. 462–3.
51. D.W. Bebbington, *Evangelicalism in Modern Britain: A History from the 1730s to the 1980s* (London: Unwin Hyman, 1989), pp. 10–12, 36, 42–63. See also Cragg, *Church*, pp. 153–6; David Hempton, *Methodism and Politics in British Society 1750–1850* (London: Hutchinson, 1984), pp. 22–8; Alec R. Vidler, *The Church in an Age of Revolution*, repr. (Harmondsworth: Penguin Books, 1990), pp. 36–40.
52. Mary Chandler, *The Description of Bath: A Poem Humbly Inscribed to Her Royal Highness the Princess Amelia, with Several Other Poems*, 6th edn (London and Bath: James Leake, 1744), p. 4.
53. This phrase was used by Charles Wesley. See Bruce Crofts (ed.), *At Satan's Throne: The Story of Methodism in Bath over 250 Years* (Bristol: White Tree Books, 1990), p. 13.
54. John Wesley, *The Journal of John Wesley*, ed. Nehemiah Curnock, 8 vols (London: Charles H. Kelly, undated), vol. 2, pp. 211–12.
55. Crofts (ed.), *At Satan's Throne*, pp. 16, 20, 22, 24, 31–3, 45.
56. Wesley, *Journal*, vol. 4, p. 138.
57. *DNB*, vol. 1, p. 311.

58. Wood, *Bath*, pp. 274–5. See also *Bath and Bristol Guide*, p. 17.
59. Romney Sedgwick, *The House of Commons 1715–1754*, 2 vols (London: HMSO, 1970), vol. 1: *Introductory Survey, Constituencies and Members A–D*, p. 528.
60. Falconer, *Mineral Water Hospital*, p. 11; Bryan Little, *Selina: Countess of Huntingdon* (Bath: Huntingdon Centre, 1989), p. 5.
61. Vincent J. Liesenfeld, *The Licensing Act of 1737* (Madison: University of Wisconsin Press, 1987), pp. 28–30, 124, 138. Jekyll was also involved in the regulation of gin consumption. William Pulteney, who laid the foundation-stone of the General Hospital, opposed his proposals – albeit on economic rather than moral grounds. See *DNB*, vol. 29, p. 288; Lee Davison, 'Experiments in the Social Regulation of Industry: Gin Legislation, 1729–1751', in L. Davison, T. Hitchcock, T. Keirn and R.B. Shoemaker (eds), *Stilling the Grumbling Hive: The Response to Social and Economic Problems in England 1689–1750* (Stroud: Alan Sutton, 1992), pp. 29, 33, 34.
62. *Proposals for a National Reformation of Manners* (1694), quoted in Shoemaker, 'Reforming the City', p. 101.
63. Wood, *Bath*, p. 288.
64. John Brown, *On the Pursuit of False Pleasure, and the Mischiefs of Immoderate Gaming* (Bath: James Leake, 1750), pp. 8–9.
65. Brown, *False Pleasure*, pp. 1–2.
66. Andrew, *Philanthropy and Police*, p. 14.
67. Dalton, *Religious Use*, pp. 17–8.
68. Leyborne, *Charity Conducive*, p. 26. See also Dalton, *Religious Use*, p. 18. The committee of the Leicester Infirmary put this case, faced with financial difficulties in 1792:

    > May not the opulent manufacturers, with the greatest propriety be called upon to support this noble edifice, which opens wide its doors for the reception of those very poor, by whose labours *they* are enriched? For to whom may the infirm and diseased artificers look up for aid, with so much reason, as to those, in whose service they have spent their strength?

    See Frizelle and Martin, *Leicester Royal Infirmary*, p. 70.
69. For more detailed discussion of the relationship between civilization and disease, see Roy Porter, 'Civilization and Disease: Medical Ideology in the Enlightenment', in Jeremy Black and Jeremy Gregory (eds), *Culture, Politics and Society in Britain 1660–1800* (Manchester: Manchester University Press, 1991); Roy Porter, 'Reforming the Patient in the Age of Reform: Thomas Beddoes and Medical Practice', in R. French and A. Weir (eds), *British Medicine in an Age of Reform* (London: Routledge, 1991).
70. Warburton, *Sermon* [1742], pp. 20–22. See also Dalton, *Religious Use*, pp. 17–18; Leyborne, *Charity Conducive*, p. 26.
71. Bayly, *Sermon*, pp. 15, 18.
72. Dalton, *Religious Use*, pp. 16–17.
73. Brown, *False Pleasure*, p. 20.
74. Leyborne, *Charity Conducive*, pp. 29–30. See also Bayly, *Sermon*, p. 7; Olive, *Particular Excellence*, p. i.

75. Leyborne, *Charity Conducive*, pp. 35–6.
76. Brown, *False Pleasure*, pp. 16–17. See also p. 21.
77. Bayly, *Sermon*, pp. 13–14, 20–22.
78. Schama, *Embarrassment*, pp. 327–8.
79. Andrew, *Philanthropy and Police*, pp. 21, 36, 38; Baugh, 'Poverty', p. 73; W.S. Lewis and Ralph M. Williams, *Private Charity in England, 1747–1757* (New Haven: Yale University Press, 1938), p. 11; Porter, 'Gift Relation', p. 162. For a discussion of sensibility in relation to the Royal Humane Society, see Carolyn D. Williams, '"The Luxury of Doing Good": Benevolence, Sensibility and the Royal Humane Society', in Roy Porter and Marie Mulvey Roberts (eds), *Pleasure in the Eighteenth Century* (London: Macmillan, 1996), pp. 77–107.
80. Minute Book, 16 February 1738, 'Plan and Elevation'.
81. *DNB*, vol. 2, 38–9; Falconer, *Mineral Water Hospital*, pp. 44–6.
82. Murch, *Biographical Sketches*, p. 246. Similar sentimental stanzas on benevolence and charity were published in the local press. See *Bath Journal*, 16 January 1786.
83. Minute Book, 14 December 1785.
84. *Improved Bath Guide*, pp. 95–6.
85. *Manners and Morals, Hogarth and British Painting 1700–1760*, introduced by Elizabeth Einberg (London: Tate Gallery, 1987), pp. 15–16. See also David Bindman, *Hogarth* (London: Thames and Hudson, 1981), pp. 167, 178, 180, 183.
86. Winton Dean, *Handel* (London: Macmillan, 1982), pp. 55–6.
87. John Brewer, *The Pleasures of the Imagination: English Culture in the Eighteenth Century* (London: HarperCollins, 1997).
88. Barrell, *Political Theory*, pp. 11, 16; Borsay, *English Urban Renaissance*, pp. 265–6; Simon McVeigh, *Concert Life in London from Mozart to Haydn* (Cambridge: Cambridge University Press, 1993), pp. 36–7.
89. *Bath Journal*, 23 December 1751.
90. Mark 12: 31.
91. Andrew, *Philanthropy and Police*, pp. 15, 22; Baugh, 'Poverty', pp. 73–4; Robert M. Page, *Altruism and the British Welfare State* (Aldershot: Avebury, 1996), p. 17; Alec Pemberton, 'Rescuing the Good Samaritan: An Exposition and Defence of the Samaritan Principle in the Welfare State', *Journal of Social Policy*, 19 (1990), pp. 281, 287–8; Porter, 'Gift Relation', p. 162.
92. Warburton, *Sermon* [1742], p. 15.
93. Cartwright, *Social History of Medicine*, p. 21.
94. Bayly, *Sermon*, p. 19.
95. Dalton, *Religious Use*, pp. 16–17.
96. Brown, *False Pleasure*, pp. 5, 19–20.
97. Bayly, *Sermon*, pp. 18–19.
98. John Brown was a well-known critic of superficial politeness, authoring both an essay on the Earl of Shaftesbury and a popular *Estimate of the Manners and Principles of the Times*. See *DNB*, vol. 7, p. 11. Isaac Maddox and John Waugh, preaching for the Worcester Infirmary in 1748 and 1752 respectively, likewise argued that charity was a source of enduring pleasure. See McMenemey, *Worcester Royal Infirmary*, pp. 53, 111.
99. Brown, *False Pleasure*, pp. 3–7, 9–10, 16–17, 21.

100. Hunter, *Ameliorated Condition*, pp. 9, 11, 14, 16–18, 22, 24.
101. Brewer, *Pleasures*, pp. 120–22. The emergence of harsher attitudes to the poor and their implications for the administration of charity are considered in Chapter 7.
102. Hunter, *Ameliorated Condition*, pp. 10–12, 20, 23, 25.
103. *DNB*, vol. 48, p. 426.
104. Hunter, *Ameliorated Condition*, pp. 6–7.
105. Louis Simond, *An American in Regency England: The Journal of a Tour in 1810–1811*, ed. Christopher Hibbert (London: Robert Maxwell, 1968), p. 20.
106. *The Letters of Hannah More*, ed. R. Brimley Johnson (London: John Lane, 1925), p. 80.
107. Trevor Fawcett (ed.), *Voices of Eighteenth-Century Bath: An Anthology* (Bath: Ruton, 1995), p. 138.
108. Wilson, 'Shropshire lady', p. 101.
109. Graham Davis, 'Entertainments in Georgian Bath: Gambling and Vice', *Bath History*, 1 (1986), pp. 12–13.
110. Mainwaring, *Annals*, p. 262. A late nineteenth-century commentator similarly observed that with a permanent population came 'the influx of men of large minds and cultured intelligence' who improved the quality of municipal government. See King, 'Bath', pp. 90–91.
111. *Improved Bath Guide*, p. 45. See also *The New Bath Directory* (Bath: J. Browne, 1805), p. 146.
112. Cragg, *Church*, pp. 153–6; Vidler, *Church*, pp. 36–41; Fawcett and Bird, *Bath*, pp. 79–80; Davis and Bonsall, *Bath*, p. 63.
113. Roy Porter has drawn a similar distinction between guilt and pleasure. See Porter, 'Gift Relation', pp. 162–3.
114. John Dalton, *A Sermon Preached ... Before the Governors of the Middlesex Hospital* (London: John Whiston, Benjamin White and S. Baker, 1751), pp. 9–11.
115. Dalton, *Religious Use*, pp. 5–7. Similarly, William Warburton, who maintained in his Bath sermon that justice required the better off to assist the sick poor, articulated no such obligation when he preached on behalf of the London Smallpox Hospital. See Warburton, *Sermon* [1742], p. 20; William Warburton, *A Sermon Preached Before ... Governors of the Hospital for Smallpox* (London: H. Woodfall, 1755).
116. Andrew, *Philanthropy and Police*, p. 88.
117. Donna T. Andrew, 'On Reading Charity Sermons: Eighteenth-Century Anglican Solicitation and Exhortation', *Journal of Ecclesiastical History*, 43 (1992), p. 586.

CHAPTER SEVEN

From Mercantilism to *Laissez-Faire*

In the last chapter, we traced the weakening of paternalist obligation over the long eighteenth century, tying the growth of charity as a voluntary expression of civility to the displacement of civic humanism by a polite code of moral sensibility and the shift from mercantilism to a *laissez-faire* philosophy. But as well as underwriting the decline of the tributary relationship, the economic individualism of Adam Smith both snapped the connection between population and prosperity which had been central to later mercantilist thought, and encouraged a confidence in the capacity of the market to meet all needs. The combined effect was to leave the poor wide open to moral disapprobation at a time when traditional paternalism was retreating. In Chapter 7, we consider the consequences of these developments for the Georgian Bath Infirmary. First, the application of economic ideas is explored with reference to the mortality and morbidity of patients, and their age, sex and family characteristics. Secondly, the impact of economic individualism is assessed, taking into account the changing nature of philanthropy and the ability of the General Hospital to come to terms with this new charitable environment. The chapter concludes by pulling together themes from economic and ethical thought to sketch a moral economy of Georgian medicine.

Population, health and prosperity

The protectionist features of mercantilism dominated economic thinking from the late-sixteenth to the mid-eighteenth centuries, but the post-Restoration period witnessed a move away from the initial focus on bullion and currency towards an emphasis on the role of industry and employment in the generation of wealth. Under this scenario, population acquired unprecedented prominence. Mere numbers, a political asset in international affairs, were also linked to prosperity through the size of the workforce, each pair of hands adding concrete worth to the national product.[1] In John Bellers' words: 'Regularly labouring people are the Kingdom's greatest treasure and strength, for without labourers there can be no lords; and if the poor labourers did not raise much more food and manufacture than what did subsist themselves, every gentleman must be a labourer and every idle man must starve.'[2] Paradoxically, this new 'social mercantilism' coincided with demographic stagnation. A slackening in the rate of increase between 1650 and 1750, allied to high mortality in the second quarter of the eighteenth century, led to population expansion of just half a million. In contrast, growth during the preceding century had been in excess of two millions. Furthermore, when the death rate began to abate during the 1740s, international instability continued to arouse demographic anxieties, French forces far outstripping British military personnel.[3] Extant pamphlet literature, such as the *Essay or ... Modest Proposal ... to Increase the Number of People and Consequently the Strength of the Kingdom* (1693), confirm contemporary worry about population size.[4] However, it was the inflation of real wages between 1660 and 1740 that imposed itself most forcefully; for according to the mercantilist philosophy, demographic pressure was crucial, not just to enhance economic output but also to restrain wage levels and to ensure industry rather than indolence among the workforce.[5]

Although the Hanoverians responded to their perceived population problem with a variety of initiatives which included workhouses and charity schools,[6] medicine was particularly relevant to the concerns of social mercantilism. First, ill health squandered poor relief, leaving sick workers and their families dependent at a time when the bill for state assistance had been rising sharply.[7] Equally supportive of medicine was the tradition of political arithmetic which from the later sixteenth century began to seek legitimation for charitable and statutory intervention in measures of 'social utility'.[8] The Scientific Revolution nourished this science of society. Therefore, by the early 1700s, the economic costs of disease and premature death were well appreciated. As John Bellers estimated, 'a hundred thousand ... die yearly of curable diseases; for want of timely advice, and suitable medicines'. 'Every able industrious labourer', he went on, 'that is capable to have children, who so untimely dies, may be accounted two hundred pounds loss to the kingdom.'[9] The voluntary hospital was put forward as one means of staunching this wastage of national resources, thereby gearing the Enlightenment faith in medical progress to the achievement of economic advance.[10] At Bath, publicity granted a conspicuous place to the creation of healthy workers supporting families emancipated from poor relief. Consequently, the text of the 1738 'Plan and Elevation' stressed the restoration of future patients 'from misery to ease, from impotence to strength, and from beggary and want, to a capacity of getting an honest livelihood, and comfortable subsistence'. Few parishes escaped those who ' by the loss of their limbs, are ... a burden to themselves and their neighbours'. Yet most overseers preferred an indefinite 'small allowance at home' and were unwilling or unable to pay for such 'poor cripples' to stay privately at Bath 'long enough to receive a cure'. With the Infirmary in operation, the trustees believed that this difficulty would be overcome. Upon payment of their caution money, long-term dependants would receive, free of charge, the unique assistance of the spa; and if their health revived as a result, they might once more become 'profitable to the public'.[11] Charity sermons also tapped into this theme, powerfully evoking the plight of the sick poor man and his relatives. 'Figure to yourselves', beseeched the Reverend John Brown, preaching at Bath Abbey in 1750:

> an industrious family, once maintained in decency by a father's labour, and a mother's care, but now reduced to penury, by an inflicting distemper fallen on him, who was late its comfort and support: By your timely generosity he partakes of these medicinal waters, and returns home, blessed with health and strength. Could this world afford you a sincerer pleasure than to see his smiling infants welcome his happy return, and bless and pray for the generous hand that had restored their fond parent to his health, and enabled him once more to provide them with their daily bread?[12]

Propaganda emanating from voluntary hospitals, old and new, preserved elements of the mercantilist rationale beyond the mid-century drift towards *laissez-faire*. There are several reasons. The soaring cost of poor relief, which more than doubled between 1748 and 1775, and almost quadrupled between 1785 and 1817,[13] ensured that the financial burden of sickness remained an acute anxiety not exclusive to mercantilism. The economic benefits of a fit and healthy workforce also retained their force. '[T]he flourishing state of this nation is derived from the labours of the poor', argued the *Annual Report* of the Manchester Infirmary in 1777/78, 'and ... these labours depend greatly upon the health and strength which these useful members of the community enjoy'.[14] After 1750, however, population growth began to ease the wage pressure which had especially awakened the Hanoverians' demographic disquiet;[15] and from the 1770s that growth, running at 6.5 per cent per decade in the 50 years after 1740, was increasingly regarded more as a symptom than a cause of national prosperity, beneficial only if based on sound economic foundations.[16] Therefore, the mercantilist link between population and prosperity was severed as it became recognized that, in the words of an 1816 report from the Huddersfield Dispensary, 'the genuine Wealth of Nations consists not more in a numerous than in a healthy population'.[17] Medical charities at Bath were not exempt from this reorientation of economic thinking. Thus, the broadsheet announcing the foundation of the City Infirmary and Dispensary in 1792, whilst noting that 'many lives are lost by the want of a proper asylum to receive the sick-poor', did not go on to construe these deaths as a drain on national prosperity. Furthermore, preventing financial dependency was given precedence over treating illness:

> by affording early and effectual medical relief to the heads of families, and to other persons by whose labour numbers are supported, not only diseases are shortened and lives saved; but that whole families may be prevented from becoming a burden on their respective parishes, and thus the pecuniary charges upon the occupiers of houses in those parishes would be eventually diminished.[18]

Poor relief was not only a preoccupation for the City Infirmary and Dispensary. In its entry for the General Hospital, *The Improved Bath Guide* of 1812 likewise drew attention to 'the happy effects [for parishes] of this benevolent institution, in the restoration of many of their most useful inhabitants from a state of the utmost misery and decrepitude to perfect health and vigour'.[19] But how justified was this bold claim of clinical efficacy? And to what extent was the transfer from mercantilism to *laissez-faire* reflected in the economic rationale of the Infirmary?

Mortality and morbidity

The need to use home-grown statistics stipulates a wary approach to the assessment of mortality and morbidity because institutions reliant upon voluntary contributions, and hence keen to project a curative image, may have been tempted to 'cook the books', whether by discharging patients on the brink of death or by exaggerating the extent to which their health had benefited.[20] At Bath, it is possible that the virtual disappearance of the 'incurable' category during the third quarter of the eighteenth century, and the contemporaneous increase in the number of cases deemed 'improper', may have reflected a reluctance to concede that after appropriate medical consultation any ailment failed to improve with spa therapy.[21] When the Hospital published a *Narrative on the Efficacy of the Bath Waters* in 1787, however, it naturally stressed the sincerity with which treatment outcomes were determined. Before being presented to the weekly committee, patients ready for discharge were examined by their own physician and by the medical faculty as a whole. Physicians were instructed to be conservative in their judgements:

> In order that the effects of the waters may not be magnified or misrepresented ... it is a rule with the physicians never to set down any patient as *cured*, whilst he has any degree of the disorder for which he was admitted remaining; if the slightest degree be left, he is only set down as *much better*. None are ever discharged as *much*

> *better,* unless their amendment be very considerable. In doubtful cases, it is usual to attribute too little, rather than too much, to the efficacy of the waters.[22]

Clinical records for the early years of the Infirmary allow us to make comparisons with the patient statistics published in the *Annual Reports*: a series which, like the financial accounts, ran from 1 May to 30 April. Two clinical documents survive: an Admissions Register for 1742 to 1752 with 1 643 entries, and a Casebook containing 1 618 annotated letters of recommendation for patients admitted between 1750 and 1758. Whereas the Register was an official document defined by the Hospital rules as a complete list of all patients,[23] the status of the Casebook is unclear. For the overlapping years from 1750 to 1752, it was far from comprehensive. Whether the selection was deliberate or arbitrary is nowhere specified, but even if the eight-month gap which separates the first and second entries is ignored, the number of inmates included in the Casebook was just 44 per cent of those listed in the Admissions Register. Therefore, only the Admissions Register has been used for the comparative exercise (Table 7.1). The Register recorded fewer discharges because the last entry is dated 10 May 1752 and so both the final year, and 1751/52, are incomplete. Generally speaking, however, the divergence between the two sets of figures is small enough to attribute either to clerical error or to the missing Register entries. Although the *Annual Reports* recorded a slightly higher death rate, they described patients as 'no better' less frequently and applied the label 'great benefit' with more liberality than the Register used the classification 'much better'. Semantic differences – albeit with public relations advantages – may partly explain this last inconsistency, especially since it practically disappears when patients who improved after treatment are added to those receiving considerable benefit. The higher proportion of patients whom the *Annual Reports* log as leaving at their own request may be due to smallpox cases in the latter part of 1752.[24] The relatively minor nature of these discrepancies, when allied to the disclosure of significant performance variations in *Annual Reports* throughout the Georgian period, suggest that routine records were not massaged in a sustained and systematic way to misrepresent the Hospital's therapeutic impact.

The broad integrity of patient statistics for Bath warrants their application to an analysis of mortality and morbidity. Mortality levels at the General Infirmary do not support McKeown and Brown's thesis that voluntary hospitals were 'gateways to death' during the eighteenth century.[25] The published annual death rate at five-yearly intervals between 1742 and 1759 averaged 4.5 per cent (Table 7.2), ranging from a high of 6.01 per cent in 1750/51 to a low of 2.95 in 1755/56 (Appendix A). After

Table 7.1 Bath General Hospital: the condition of patients at discharge, 1742–52

(a) Admissions Register

	Patients discharged 1742–52	
Condition at discharge	No.	%
Cured	364	22.15
Much better	340	20.69
Better	364	22.15
Little better	24	1.46
No better	126	7.67
Incurable	137	8.34
Dead	61	3.71
Improper	87	5.30
Hectical	14	0.85
At own request	16	0.97
Misbehaviour	14	0.85
Other	10	0.61
Unrecorded	86	5.23
Total	1 643	100.00

(b) Annual Reports

	Patients discharged 1742–52	
Condition at discharge	No.	%
Cured	424	24.37
Great benefit	793	45.57
Better	—	—
No better	22	1.26
Incurable	142	8.16
Dead	77	4.43
Improper	125	7.18
Hectical	—	—
At own request	142	8.16
Misbehaviour	11	0.63
Eloped	4	0.23
Total	1 740	100.00

Note: Percentages have been rounded up or down and so do not always total exactly 100.00.

Sources: Admissions Register; *Annual Reports*.

Table 7.2 Bath General Hospital: the condition of patients at discharge, 1742–59 and 1760–1830

(a) 1742–59 (five-yearly samples)

Condition at discharge	*Patients discharged* No.	%
Cured	191	27.72
Great benefit	243	35.27
Better	37	5.37
No better	17	2.47
Incurable	52	7.55
Dead	31	4.50
Improper	33	4.79
Hectical	3	0.44
At own request	71	10.30
Misbehaviour	9	1.31
Eloped	2	0.29
Total	689	100.00

(b) 1760–1830 (five-yearly samples)

Condition at discharge	*Patients discharged* No.	%
Cured	1 334	28.91
Much better	2 291	49.65
Incurable	258	5.59
Improper	576	12.48
Irregular	49	1.06
Dead	106	2.30
Total	4 614	100.00

Note: Percentages have been rounded up or down and so do not always total exactly 100.00.

Source: *Annual Reports*.

1760 the figures were compiled in a more standarized format. Quinquennial analysis of these later returns up to 1830 indicates that hospital mortality remained low, averaging a mere 2.3 per cent in the sample years (Table 7.2) and peaking at 5.78 per cent in 1805/06 (Appendix A). This experience matches that of other provincial infirmaries, where generally under 10 per cent of patients died in residence; at Shrewsbury and Liverpool, for example, where institutions opened in the later 1740s, inmate mortality only rarely exceeded seven per cent over the long eighteenth century.[26] It seems that the continuation of spa therapy at Bath, without major surgical intervention, did not lead to significantly lower mortality after 1800. In the absence of reliable local statistics or national data disaggregated according to age and sex, these deaths in hospital cannot be related to general demographic trends; nor is this a very meaningful exercise, given that inmates were a distinctive group by virtue of their ill health.[27] What can be evaluated is the thesis that voluntary infirmaries boosted the population. Even at the turn of the century, there were only an estimated 4 000 hospital beds available country-wide: too few to make a noticeable mark.[28] As a result, diet, sanitation, housing, epidemiological change and the development of other medical facilities all exerted more influence in the mortality matrix.[29] Added to these factors is the dominant thrust of fertility in Georgian demography; Wrigley and Schofield may have misjudged the importance of improving background death rates, but their overall conclusion that earlier and more frequent marriage fired population change is still intact.[30] For these reasons, voluntary hospitals, if not the death-traps that their critics alleged, contributed little to demographic expansion.

Over and above population growth, medical care pursued the more effective use of existing labour. Idleness among the poor, who constituted the great bulk of the workforce, was regarded with particular alarm, whether its cause was ill health or moral turpitude. Consequently, infirmaries were welcomed as a vehicle for returning the sick poor to physical and moral fitness. The moral reform of the masses will be considered in Chapter 10; at this juncture, we turn to morbidity. The extent to which the Bath Hospital healed its patients is difficult to gauge. Between 1742 and 1759, the *Annual Reports* recorded cures for 27.72 per cent of inmates (Table 7.2), the yearly level generally ranging from a fifth to a third. The average for the sample years after 1760 was slightly higher at 28.91per cent (Table 7.2) and the variation was also less pronounced with figures rarely dropping below a quarter. That these treatment outcomes compare unfavourably with those of sister institutions vouches for their essential accuracy: the Salop Infirmary normally reported a minimum success rate of 50 per cent; while at Liverpool eight out of ten patients were regularly described as cured, at least until the second decade of the nineteenth century.[31] However, the term 'cured' is itself misleading because in the context of Georgian medicine it implied reverting to a healthy equilibrium rather than mending a defective organ or bodily function.[32] Therefore, combining the 'cured' and 'relieved' categories makes sense, particularly for spa therapy which rested on holistic principles. Only when this is done does the proportion of patients emerging from the Bath Hospital with some improvement in their health climb to over 70 per cent (Table 7.2).

The Bath governors were conscious that their institution offered more relief than cure and attempted to offset criticism in publicity material. Their case rested on the position of the spa as a place of last resort for chronic disorders. During the 1740s and 1750s, the accounts of the Infirmary attached to printed charity sermons pointed out that: 'we have few persons sent to us but such as labour under leprosies, palsies, old inveterate rheumatisms or lameness, many of them contracted long ago'. Physicians were appealed to: they knew 'how difficult of cure these distempers are in their most recent state'; but how much more stubborn they were rendered when the administration of the waters was delayed until 'all [other] methods have been tried upon them'.[33] From 1760/61, the *Annual Report* picked up this message, informing contributors that the 'objects' of 'this useful charity' were 'very frequently those miserable patients who have been discharged from other Hospitals, as not to be relieved, or incurable'. The matter resurfaced in the 1780s. Not only did leaflets designed to raise money from parishes and charity services stress the 'happy effects of the Bath waters, in relieving various disorders incident to mankind, when all other means have proved ineffectual',[34] but a statement was added to the *Annual Report*, specifying the number of patients who had benefited at Bath after being dismissed as incurable from other infirmaries.[35] The mid-century Admissions Register and the Casebook substantiate the chronic disease profile of patients at the General Hospital. Approximately 70 per cent of cases listed in each document were suffering from rheumatism, paralysis, or another musculoskeletal or neurological disability, while one in ten had skin complaints (Table 7.3). The *Annual Reports*, which after 1760 classified discharges according to clinical condition as well as degree of improvement, confirm that a similar pattern prevailed up to 1830. Though there were differences between the sample years, over the seventy-year period in its entirety rheumatism and paralysis both accounted for a quarter of all patients; lameness for 15 per cent; and leprosy, 'hip cases' and colica pictonum for 10 per cent each (Table 7.4).

The letters of recommendation contained in the Casebook put flesh on these bare bones, its personal histories illustrating how ineffective treatment caused patients to run the gauntlet of medical care. Both unorthodox and regular practitioners were consulted. James Willcox, aged 16, had 'for about two years since been afflicted with a stiffness and pain in the locking of the left hip, without the least swelling or dislocation'. His family had 'applied to some good old woman, in the neighbourhood [of Hentland in Herefordshire], but without success'.[36]

Table 7.3 Bath General Hospital: the disease profile of patients, 1742–59

Disease category	*Admissions Register (1742–52)* No.	%	*Casebook (1750–59)* No.	%
Genitourinary diseases	5	0.30	4	0.25
Surgical infections	26	1.58	23	1.42
Diseases of the digestive system	65	3.96	71	4.39
Musculoskeletal disorders				
Rheumatism	245	14.91	251	15.50
Sciatica	28	1.70	27	1.67
Hip cases	59	3.59	42	2.59
Contraction	26	1.58	34	2.10
Weakness/lameness	158	9.62	150	9.26
Other musculoskeletal disorders	82	4.99	67	4.14
Neurological and mental disorders				
Paralysis/palsy	293	17.83	193	11.92
Hemiplegia	62	3.77	127	7.84
Epilepsy, etc.	7	0.43	3	0.19
Lost the use of limbs/numbness	124	7.55	234	14.45
Other neurological/mental disorders	42	2.55	50	3.09
Traumatic conditions	8	0.49	17	1.05
Skin diseases	167	10.16	192	11.86
Scrofula	7	0.43	2	0.12
Tumours	4	0.24	4	0.25
Miscellaneous conditions	43	2.61	19	1.17
Unclassified	192	11.69	109	6.73
Total	1 643	100.00	1 619	100.00

Note:

1. The disease categories used in this table are based on the adaptation of William Cullen's nosology developed in Chapter 3 of Guenter B. Risse, *Hospital Life in Enlightenment Scotland: Care and Teaching at the Royal Infirmary of Edinburgh* (Cambridge: Cambridge University Press, 1986). Muscoloskeletal and neurological disorders have been broken down to accommodate the clinical profile of Bath patients. Given the briefness of entries in the Admissions Register and the variable nature of the medical recommendations in the Casebook, the outcome of the exercise is inevitably tentative.
2. Percentages have been rounded up or down and so do not always total exactly 100.00.

Sources: Admissions Register; Casebook.

Table 7.4 Bath General Hospital: the disease profile of patients, 1760–1830 (five-yearly samples)

Disease category	*No.*	%
Rheumatic	1 236	26.79
Paralytic	1 215	26.33
Lameness	675	14.63
Leprosy	484	10.49
Colica pictonum	452	9.80
Hip cases	430	9.32
Distorted vertebrae	96	2.08
Biliary/visceral/jaundice	26	0.56
Total	4 614	100.00

Note: According to eighteenth-century nosology, leprosy was a generic term which covered a variety of skin conditions. Colica pictonum was a form of lead poisoning where paralysis was accompanied by gastro-intestinal pain, fever, vomiting and costiveness. The hip case was a rheumatic condition in which the joint and its surrounding muscles became stiff and painful.

Source: *Annual Reports*.

Southampton resident, Thomas Phillips, in middle age 'troubled with a nervous weakness which appears to threaten a palsy', had 'spent the greatest part of his substance upon quacks to no purpose';[37] while Richard Orpwood of Ardington in Berkshire had turned to the sea:

> about forty years of age, [he] has for four years been afflicted with an asthmatical complaint, proceeding ... from a scorbutic habit which formerly shewed itself on the surface of the skin ... he has taken many medicines by Dr Pitt's advice and last summer drank and bathed in sea water, which greatly relieved him for the time, but since the disuse of it his complaints are the same.[38]

Water was blamed for the condition of Silvanus Blackbourn, a 41 year old ex-mariner. After falling asleep on board ship in wet clothing, he had

> caught an ague and fever which held him at different times for near a year, with violent flying pains in every part of his body and limbs. By the use of the bark he got rid of his ague but his pains still continue. He has been under the care of several physicians in the country for two years past and was in St Thomas' Hospital for two months without receiving much benefit.[39]

Another London institution had discharged William Thomas, a young man 'jammed between the seat of a caravan and the gateway of the Bell

Inn, Holborn ... by which accident he was very much bruised in the small of his back, his hips and thighs. He was immediately conveyed to St Bartholomew's Hospital: there, he remained 25 weeks and then was turned out as by then deemed incurable. Yet', concluded the apothecary writing the medical report, 'they recommended his case to the use of the Bath'.[40]

Silvanus Blackbourn and William Thomas were not alone among the Casebook patients in having prior encounters with other infirmaries. One in ten letters mentioned contact with a medical institution and in 68 cases there was a direct referral. Whilst appreciating that the spa was the remedy to be tried when all else had failed, the governors of the Bath Hospital propounded the therapeutic rationale of their institution and challenged the assumption that it was a hostel for the hopeless. First and foremost, the admissions policy guarded against the injustice of 'letting an incurable eat the bread of one who might find a cure'.[41] Since donors and subscribers obtained no sponsorship rights and prospective patients submitted details of their ailments drawn up by a neighbourhood 'physician or person of skill', the honorary physicians and surgeons were spared the pressure of lay patronage and so empowered – in theory if not in practice – to select only those cases receptive to the healing qualities of the Bath waters.[42] Once admitted, residence could be protracted. Whereas most hospitals usually discharged their patients after two or three months unless there were exceptional circumstances,[43] the General Infirmary was initially flexible and then introduced a six-month rule from 1747.[44] The mid-century Admissions Register and the Casebook record mean stays of 149.54 and 133.66 days respectively – longer than the 43 days clocked up by the average near-contemporary patient at the Bristol Infirmary, or even the 105 days at Northampton.[45] Though the 1787 *Narrative* on clinical efficacy maintained that 'Much the greatest part of those who received a cure, or any considerable benefit, remained in the house from three to nine months and upwards',[46] this assertion has to be questioned in the light of evidence from the earlier Register and Casebook (Table 7.5). Most patients in the shortest category of stay were indeed unlikely to show major improvement and some six out of ten were dismissed as 'improper' for spa therapy. Eight to ten months was also the optimum period for receiving benefit, but after 40 days there was no straightforward correlation between length of residence and treatment outcome. Shorter stays are implied by the higher annual turnover of patients in the third decade of the nineteenth century when the number of beds in commission was constant: in the sample years between 1760 and 1820, an average of 296 were discharged from (or died in) the Hospital annually; in 1825 and 1830, the throughput was over 380.[47] From an

Table 7.5 Bath General Hospital: length of stay and condition at discharge, 1742–59

	Admissions Register (1742–52)						*Casebook (1750–59)*					
	Cured		*Much better*		*Cured or much better*		*Cured*		*Much better*		*Cured or much better*	
Length of stay (days)	No.	%	No.	%	No.	%	No.	%	No.	%	No.	%
1–40	16	8.47	11	5.82	27	14.29	30	17.05	8	4.55	38	21.60
41–80	67	25.38	41	15.53	108	40.91	73	29.56	34	13.77	107	43.33
81–120	80	32.39	41	16.60	121	48.99	72	28.13	60	23.44	132	51.57
121–160	64	28.44	52	23.11	116	51.55	71	30.87	72	31.30	143	62.17
161–200	43	20.48	55	26.19	98	46.67	50	25.64	83	42.56	133	68.20
201–240	28	18.42	53	34.87	81	53.29	31	22.30	54	38.85	85	61.15
241–280	31	30.39	30	29.41	61	59.80	24	24.00	52	52.00	76	76.00
280 +	35	20.35	57	33.14	92	53.49	30	21.74	65	47.10	95	68.84
Total	364		340		704		381		428		809	

Sources: Admissions Register; Casebook.

early stage, however, publicity material underlined that patients were dismissed 'as soon as the physicians and surgeons tell they can receive no further benefit'.[48] More than that, they were frequently released 'quite restored or greatly relieved',[49] as was 'apparent from the many crutches left behind' by those who 'without the benefit of the Hospital, would have had for many tedious years only an uncomfortable, useless existence'.[50]

Age, sex and family status

The extent to which patients took up 'useful' employment upon return to the community is impossible to tell because there was no follow-up procedure. However, the Casebook letters, together with the age-sex characteristics which they and the Admissions Register reveal, intimate that at mid-century the Hospital was able to retain a therapeutic image and hence use the rehabilitation of the sick poor to legitimate a mercantilist ideology. Medical recommendations despatched to the Bath Infirmary were expected to enumerate patients' symptoms and specify their sex.[51] In a number of letters, however, information designed to strengthen the application complemented the basic ingredients. Among these embellishments was mention of the effects of ill health for socio-economic function at work and at home, volunteered in nearly 10 per cent of cases. Sickness had already driven some applicants from their occupations and reduced them to poverty. Robert Gilman, for example, aged 57, from Grosvenor Mews in London, had 'long been afflicted with the gout and rheumatism ... and disabled ... from following his employment which is that of a coachman'.[52] Likewise, Newton Highhorn, a 20-year-old printer from Bloomsbury, had been 'greatly afflicted with the colic or dry gripes and has so far lost the use of his hands as to be disabled from working at his trade or earning his bread'.[53] In other instances, the prevention of economic inactivity was used to plea for admission. Nineteen-year-old Richard Uddal from Netherbury in Dorset had 'for 2 or 3 years laboured under great weakness and relaxation of the right knee attended with violent pains and crookedness of the joint ... as he is poor in circumstances he is likely to be deprived of the means of subsistence unless the Bath afford him relief'.[54] The exceptional nature of the patient's current ailments was used to affirm the potential for such benefit. John Bryers, a middle-aged man from Hanover Square in London, was 'in perfect health' before being 'seized on a sudden' with St Vitus' Dance;[55] Abraham Woods, aged 23 from Swallowfield in Berkshire, had 'enjoyed a very good state of health till last summer ... when being heated with exercise and in a very great sweat imprudently went into the river the consequences of which was a violent fever which ended in a scorbutic eruption all over him';[56] while applicants like the teenager, Ann Brown of Stalbridge in Dorset, were described as of a robust constitution. Apart from losing the use of her legs, she was 'in other respects in perfect health, eats, digests and sleeps as well as ever, and has her monthly periods regularly'. In the opinion of her medical sponsor, 'She will in all likelihood find relief from bathing, drinking the waters and your good assistance'.[57]

Though the Bath Infirmary openly expressed its commitment to rendering the sick poor productive for the community, the age and gender implications of this mission were not acknowledged. As the Casebook demonstrates, however, family dynamics intruded the application process. First, letters of recommendation reflected the centrality of the male breadwinner to the household economy. John Wilkins had 'lately been seized with a stroke of the palsy which has deprived him of the use of one of his arms ... [and] rendered him incapable of assisting his family which consists of a wife and five small children'.[58] James Nash of Nublegin in Somerset, aged 41, was a widower supporting 'himself and three young children by renting £37 per annum'. He had 'lost the use of his hands, by a fit of the colic; [and] he and his children must soon be on the parish if he can't get the use of his hands restored'.[59] Marital status featured more commonly in applications for women, an indication of how far their 'work rhythms were ... determined ... by individual biological and social events such as marriage, motherhood, and widowhood'.[60] Depicting Elizabeth Fry of Wells as a widow[61] or Frances Leadbetter of Long Compton in Warwickshire as a spinster[62] thus flagged their financial vulnerability in the face of illness. However, socio-economic responsibilities for kin were also deployed in the cause of female patients. For example, the letter recommending an adolescent from Brecon called Mary Williams not only noted that for three years she herself had 'been altogether sickly and incapable of doing any work', but observed that her mother too was 'greatly afflicted with scurvy and rheumatism'.[63] The incumbrance of an incapacitated wife was also articulated. Ann Hayter, aged 35 from Gillingham in Dorset, had 'for near three years laboured under the affliction of a decaying and lingering illness having nothing to rely on ... but her husband's labour ... by which means ... they are reduced to very low and mean circumstances'.[64] Moreover, in the case of 32 year old Mary Coombs of Buckland Denham, the input of married women to the household economy was directly recognized: suffering from severe rheumatic pains for the past six months, she was 'now in a great measure disabled and incapable of performing the usual labour for the support of her family'.[65]

Systematic analysis of the Casebook letters and the Admissions Register produces a more comprehensive age and sex profile for Bath patients.

Since the Infirmary had a wide catchment area, comparison with the population 'tree' for England as a whole raises fewer problems of urban and regional variation than where an institution served a particular locality.[66] When this exercise is carried out, it becomes clear that children and old people were under-represented at the Bath Hospital.[67] No more than 8 per cent of inmates, but a third of the English population, were juveniles, whilst at the other end of the spectrum the proportion of elderly patients was under half the national average (Table 7.6). Investigating the Bristol Infirmary later in the Georgian period, Mary Fissell discovered a similar configuration of ages. More young people under 15 and more elderly people over 60 were treated at Bristol than at Bath, and fewer patients fell into the big 25 to 59 age category; but an orientation towards young adults was evident at both institutions (Table 7.7). Superimposed upon the age structure of hospital constituencies was the balance between the sexes. The Bristol Infirmary 'treated about equal proportions of men and women, with a slight tendency towards increasing numbers of men' and a marked tendency in the young adult

Table 7.6 Bath General Hospital: the age profile of patients, 1742–59

	England		*Bath General Hospital*			
			Admissions Register (1742–52)		*Casebook (1752–58)*	
Age group (years)	*1741* %	*1756* %	No.	%	No.	%
0–4	12.91	13.04	6	0.69	12	1.02
5–14	19.90	20.09	70	8.03	79	6.71
15–24	17.87	18.48	198	22.71	282	23.96
25–59	41.21	40.02	567	65.02	757	64.32
60 +	8.11	8.37	31	3.56	47	3.99
Total	100.00	100.00	872	100.00	1 177	100.00

Notes:
1. The total for the Admissions Register excludes 771 cases for whom no age information was available.
2. The total for the Casebook excludes 441 cases for whom no age information was available.
3. Percentages have been rounded up or down and so do not always total exactly 100.00.

Sources: Admissions Register; Casebook; E.A. Wrigley and R.S. Schofield, *The Population History of England 1541–1871: A Reconstruction* (London: Edward Arnold, 1981), p. 529, Appendix A3.1.

Table 7.7 Bath General Hospital and Bristol Infirmary: patients by age group and sex

	Bath General Hospital				*Bristol Infirmary (1771–1805)*	
	Register (1742–52)		*Casebook (1750–58)*			
Age *group*	*Male %*	*Female %*	*Male %*	*Female %*	*Male %*	*Female %*
0–4	0.40	0.84	1.25	0.66	1.00	3.30
5–14	6.18	10.89	6.38	7.27	13.90	9.70
15–24	21.31	24.86	21.22	28.19	23.20	30.90
25–59	67.13	61.73	66.16	61.89	53.70	49.60
60 +	4.98	1.68	4.99	1.98	8.20	6.50
Total	100.00	100.00	100.00	100.00	100.00	100.00

Note: Percentages have been rounded up or down and so do not always total exactly 100.00.

Sources: Admissions Register; Casebook; Fissell, *Patients*, p. 103, table 5.1.

category towards females.[68] At the Bath Infirmary too a higher proportion of women were under 20 years old, and when we adopt narrower bands for the middle years the same trend pertains up to 40 (Table 7.8). Mean age was correspondingly low, at 28.86 years for women listed in the Admissions Register and 30.31 years for those in the Casebook.[69] This suggests that female patients at Bath may have been older than the women patients at Bristol who were so prominent in the 15 to 24 category. The implications for marital status are complicated by the fall in mean age of marriage for women during the eighteenth century[70] but, in all probability, females who gained entry to the Bath Hospital were less likely to have been single and unsupported than their Bristol counterparts. Marital status aside, women admitted to the Bath Infirmary did not match the percentage at Bristol. Females were more geographically mobile during the early modern period, albeit over shorter distances.[71] Sex ratios at burial had also been rising, and hence the proportion of women falling.[72] Yet the Register and Casebook show that between 1742 and 1758 almost two-thirds of patients travelling to the General Hospital were male. Though more men than women were over 40, their average age, calculated from the Admissions Register and the Casebook, was only 34.08 years and 33.99 years respectively because the majority were younger. Wartime demand for military manpower may partly explain this sex/age bias in the same manner that it

Table 7.8 Bath General Hospital: patients by age category and sex

	Admissions Register (1742–52)				*Casebook (1750–58)*			
	Male		*Female*		*Male*		*Female*	
Age Category	*No.*	*%*	*No.*	*%*	*No.*	*%*	*No.*	*%*
0–4	2	0.40	3	0.84	9	1.25	3	0.66
5–9	12	2.39	12	3.35	18	2.50	14	3.08
10–14	19	3.78	27	7.54	28	3.88	19	4.19
15–19	34	6.77	29	8.10	58	8.04	57	12.56
20–24	73	14.54	60	16.76	95	13.18	71	15.64
25–29	67	13.35	68	18.99	93	12.90	65	14.32
30–39	114	22.71	94	26.26	158	21.91	109	24.01
40–49	84	16.73	40	11.17	123	17.06	71	15.64
50–59	72	14.34	19	5.31	102	14.15	36	7.93
60 +	25	4.98	6	1.68	37	5.13	9	1.98
Total	502	100.00	358	100.00	721	100.00	454	100.00

Note: Percentages have been rounded up or down and so do not always total exactly 100.00.

Sources: Admissions Register; Casebook.

popularized the Marine Society's recruitment of destitute boys for the navy.[73] But what the disparity indicates above all is the apparent primacy afforded to male heads of household with dependent kin.

Neither the Casebook nor the Admissions Register regularly noted marital status, but we can explore the consequences of the domestic economy for the male:female balance by continuing with the comparison of institutions. The predominance of men over women at Bath was in line with the position at the late eighteenth-century Edinburgh Infirmary and indeed at other voluntary hospitals.[74] Fissell correctly attributes the Edinburgh ratio to the admission of soldiers and sailors under contract and the devotion of up to one hundred beds to clinical teaching purposes.[75] Though neither condition applied at the General Infirmary, its system of medical recommendation without the formal patronage of governors may have granted physicians and surgeons more control of the admissions procedure. However, in accounting for the different balance between the sexes at Bath and Bristol, the social networks of patients are of greater importance. Fissell argues strongly that at Bristol 'unremitting primary poverty [was not] the key to an individual's encounter with "institutional" health care' because occupations differed little from those of neighbours. Rather, in-patients as a group were characterized by the lack of family and community resources when illness struck, young single women being especially vulnerable. From residents of Bristol, the Infirmary asked for no caution money; and from those outside the city only 10 shillings. Therefore, it offered a relatively easy route to assistance in times of medical trouble, particularly as surgeons wrenched control of entry from lay patrons.[76] Conversely, access to the Bath Hospital was tortuous in the extreme, with applicants requiring not just a substantial deposit of £3.00, but a clinical report and a statement of their circumstances which were then scrutinized by medical staff and governors. To gain admission, therefore, patients had to pass through a local filter as well as vetting by the Infirmary.

At both levels, there was opportunity for the socio-economic role of women to come into play and skew the procedure against them. Although the family was no longer a self-contained unit of production by 1750, the household economy had not disintegrated, and husbands and wives continued to engage in 'working partnerships' less rigid than the sexual division of labour associated with the later advance of mechanization and industrialization. Furthermore, in a society which had to exploit its limited resources to the full, 'careful housewifery' was highly valued and women in rural as well as urban areas also participated in manufacturing industry, combining this work with agricultural jobs and domestic duties.[77] However, as Merry Wiesner has argued:

> All economies need both structure and flexibility, and during the early modern period these qualities became gender-identified: male labor provided the structure, so that it was regulated, tied to a training process, and life-long; female labor provided the flexibility, so that it was discontinuous, alternatively encouraged or supressed, not linked to formal training, and generally badly paid.

Women's work, she concludes, though 'irreplaceable' was also 'marginal'.[78] It was the priority given to male employment which underpinned the sex distribution of hospital patients. Paradoxically, the same economic marginality which predisposed young single women to admission under the more open system at Bristol mitigated against them obtaining a place under the more closed system at Bath. Governors at both institutions were dedicated to assisting productive men in the temporary grip of illness, thus permitting them to resume their family obligations.[79] At the General Infirmary, however, they were aided in the implementation of this policy by the local selection of prospective patients. Women's work was not perceived as structural to the economy and dependency within the household unit was assumed to be the norm, particularly after marriage. Men, conversely, were expected to achieve financial independence for themselves and their families; and hence communities were likely to show greater readiness to invest in the cost of transport and caution money. Unlike the early Georgian workhouses,[80] therefore, the Bath Infirmary in the 1740s and 1750s was not essentially a receptacle for women and children; despite its chronic disease profile, demand from patients and their sponsors led men to be more mobile in search of medical care for longer in the life cycle.

Detailed documentation similar to the early Register and Casebook do not survive for later periods because most of the Hospital's clinical records were destroyed after it was bombed during the Second World War.[81] However, it seems that male recruitment remained a priority. In 1789, a committee was set up to consider 'whether it be practicable to admit for the present a greater number of men patients into the House, the number now upon the list being thirty five',[82] and with the opening of a new extension six years later, twenty beds in two wards were reserved for male occupation.[83] Moreover, when in the 1820s the *Bath Journal* began to print partial listings of treatment outcomes, men continued to outnumber women. During 1825, for example, no figures were published in October, but in the remaining 11 months a total of 247 patients were discharged having been cured or relieved. Of these, 142 were men and only 85 were women. Twenty cannot be classified as male or female because no Christian names were given.[84] This heavy recruitment of male patients identified with economic productivity played to the therapeutic concerns which characterized both mercantilism and *laissez-faire*. Therefore, irrespective of its real impact on mortality and morbidity, the Georgian Bath Infirmary was able to symbolize the physical rehabilitation of the sick poor and extol the virtues of preserving them from idleness.

Rational benevolence

If the changing economic ideology produced a consistent gender profile, it helped to transform the nature of philanthropy, intensifying charitable discrimination and fostering new types of organization to put this ideal into practice. By the early eighteenth century, discrimination in giving had already undergone a series of mutations. Not only had the decline of traditional hospitality post-1500 brought about a division between conviviality for the affluent and alms for the poor, but under the influence of civic humanism and the Protestant Reformation, a new commitment to public relief aimed to reform the whole gamut of support for the lower orders by replacing casual alms-giving with a more rational, directive approach which selected on the basis of personal merit rather than indulging the donor's wish for deliverance or self-satisfaction.[85] The Enlightenment gave added stimulus to this rationalization process. Moreover, from the late seventeenth century, the risk of abuse to which posthumous giving was liable popularized the associated model of philanthropy, in which contributors oversaw the execution of their charitable objectives. Applied to voluntary hospitals, associated philanthropy exemplified rationality in two key respects. First, infirmaries were presented as a rational use of resources on the grounds that it was cheaper to offer the sick poor institutional relief than private charity at home. 'It has been laid down as a matter of fact, confirmed by experience', declared the first *Annual Report* of the Nottingham General Hospital in 1782, 'that distressed objects are taken care of in infirmaries, for a tenth part of what must necessarily be spent for them at their own habitations'.[86] The voluntary infirmary aimed, secondly, to fend off pauperization by rationalizing the distribution of medical aid. For patients, this was achieved by lay recommendation and professional scrutiny, which meant that it was 'a charity subject to no imposture, but what must be discovered by the physicians and surgeons'. By removing 'their most plausible reasons for begging', however, hospitals also prevented the squandering of charity on vagrants peddling 'the specious pretence of sick relations or friends'.[87] The capacity of associated philanthropy to discriminate between genuine and bogus 'cases of distress' impressed contemporaries, who were often highly critical of public welfare;[88] indeed, Bishop Warburton went so far as to suggest that the development of voluntary hospitals alone might eventually obviate the need for a statutory Poor Law and so 'put some stop to the growing mischiefs of that provision'.[89]

Related by marriage to Ralph Allen, William Warburton was a regular visitor to Bath. In the sermon which he preached for the General Infirmary in 1742,[90] there were no traces of his aspirations for the hospital movement, but the rationalization of philanthropy was worked through in the city and shaped by local circumstances. Eighteenth-century Bath gained a reputation for extravagant private giving, which owed much to Master of Ceremonies, Richard 'Beau' Nash, whose munificence was made legendary by Oliver Goldsmith's biography:

> A gentleman of broken fortune, one day standing behind his chair, as he was playing a game of picquet for two hundred pounds, and observing with what indifference he won the money, could not avoid whispering these words to another who stood by, 'Heavens! how happy would all that money make me!' Nash, overhearing him, clapped the money into his hand; and cried, 'Go and be happy.'

Nash's personal charity was not confined to fellow gamblers who had fallen on hard times. During the severe winter of 1739, he allegedly 'entered the houses of the poor, whom he thought too proud to beg, and generously relieved them'.[91] That Bath eulogized such 'thousand instances'[92] of Nash's benevolence was not surprising, given the ambivalence that surrounded the leisure and luxury which the city marketed. Alongside this private random charity, however, there developed rational forms of associated philanthropy, the flagship being the General Infirmary of which Nash himself was an active governor. The cost effectiveness argument was given a local gloss when the Revd Robert Leyborne, in his sermon of 1754, noted that since medicines were dispensed 'by the most skilful hands', the charity afforded patients cure rather than 'momentary refreshment, like those distilled waters, in which too often are spent the alms thrown away on common street-beggars'; like the poor whom Ezekiel described, their 'dry bones' would be covered with sinews, flesh and skin, and their bodies filled with breath, so that they would know the Lord and be resurrected to 'a better life'.[93] More fundamental to the moral economy of the Bath Hospital, however, was the rational classification of the poor as worthy or unworthy of assistance.

The discrimination imposed through the General Infirmary was applied to the indigenous population was well as to patients. Central to the Hospital's rationale was the eradication of vagrancy because in an elegant city dedicated to fashionable pleasures the presence of beggars was incongruous and menacing. The problem was aggravated by a section of the Elizabethan Poor Law which gave 'the diseased, impotent, poor people of England' a right to travel to Bath and obtain free use of the waters under licence from their local Justices of the Peace.[94] After the relevant Act expired in 1714, illegal immigrants were exposed to the full vigour of the vagrancy laws, but 'the beggarly stream still continued to flow'[95] and tease 'people of fashion for relief'. It was to stem this influx that the 1723 proposal for a Hospital was framed. Contributors called upon the magistrates of Bath 'to expell and punish vagrants and impostors'; in return, their Charity would support and treat genuine cases whose poverty prevented them from coming to the waters.[96] In other words, 'undeserving' beggars could be suppressed without conscience because 'deserving' sick and disabled people were being sheltered. The 'certificate of the poverty or circumstances', which accompanied the medical statement and was 'attested by the Minister and Church-wardens ... or other creditable persons',[97] was intended to ensure that patients admitted to the Hospital were financially worthy of treatment. The mid-century Casebook bears out their penury. James Ward, a 50-year-old surgeon from Bodmin, had 'the misfortune of being greatly reduced in his circumstances'. In bad health for many years due to 'a gouty habit', he had been unable to walk since more recently breaking his leg and 'now imagines that the Bath would do him great service but can't ... [carry] the expense unless he might have the favour of being admitted into the Hospital'.[98] In the case of John Freeman, a plumber and glazier who 'six years since' had 'lost the use of his limbs', poverty had arisen as a direct result of impairment, leading him to spend 'all his substance by endeavouring to get help'.[99] With Mary Tuck of Sopley in Hampshire, it was her husband who was impoverished by the bill for her paralytic disorder; 'by this misfortune of his wife and the dearness of provisions ... [he was] rendered unable to procure medicines proper for her even to maintain her and 3 poor small children'.[100] Supporters of the Bath Infirmary remained convinced that its admissions procedure identified the righteous sick who were financially deserving. As Joseph Hunter told his congregation at the local Presbyterian Chapel in 1810: 'your bounty is defended from the encroachments of the bold and forward, who in many other modes of bestowing relief often seize upon that which ought to fall into the hands of the more necessitous, but more modest poor'.[101] By the later Georgian period, however, rational benevolence was being redefined. No longer was the mere exclusion of cheeky impostors enough; charity was also expected to drive the worthy poor towards personal independence.

Scientific philanthropy

At the core of this 'new medicine for poverty'[102] was the economic individualism of Adam Smith's *Wealth of Nations*. Smith himself believed that the co-operative qualities of the free market produced a moral social system; 'The wise and virtuous man', he contended, 'is at all times willing that his own private interest should be sacrificed to the public interest of his own particular order or society.'[103] This public good embraced the needs of the meritorious lower orders, whom Smith regarded as ill-treated under the old economic regime. Mercantilists advocated low wages to tame the feckless poor; he assumed that the majority were sober and industrious workers who shared the moral values of society as a whole. Therefore, he subscribed to a subsistence income on the grounds that the 'liberal reward of labour' would render 'the common people' both fit and assiduous, as they applied their inherent moral qualities to self- (and hence social) betterment.[104] Smith's consequent endorsement of a continuing role for state support, pointed towards that minority of the poor who were genuinely unable to maintain themselves,[105] was challenged by T.R. Malthus's demand for the repeal of the Poor Laws when the first edition of his *Essay on the Principle of Population* was published in 1798. Underpinning this prescription was a derogatory view of the mass of mankind. 'Man as he really is', wrote Malthus, was 'inert, sluggish, and averse from labour, unless compelled from necessity'. The availability of a safety net 'diminish[ed] both the power and the will to save ... and thus ... weaken[ed] one of the strongest incentives to sobriety and industry, and consequently to happiness'. Therefore, it was the duty of society to dismantle a statutory system of poor relief which killed self-reliance and threatened the very survival of humanity by destroying 'moral restraint' in family reproduction.[106]

Donald Winch has wisely cautioned against allying Smith with 'Enlightenment optimism' and Malthus with 'post-Enlightenment pessimism'.[107] It is the case that whereas the 'psychological premiss' of the *Wealth of Nations* was self-interest, the Malthusian scenario emphasized the 'economic conscience' – 'innate ... yet needing to be nurtured into a habitude through the mechanism of the free market, with its constant operation of temptation, trial and exemplary suffering'.[108] However, even before the French Revolution brought the Enlightenment formally to a close in 1789, Rousseau's ideas were bursting the bubble of man's perfectability.[109] The political climate was also chilly. The American War of Independence had cost Britain prestigious North Atlantic colonies and prompted a campaign for the reform of government that was only temporarily distracted by the violence of the Gordon Riots in 1780.[110] Come the turn of the eighteenth century, Britain was embroiled in the lengthy Napoleonic Wars with France. Inflation was surging. Popular radicalism was on the boil. And the first Census was about to discredit the longstanding view that population growth was slow. It was in this ferment that the Evangelical Revival gathered momentum. Highly critical of 'the traditional social order for resting on a weak state' and tolerating popular unrest, Evangelicals used moral self-reproach to generate social projects which aimed to rehabilitate the sinful but retrievable poor.[111] Malthusianism reinforced this agenda. Therefore, Adam Smith's belief in the moral responsibility of the labouring classes always occupied a hostile environment, his faith in the capacity of the market economy to provide for the industrious and diligent easily transmuted into the conviction that only the idle and feckless sought relief.[112]

The roots of the new morality in economic individualism and Evangelical religion associated it closely with the middle orders to whom these values particularly appealed as a means of establishing an identity distinctive from that of the landed élite.[113] This bonding with the professional and commercial classes led to a complex political response.

The exact chronology of paternalism's demise is disputed. David Cannadine may be exaggerating when he speculates that Malthus was 'the champion of the revised aristocratic, paternal ideal of the 1820s'.[114] But if the 'ideological break' occured at the end of the eighteenth century,[115] paternalism did not disappear without trace in the 1790s and the free market economists were not tied unequivocally to the Whigs. Consequently, mutual obligation continued to inform, if not determine, the workings of rural poor relief up to 1834,[116] and the notorious Poor Law Amendment Act was passed with the support of Liberal Tories as well as Whigs. For them, '*paternalism* stopped short at moral exhortation and education'. Only 'High Tories ... were appalled by the inhumanity of the ... legislation'.[117]

The penetration of the Tory Party by *laissez-faire* ideas is indicative of the extent to which the landowning classes were adapting to the political demands of a middling sort growing in power. Given the state's lingering attachment to paternalism, however, and their own exclusion from parliamentary politics, these middle men turned to voluntary organizations in their bid to steady a society put on tenterhooks by urbanization and industrialization, internal unrest and an external enemy.[118] Their methods were inspired by the materialist psychology of the Enlightenment. A leading exponent of this school was David Hartley, an honorary physician at the Bath Infirmary between 1744 and 1748. Starting from the epistemology of Hobbes and Locke, Hartley maintained that ideas arose from external objects which acted on the senses and became associated together through physiological processes seated in the brain. It followed from this integration of mind and body that morality was not innate but learned, and that moral and hence social improvement was therefore possible through a regulated physical environment. Hartley was imbued with the progressive ethos of the Enlightenment; for him, God oversaw over the association principle, constructing a kindly world in which individuals were responsive to the needs of others. Such optimism did not survive the political turmoil of the late eighteenth century. But from the contemporary velocity of the Evangelical Revival came the moral imperative that depraved members of humanity should be given the opportunity to change. Furthermore, the rational science of man which materialism offered was now being toughened by the utilitarianism of Jeremy Bentham: social policies were to induce the appropriate behavioural responses by exploiting the propensity of men and women to seek pleasure and avoid pain.[119] Though this theory found its ultimate expression in Bentham's grand plans for the criminal and impoverished, they were also more widely applied in domiciliary schemes to discipline the non-criminal poor. Therefore, even the most deserving applicants for charitable help had to be subjected to thorough inspection. The personal contact which this involved conformed to the new code of moral sensibility, emotionally engaging benefactors in the act of giving.[120] But such scrutiny was also essential to ensure that recipients were capable of self-improvement, and that their aid, allocated on a temporary and intermittent basis, was evincing the desired good conduct.[121] Furthermore, 'information respecting the circumstances and situation of the poor, and the most effectual means of ameliorating their condition' was to be collected carefully and analysed scientifically so that the results could be used to promote the happiness of the lower orders and 'add to the virtue and morality of ... [the] nation'.[122]

Though this was a science of self-help rather than an all-encompassing sociology of the sort that arrived in the later nineteenth century, its emergence created a new context for voluntary hospitals born of traditional paternalism. Their *laissez-faire* credentials were first seriously questioned in the 1770s when the acceleration of the dispensary movement led to complaints that institutional provision was an extravagant response to medical need which not only exposed the sick poor to the risk of fever but also encouraged in them an unhealthy dependency; with all requirements satisfied regardless of effort, the long-term incentive to labour was jeopardized.[123] Setting up or expanding out-patient clinics and home visiting schemes helped voluntary hospitals to deflect the criticisms of the dispensary movement;[124] and corporate subscriptions also created a chance for mutual reliance within friendly societies and Nonconformist congregations, as well as a cheap means of treating the parish poor.[125] According to the criteria of scientific philanthropy, however, moral assessment by the lay patrons who sponsored individual patients was amateurish. Clinical judgement, on the other hand, conformed to the scientific standard. Therefore, change within the charitable sector consolidated the growing prestige of medical knowledge which was enabling doctors to gain greater control over admissions, therapies and discharge.

For the Bath Infirmary, adaptation was more problematic. Out-patient clinics were not a viable answer to the dispensary, given a national catchment area and the ban on city residents. The cultivation of self-help through corporate subscription was likewise frustrated by the Hospital's terms of reference; local groups of the provident poor had little incentive to subscribe when entry by medical recommendation was added to the exclusion of the immediate community. Yet the admissions procedure itself was unable to deliver adequate scientific discrimination. The Casebook letters show that self-help was a force for admission, even during the 1750s. In attempting to cure his dislocated shoulder, for example, Nathanial Workman from Bisley in Gloucestershire had 'made use of all means that his circumstances would admit of but to no purpose',[126] while Samuel Arris, a Birmingham journeyman printer with 'a weakness in his hands' had 'been at Bath for two months upon his own expenses, and received some benefit, but cannot support himself here any longer'.[127] Arris was proposed by a former physician to the Infirmary, other patients by current incumbents of honorary posts; but in the majority of cases, medical and moral assessment was second-hand. Therefore, the investigative potential of clinical recommendation was more apparent than real. Medical screening dominated the selection process, but patients were normally examined only after their arrival; in deciding whom to admit, doctors and governors relied on the judgements contained in clinical reports, the quality of which they not infrequently berated. When this failure to inspect patients closely prior to admission is added to the declining credibility of spa water therapy within mainstream medicine, it becomes clear that the Bath Hospital had some difficulty in meeting the requirements of scientific charity.

The hierarchy of charities

The relationship of the Bath Infirmary to developments in philanthropy was ultimately to affect its position in the hierarchy of local benevolence. At the beginning of the eighteenth century, the city possessed a number of endowed institutions. St Catherine's and St John's Hospitals each accommodated about a dozen poor Bath inhabitants, while Bellot's Hospital, open during the summer months, offered free lodging and bathing, medical assistance and a weekly allowance to ten male visitors seeking help from the waters.[128] In 1711 a Blue-Coat Charity School was inaugurated in Bath, complementing the educational services of the public grammar school founded by Edward VI.[129] Being a piece of associated philanthropy, this charity school competed with the General Hospital for funds, but its expenditure in the 1750s was only in the region of £200 per annum and charity services on its behalf generated under £100 each year – far less than the sums raised for the Infirmary.[130] In 1747, a medical subscription was opened to supply the sick poor of the city and its neighbourhood with free assistance. Under this Pauper Scheme, physicians and surgeons of the General Hospital gave advice to those ineligible for poor relief and sent directions to an approved apothecary who dispensed the medicines. Even the needs of vagrants were acknowledged; though the Charity had no wish to 'encourage ... common beggars ... the maladies even of these are in some cases so evident and urgent, as to call for a compassionate assistance in a medical way'.[131] The involvement of the Infirmary doctors hints at an attempt to defuse disapproval of its exclusionary brief, but a plan in 1750/51 to build a hospital for local residents apparently floundered and in the early 1760s the system of outdoor medical assistance ran into debt.[132] This crisis provoked a reappraisal and by 1764 the Pauper Scheme was describing itself as 'enlarged'; indeed, the *Bath Journal* in December of that year reported that the subscribers were seeking proposals from any person with a four-bedded house who was willing to nurse surgical patients and supply them with the provisions directed by the attending physicians and surgeons.[133] Until remodelled in the 1790s, however, the hallmark of the Pauper Charity was its non-institutional character. Each month the number of patients relieved was proudly announced in the local press,[134] and at the end of each financial year the modest cost of this impressive workload was trumpeted: in the late 1750s, for example, more than 1 000 patients were relieved annually for just over £100.[135] After 1785, sick paupers had access to a Poor Law dispensary[136] and in 1792 the Pauper Scheme itself was expanded to become the Bath City Infirmary and Dispensary,[137] but it was 1829 before another charitable dispensary was founded in the town and 1831 before its facilities became available to men.[138]

The expansion of the Pauper Charity in the 1790s was a manifestation of the philanthropic bonanza which swept across Britain in response to the popular unrest and moral disquiet of the later Georgian period.[139] At Bath, educational charities started the ball rolling with a subscription for Sunday Schools in 1785.[140] Three years later, a Casualty Hospital was opened for the treatment of accident victims.[141] In 1805 a Female Penitentiary and Lock Hospital was founded, together with the Bath Society for the Suppression of Common Vagrants and Impostors, Relief of Occasional Distress, and Encouragement of Industry. An Eye Infirmary followed in 1811 and in 1823 the Casualty Hospital merged with the City Infirmary and Dispensary to become the Bath United Hospital.[142] As well as catering for the local population in a way that the General Hospital did not, these charities practised inspection and scrutiny in the name of self-help. The Society for the Suppression of Common Vagrants best epitomized the strictures of scientific philanthropy. In an effort to stamp out 'promiscuous donations to common beggars', tickets were issued to the nobility and gentry, who were asked to distribute these rather than alms when approached for assistance. Recipients then reported to the Society, where they were subjected to 'strict investigation ... to distinguish between fraud and real distress'. The resident poor were similarly examined, with visitors calling at the homes of applicants and enquiring into their means and character.[143] Charities of a quasi-medical nature also celebrated their discriminatory prowess. Thus the Bath Penitentiary and Lock Hospital declared in 1824 that 'The experience of four years has enabled the Ladies' Committee to select with better judgement, from among the applicants, those who offer the greatest hopes of reformation'.[144]

The expansion of the Pauper Scheme into a hospital was both medical and moral in motivation. The publicity broadsheet that announced its upgrading recognized a clinical demand for in-patient facilities. Assisting the sick poor was 'often ... entirely frustrated, while they either live widely dispersed, or have no fixed place of abode. Moreover, in acute and critical diseases, medical advice, attendance, drugs, and other necessaries, ... [could] only be administered with certain advantage, when the patients ... [were] properly accommodated and collected together'. Prefacing this argument, however, was the case for more accurate selection. By the early 1790s, the expansion of Bath, with a disproportionate increase in its poor inhabitants, was hindering the provision of 'adequate relief to the numerous objects' who sought help from the dispensary. Therefore, the subscribers had 'determined to revise and new-model' their institution in order 'to confer the benefits of their charity, in urgent cases, with better effect; to guard against bestowing them on improper objects; and to rectify some other abuses and misapplications'.[145] In short, institutional facilities were added to outdoor relief to tighten the exercise of discrimination.

The flowering of medical charity in late Georgian Bath and the appearance of self-help societies which embodied the principles of scientific philanthropy were delayed in their impact upon the General Hospital. Rival charities made ambitious claims for their endeavours. Though conceding that only a quarter of its patients recovered, the Penitentiary was adamant that this exceeded most expectations given the magnitude of rescue from 'an existence soiled and contaminated by all that can degrade and debase the human character'. Other institutions recorded higher success rates that the General Infirmary was unable to equal. All 17 patients discharged from the Lock Hospital in 1818/19 were cured.[146] The Eye Infirmary reported in 1815 that 92 per cent of patients had been cured and a further 5 per cent relieved.[147] Even the Bath City Infirmary and Dispensary claimed to have cured 72 per cent of its in-patients between 1792 and 1794, and relieved another 15 per cent, despite dealing with a wide range of clinical conditions.[148] Yet though faring badly in terms of these performance indicators, the General Hospital remained the premier charity in Bath, heading the parade of philanthropic enterprises listed in Georgian and Victorian guidebooks to the city.[149] Size was a major factor. The City Infirmary and Dispensary opened with just 18 beds in 1792 and the Eye Infirmary had only 12 as late as 1888.[150] The General Infirmary, on the other hand, was built to accommodate over 100 in-patients and by the later Georgian

The different hospitals

period was normally full. Income and expenditure reflected this differential. Even the Penitentiary and Lock Hospital, perhaps the nearest competitor until the United Hospital was founded in 1823, operated with an average budget only half that of the General Infirmary between 1817 and 1823 (Table 7.9).

It was this degree of financial disparity which underpinned the Parish affair in 1819. In alleging profligacy, Mr Parish was angered by the refusal to grant the Penitentiary and Lock Hospital an 'annual recommendation' from the pulpits of local churches, 'lest it should affect the interests of the Bath Hospital, already enjoying the exclusive privilege of two annual sermons'.[151] His campaign to win the Penitentiary a permanent place in the religious calendar failed,[152] but in 1827 the United Hospital did take over one of the two slots previously occupied by the General Infirmary. This concesson – made at a time when paternalism was resurging – heralded a small but significant change in the status of the Bath institution which best represented traditional obliga-

Table 7.9 Bath Charities: income and expenditure

Charity	*Year(s)*	*Income £*	*Expenditure £*
General Hospital	1790–91	2 907.30	2 160.55
	1825–26	3 362.25	3 507.15
City Infirmary and Dispensary	October 1792–December 1793	857.00	918.55
Casualty Hospital	1793	459.20	305.75
Eye Infirmary	1815	83.05	112.10
Penitentiary and Lock Hospital	1817–23	Maximum: 2 660 Minumum: 680 Average: 1 629	Maximum: 2 100 Minimum: 780 Average: 1 214

Sources: Bath General Hospital, *Annual Reports*, 1790/91 and 1825/26. For five-yearly income and expenditure figures, see Chapter 3; *State of the Bath City Infirmary and Dispensary* ... (Bath: Crutwell, 1794), pp. 20–21; *The Sixth Year's State of the Casualty-Hospital in the City of Bath* ... (Bath: R. Cruttwell, nd), p. 14; *Bath Infirmary for the Cure of Diseases of the Eye ... Fourth Annual Report* ... (Bath: Richard Cruttwell, 1816), p. 16; *The Collective Reports of the Bath Penitentiary and Lock Hospital, from 1816 to 1824* (Bath: Wood, Cunningham and Smith, 1824), pp. 202, 207. The average income figure for the Penitentiary and Lock Hospital includes a legacy of £1 500 from the Chairman which is not associated in the accounts with any particular year.

tions. For a spa resort, with a residential population latterly swollen by the immigration of past visitors, an institution dedicated to balneology for strangers retained huge symbolic significance. By the end of the Georgian period, however, the inability of the General Infirmary to apply an effective clinical filter to patients was alienating it from the dominant ethos of scientific philanthropy. Under these circumstances, the presence of the United Hospital, supplying the local community with a conventional service more able to practice medical discrimination, began to erode the hegemony that the General Infirmary had enjoyed throughout the eighteenth century. Charity coverage in the local press, though difficult to interpret, is not at odds with this hypothesis. During the early Georgian period, an account of the May general court, together with incidental items relating to the General Hospital, featured in the *Bath Journal*.[153] In the 1820s patient discharges were added,[154] and the sums raised by church collections continued to be published,[155] but it was the recent foundations that dominated reporting – the Bath Sunday School Union, the Asylum for the Maintenance and Instruction of Young Females in Plain Household Work, the Strangers' Friend Society, the National Society for the Education of the Poor, the Penitentiary, and the Mechanics Institute.[156] Reaching a firm conclusion is impossible, given the uncertainties which surround the submission and editing of news. But to the extent that the *Bath Journal* reflected local priorities, we can surmise that the General Infirmary was losing ground in an increasingly competitive arena of benevolence.

In this chapter, we have considered how the Bath Infirmary was affected by the gravitation from social mercantilism to *laissez-faire*. Voluntary infirmaries founded in the early Georgian period articulated the mercantilist view that population spelt prosperity, claiming to cut mortality and morbidity as well as the cost of poor relief. These objectives were manifest in the bias towards young male patients with economic potential and family commitments. From 1750, the parameters of the demographic debate altered, as population increase reduced wage pressure and queried the premiss that more people inevitably produced more wealth. With the triumph of *laissez-faire* ideas, a healthy workforce became coupled with higher wages; but this formula was dependent upon a view of the poor as responsible moral agents which was tenuous and failed to withstand the blast of Malthusian political economy. From the late eighteenth century, the assumption that the lower orders were for the most part morally degenerate combined with materialist psychology to usher in a model of scientific philanthropy. Whereas rational benevolence had been defined as the exclusion of impostors, under the new regime even the worthy poor had to be subjected to minute inspection to ensure that they were progressing towards personal independence. It was the interaction of these free-market charitable objectives with the passing of paternalism which moulded the later Georgian moral economy. The Bath Infirmary was taxed by the *laissez-faire* conditions. Out-patient clinics and corporate subscriptions which encouraged self-help among the poor were impractical; and, at a time when the efficacy of spa treatment was losing clinical respectability, long-distance recruitment remained an impediment to the effective moral and medical appraisal of those whom treatment would benefit. Being out of step with the new moral economy for the labouring classes alienated the Hospital from those mores of the middling sort that were making incursions against paternalism. But if a breakdown of the consensus over managing the poor generated dissonance on the patient front, the ethics of giving increasingly harmonized with the values of the middle orders. As we saw in Chapter 6, the mutual obligations of the tributary relationship, based on land ownership, were overtaken during the later Georgian period by a more open, proprietary relationship in which charity was reduced to voluntary acts of benevolence signifying the donor's civility. The Bath Infirmary was well equipped to bestow this moral sensibility because its status as the leading local charity and its historical association with the philanthropy of fashionable visitors endowed deep reserves of politeness. At a time when the former stewards of prosperity were being absolved of their paternalist responsibilities, this was a valued service. Earlier the Hospital had purged the embarrassment of riches. Now it was excusing a harsher attitude towards the poor by validating a selective moral sensibility which appeased the ambivalence arising from the class relations of a market economy. Therefore, despite the advent of organizations better personifying scientific philanthropy, the General Infirmary remained the colossus of Bath charity until the very end of the Georgian period, its pre-eminence secured by a dynamic social and political agenda.

Notes

1. Andrew, *Philanthropy and Police*, pp. 23–4; Wilson, *England's Apprenticeship*, pp. 353–5, 384.
2. Bellers, 'Essay', p. 204. See also Nelson, *Address*, p. 211.
3. Andrew, *Philanthropy and Police*, p. 56; R.A. Houston, *The Population History of Britain and Ireland 1500–1750* (London: Macmillan, 1992), p. 28; Langford, *Polite and Commercial People*, p. 145; Porter, *Disease*, p. 61.
4. Andrew, *Philanthropy and Police*, p. 24.

5. Baugh, 'Poverty', p. 82; Lewis and Williams, *Private Charity*, pp. 2–3. The development of hospitals in Renaissance Florence has also been linked to rising wages provoked by the labour shortages which followed recurrent plague outbreaks. See Katharine Park, 'Healing the Poor: Hospitals and Medical Assistance in Renaissance Florence', in Jonathan Barry and Colin Jones (eds), *Medicine and Charity before the Welfare State* (London: Routledge, 1991), p. 39.
6. Langford, *Polite and Commercial People*, p. 133; Wilson, *England's Apprenticeship*, pp. 231–4.
7. *Gentleman's Magazine*, **11** (1741), p. 475; Himmelfarb, *Idea of Poverty*, p. 26.
8. Heal, *Hospitality*, pp. 122–3.
9. Bellers, 'Essay', pp. 178–9.
10. See, for example, Clark-Kennedy, *The London*, pp. 140–41, 146; Hume, *Newcastle Infirmary*, p. i; McLoughlin, *Liverpool Infirmary*, pp. 17–19; McMenemey, *Worcester Royal Infirmary*, p. 21; Risse, *Hospital Life*, pp. 2–3.
11. Minute Book, 16 February 1738, 'Plan and Elevation'.
12. Brown, *False Pleasure*, p. 19. See also Bayly, *Sermon*, p. 15.
13. Andrew, *Philanthropy and Police*, p. 139; Himmelfarb, *Idea of Poverty*, p. 134.
14. Cherry, 'Voluntary General Hospitals', p. 98. See also Anning, *General Infirmary at Leeds*, pp. 3–4; Jacob, *General Hospital*, p. 18; Marland, *Medicine and Society*, p. 128.
15. Baugh, 'Poverty', pp. 90–91.
16. Andrew, *Philanthropy and Police*, pp. 146–9; William J. Hausman, 'The British Economy in Transition, 1742–1789', in J. Black (ed.), *British Politics and Society from Walpole to Pitt 1742–1789* (London: Macmillan, 1990), pp. 59–60.
17. Marland, *Medicine and Society*, p. 128.
18. *State of the Bath City Infirmary*, pp. 1–2.
19. *Improved Bath Guide*, p. 47.
20. S. Cherry, 'The Role of a Provincial Hospital: the Norfolk and Norwich Hospital, 1771–1880', *Population Studies*, **26** (1972), pp. 296–7; Risse, *Hospital Life*, pp. 230–33; Eric Sigsworth, 'A Provincial Hospital in the Eighteenth and Early Nineteenth Centuries', *College of General Practitioners Yorkshire Faculty Journal* (June 1966), pp. 28, 31;Woodward, *To Do the Sick No Harm*, pp. 140–41.
21. *Annual Report*, 1756/57–1780/81. The Edinburgh Infirmary introduced this semantic change in the 1780s. See Risse, *Hospital Life*, p. 236.
22. [Bath General Infirmary], *Narrative*, pp. vii–ix.
23. Wood, *Bath*, p. 294.
24. See Minute Book, 6 May 1752; 20 May 1752; 17 June 1752; 8 November 1752; 22 November 1752.
25. Karl F. Helleiner, 'The Vital Revolution Reconsidered', *Canadian Journal of Economics and Political Science*, **23** (1957), p. 6. See also Thomas McKeown and R.G. Brown, 'Medical Evidence Related to English Population Changes in the Eighteenth Century', *Population Studies*, **9** (1955), pp. 124–6.
26. Bevan, *Salop Infirmary*, 'A Comparative Average Statement of In and Out-Patients'; McLoughlin, *Liverpool Infirmary*, pp. 101–3, Appendix

IX. See also Berry, 'Patronage', p. 243; Fissell, *Patients*, p. 108; Lane, *Worcester Infirmary*, pp. 38–9; Risse, *Hospital Life*, pp. 46–9, 289–91; Sigsworth, 'Provincial Hospital', pp. 25–9; Woodward, *To Do the Sick No Harm*, pp. 142, 153–8.

27. Sigsworth, 'Provincial Hospital', p. 31.
28. Abel-Smith, *The Hospitals*, p. 1.
29. Cherry, 'Voluntary General Hospitals', pp. 270–71; Mary J. Dobson, *Contours of Death and Disease in Early Modern England*, (Cambridge: Cambridge University Press, 1997), p. 527–33.
30. Hudson, *Industrial Revolution*, pp. 147–9; E.A. Wrigley and R.S. Schofield, *The Population History of England 1541–1871: A Reconstruction* (London: Edward Arnold, 1981), pp. 418–19.
31. Bevan, *Salop Infirmary*, 'A Comparative Average Statement of In and Out-Patients'; McLoughlin, *Liverpool Infirmary*, pp. 101–3, Appendix IX. See also Lane, *Worcester Infirmary*, p. 41; Risse, *Hospital Life*, pp. 46–9; Woodward, *To Do the Sick No Harm*, pp. 153–9.
32. Fissell, 'Physic of Charity', p. 202. See also Porter and Porter, *Patient's Progress*, p. 163.
33. [Bath General Infirmary], 'Short Account', in Bayly, *Sermon*, p. 25. See also [Bath General Infirmary], 'Short Account', in Dalton, *Religious Use*, p. 22; [Bath General Infirmary], 'Short Account', in Leyborne, *Charity Conducive*, p. 40; [Bath General Infirmary], 'A Short Account of the Nature, Rise and Progress of the General Infirmary at Bath', in W. Warburton, *A Sermon Preached at the Abbey-Church at Bath* (London: J. Leake, 1742), p. 27.
34. Minute Book, 4 June 1783; 2 May 1785.
35. At least 20 patients typically fell into this category in each sample year.
36. Casebook, admitted 15 October 1757.
37. Casebook, admitted 20 February 1754.
38. Casebook, admitted 9 January 1756.
39. Casebook, admitted 16 May 1752.
40. Casebook, admitted 23 May 1753.
41. [Bath General Infirmary], 'Short Account', in Bayly, *Sermon*, p.25.
42. Minute Book, 7 December 1738; 12 Geo. II, pp. 575–7; [Bath General Infirmary], 'Short Account', in Olive, *Particular Excellence*, p. 31.
43. See, for example, Clark-Kennedy, *The London*, p. 109; Humble and Hansell, *Westminster Hospital*, p. 29; Pickstone, *Medicine and Industrial Society*, p. 13; McLoughlin, *Liverpool Infirmary*, pp. 33, 74.
44. Minute Book, 11 February 1747.
45. Berry, 'Patronage', p. 238. See also Bevan, *Salop Infirmary*, 'A Comparative Statement, Showing the Average Number of Days which Each Patient of the Salop Infirmary, Remained in the House at Different Periods'.
46. [Bath General Infirmary], *Narrative*, p. xiii.
47. *Annual Report*, 1760/61–1830/31.
48. [Bath General Infirmary], 'Short Account', in Olive, *Particular Excellence*, p. 32.
49. [Bath General Infirmary], 'Short Account', in Bayly, *Sermon*, p. 25.
50. [Bath General Infirmary], 'Short Account', in Olive, *Particular Excellence*, p. 32. See also Leyborne, *Charity Conducive*, p. 17.
51. 12 Geo. II, p. 575.
52. Casebook, admitted 27 January 1753.

53. Casebook, admitted 29 October 1751.
54. Casebook, admitted 23 June 1758.
55. Casebook, admitted 15 April 1753. The symptoms of St Vitus' Dance were involuntary convulsions, often on one side, which paralysed the leg and caused it to be dragged along.
56. Casebook, admitted 11 December 1753.
57. Casebook, admitted 22 May 1751.
58. Casebook, admitted 14 April 1758.
59. Casebook, admitted 10 September 1753.
60. Merry E. Wiesner, *Women and Gender in Early Modern Europe* (Cambridge: Cambridge University Press, 1993), p. 83.
61. Casebook, admitted 15 April 1752.
62. Casebook, admitted 31 October 1753.
63. Casebook, admitted 24 February 1752.
64. Casebook, admitted 13 March 1753.
65. Casebook, admitted 25 February 1754.
66. Mary E. Fissell, 'The "Sick and Dropping Poor" in Eighteenth-Century Bristol and its Region', *Social History of Medicine*, **2** (1989), p. 46.
67. The late eighteenth-century Edinburgh Infirmary, and the fever wards of the Glasgow Royal Infirmary in 1871, were also dominated by young adults. See Risse, *Hospital Life*, p. 87; Marguerite W. Dupree, 'Family Care and Hospital Care: The "Sick Poor" in Nineteenth-Century Glasgow', *Social History of Medicine*, **6** (1993), p. 204.
68. Fissell, 'Physic of Charity', pp. 177–8.
69. Similar differentials have been reported for the Bristol, Northampton, and Devon and Exeter Hospitals. See Berry, 'Patronage', p. 221.
70. The mean age of marriage for women dropped from 27.0 years in the first half of the eighteenth century to 25.4 between 1750 and 1799. See R.D. Lee and R.S. Schofield, 'British Population in the Eighteenth Century', in Roderick Floud and Donald McCloskey (eds), *The Economic History of Britain since 1700*, 2 vols (Cambridge: Cambridge University Press, 1981), vol. 1: *1700–1860*, p. 27, table 2.2.
71. Peter Clark, 'Migration in England during the Late Seventeenth and Early Eighteenth Centuries', *Past and Present*, **83** (1979), p. 67.
72. David Souden, 'Migrants and the Population Structure of Later Seventeenth-Century Provincial Cities and Market Towns', in Peter Clark (ed.), *The Transformation of English Provincial Towns 1600–1800* (London: Hutchinson, 1984), pp. 158–9.
73. Andrew, *Philanthropy and Police*, p. 130.
74. Berry, 'Patronage', pp. 218–19.
75. Fissell, 'Sick and Drooping Poor', pp. 49–50.
76. Ibid., pp. 35, 38–9, 47–9, 52, 55–7.
77. Hill, *Women*, pp. 38–40, 44–9, 53–6, 259–65. See also Mary Abbott, *Family Ties: English Families 1540–1920* (London: Routledge, 1993), pp. 88–9, 91–5, 125, 149; Berg, *Age of Manufactures*, pp. 19, 129, 317; Laurence, *Women*, pp. 116–24; Levine, 'Industrialization', pp. 175–6.
78. Wiesner, *Women and Gender*, p. 86.
79. Fissell, 'Physic of Charity', p. 91.
80. Timothy V. Hitchcock, 'The English Workhouse: A Study in Institutional Poor Relief in Selected Counties 1696–1750' (unpublished doctoral thesis, University of Oxford, 1985), pp. 194–208.

81. Minute Book, 17 June 1942.
82. Minute Book, 1 May 1789.
83. Minute Book, 4 February 1795; 4 March 1795.
84. *Bath Journal*, 10 January 1825; 14 February 1825; 14 March 1825; 11 April 1825; 16 May 1825; 13 June 1825; 11 July 1825; 8 August 1825; 12 September 1825; 14 November 1825; 12 December 1825. Duplicate entries for the same patient have been excluded.
85. Andrew, *Philanthropy and Police*, p. 22; Heal, *Hospitality*, pp. 139–40, 393; Felicity Heal and Clive Holmes, *The Gentry in England and Wales 1500–1700* (London: Macmillan, 1994), p. 286; Slack, *English Poor Law*, pp. 14–15, 49–50; Slack, *Poverty*, pp. 9, 22, 168.
86. Jacob, *General Hospital*, p. 18. See also Bevan, *Salop Infirmary*, p. 6; [Hull General Infirmary], 'General Infirmary, Kingston upon Hull', in K.J. Lowson, *Hull Royal Infirmary* (no place of publication, publisher or date); McLoughlin, *Liverpool Infirmary*, p.16.
87. 'A View of the Many Peculiar Advantages of Public Hospitals', *Bath Journal*, 14 January 1751. See also [Winchester County Hospital], 'An Account of the Establishment of the County Hospital at Winchester', in J. Woodward, *To Do the Sick No Harm: A Study of the British Voluntary Hospital System to 1875* (London: Routledge and Kegan Paul 1974), pp. 150–51.
88. Andrew, *Philanthropy and Police*, pp. 26–7.
89. William Warburton, 'Sermon Preached Before the Governors of the London Hospital in 1767', in William Warburton, *Works*, ed. by Richard Hurd, 12 vols (London: T. Cadell and W. Davies, 1811), vol. 10, pp. 255, 258.
90. Warburton, *Sermon* [1742].
91. *Miscellaneous Works of Oliver Goldsmith*, pp. 538–9.
92. *Original Bath Guide* [1840], pp. 16–17.
93. Leyborne, *Charity Conducive*, p. 17.
94. Wood, *Bath*, pp. 275–8, 282. See also Turner, *Mineral Water Hospital*, p. 6.
95. Bath Chronicle, *Hot Water Hospital*, p. 6.
96. Wood, *Bath*, pp. 279, 282.
97. 12 Geo. II, p. 575.
98. Casebook, admitted 9 June 1754.
99. Casebook, admitted 29 August 1754.
100. Casebook, admitted 15 September 1758.
101. Hunter, *Ameliorated Condition* , p. 24.
102. Tawney, *Religion*, p. 253.
103. Adam Smith, *The Theory of Moral Sentiments*, 2 vols, 9th edn (London: T. Cadell and W. Davies, 1801), vol. 2, p. 99.
104. Smith, *Wealth of Nations*, p. 37.
105. Barber, *History of Economic Thought*, p. 48; Himmelfarb, *Idea of Poverty*, pp. 61–2.
106. T.R. Malthus, *An Essay on the Principal of Population*, ed. Anthony Flew (Harmondsworth: Penguin Books, 1970), pp. 71, 93–4, 97–8, 101–2, 205; T.R. Malthus, *A Summary View of the Principle of Population*, in T.R. Malthus, *An Essay on the Principle of Population*, ed. A. Fleur (Harmondsworth: Penguin Books, 1970), pp. 238, 269–70.
107. Donald Winch, *Riches and Poverty: An Intellectual History of Political*

Economy in Britain 1750–1834 (Cambridge: Cambridge University Press, 1996), p. 13.

108. Boyd Hilton, *The Age of Atonement: The Influence of Evangelicalism on Social and Economic Thought 1795–1865* (Oxford: Clarendon Press, 1988), pp. 69–70.
109. Cragg, *Church*, pp. 169–70; Hankins, *Science*, pp. 173–5; Ludmilla Jordanova, 'The Authoritarian Response', pp. 202–3.
110. Andrew, *Philanthropy and Police*, pp. 163–4; Joanna Innes, 'Politics and Morals: The Reformation of Manners Movement in Later Eighteenth-Century England', in E. Hellmuth (ed.), *The Transformation of Political Culture: England and Germany in the Late Eighteenth Century* (Oxford: Oxford University Press, 1990), pp. 60–61.
111. Ignatieff, *Just Measure*, pp. 148–9, 211. See also Bebbington, *Evangelicalism*, pp. 70–71.
112. Wilson, *England's Apprenticeship*, pp. 351–2.
113. Evangelicalism expanded so rapidly at the end of the eighteenth century because it gained the support of the middling sort. See David Hempton, 'Religion in British society, 1740–1790', in J. Black (ed.), *British Politics and Society from Walpole to Pitt 1742–1789* (London, Macmillan, 1990).
114. David Cannadine, 'Conspicuous Consumption by the Landed Classes, 1790–1830', in Michael Turner (ed.), *Malthus and his Time* (London: Macmillan, 1986), pp. 105–6.
115. E.P. Thompson, 'Eighteenth-Century English Society: Class Struggle without Class?' *Social History*, 3 (1978), p. 163.
116. Peter Dunkeley, 'Paternalism, the Magistracy and Poor Relief in England, 1795–1834', *International Review of Social History*, 24 (1979), pp. 371–97.
117. Hilton, *Age of Atonement*, pp. 225–6. See also Winch, *Riches*, pp. 23–5.
118. Martin Daunton, *Progress and Poverty: An Economic and Social History of Britain 1700–1850* (Oxford: Oxford University Press, 1995), p. 471; Owen, *English Philanthropy*, p. 97.
119. Bynum, *Science*, p. 68; Christopher Dandeker, *Surveillance, Power and Modernity: Bureaucracy and Discipline from 1700 to the Present Day* (Cambridge: Polity Press, 1990), pp. 117–18, 138–9.; Ignatieff, *Just Measure*, pp. 60–61, 66–7; Isaac Kramnick, 'Eighteenth-Century Science and Radical Social Theory: The Case of Joseph Priestley's Scientific Liberalism', *Journal of British Studies*, 25 (1986), pp. 15–17, 24–5.
120. Joanna Innes, 'The "Mixed Economy of Welfare" in Early Modern England: Assessments of the Options from Hale to Malthus (c.1683–1803)', in M. Daunton (ed.), *Charity, Self-Interest and Welfare in the English Past* (London: UCL Press, 1996), p. 164.
121. Andrew, *Philanthropy and Police*, pp. 169, 174, 200; Fissell, *Patients*, pp. 122–5.
122. *First Report of the Society for Bettering the Conditions and Increasing the Comforts of the Poor* (London: 1797), pp. i, ii, 3.
123. Andrew, *Philanthropy and Police*, 132–3, 155–6; Bronwyn Croxon, 'The Public and Private Faces of Eighteenth-Century London Dispensary Charity', *Medical History*, 41 (1997), pp. 127, 135–9; Innes, 'Mixed Economy of Welfare', pp. 163–4; Kilpatrick, 'Living in the Light', pp. 254–7; Pickstone, *Medicine and Industrial Society*, pp. 16–17; Risse, *Hospital Life*, p. 24; Guenter B. Risse, 'Medicine in the Age of

Enlightenment', in A. Wear (ed.) *Medicine in Society: Historical Essays* (Cambridge: Cambridge University Press, 1992), pp. 180–81. Further, the 'temporal coincidence' between falling support for London voluntary hospitals and the growth of dispensaries has been linked to competition for funds. See Croxson, 'Economic Analysis', pp. 86–104.

124. A 'home-patients' scheme was introduced by the Manchester Infirmary in 1781. See Brockbank, *Royal Infirmary, Manchester*, pp. 28, 31, 44. At the Salop and Liverpool Hospitals, the annual number of out-patients increased more than fivefold between the mid-eighteenth century and the 1820s. See Bevan, *Salop Infirmary*, 'A Comparative Average Statement of In and Out-Patients'; McLoughlin, *Liverpool Infirmary*, p. 104, Appendix X.
125. See, for example, Frizelle and Martin, *Leicester Royal Infirmary*, p. 70; Marland, *Medicine and Society*, pp. 195–6; Turner, *Hampshire County Hospital*, p. 61; Berry, 'Patronage', ch. 4.
126. Casebook, admitted 25 October 1752.
127. Casebook, admitted 8 November 1753.
128. *Bath and Bristol Guide*, p. 19; British Medical Association, *The Book of Bath: Written for the Ninety Third Annual Meeting of the BMA held at Bath in July 1925* (Bath: BMA, 1925), p. 134; Wood, *Bath*, pp. 305–6.
129. Collinson, *Somerset*, pp. 50–51.
130. *Bath Journal*, 8 August 1757; 4 September 1758; 6 November 1758; 14 April 1760; 3 August 1761; 17 May 1762.
131. *Bath Journal*, 15 December 1746; 23 March 1752.
132. *Bath Journal*, 14 January 1751; 8 November 1762.
133. *Bath Journal*, 17 December 1764; 22 December 1764.
134. See, for example, *Bath Journal*, 6 March 1758; 2 April 1759; 5 May 1760; 1 June 1761; 5 July 1762; 1 October 1770.
135. *Bath Journal*, 6 February 1758; 7 January 1760.
136. Monica Baly, 'The Care of the Sick Poor in Bath from the Late Eighteenth Century to the First Half of the Nineteenth Century', p. 9. I am grateful to the author for supplying me with a copy of this undated typescript.
137. Warner, *Bath*, pp. 302–3.
138. John Ellis, *The History of the Eastern Dispensary of Bath* (Bath: W. and F. Dawson, 1855), p. 1.
139. F.K. Prochaska, 'Women in English Philanthropy, 1790–1830', *International Review of Social History*, **19** (1974), pp. 426–7.
140. William Tyte, *Bath in the Eighteenth Century: Its Progress and Life Described* (Bath: G. and F. Pickering, 1903), p. 119.
141. Kirkup, 'Bath Casualty Hospital', pp. 51, 57.
142. Mainwaring, *Annals*, pp. 41–2, 53, 114, 241–2.
143. *Bath Chronicle*, 24 January 1805; Percy Vere Turner, *'Charity for a Hundred Years': History of the Monmouth Street Society, Bath, from 1805 to 1904* (no place of publication, publisher or date), p. 25.
144. *The Collective Reports of the Bath Penitentiary and Lock Hospital, from 1816 to 1824* (Bath: Wood, Cunningham and Smith, 1824), pp. 92–3.
145. *The Pauper Charity, Hereafter to be Called Bath City Infirmary and Dispensary* (no place of publication, publisher or date), p. 1.
146. *Collective Reports*, pp. 89, 95.

147. *Bath Infirmary for the Cure of Diseases of the Eye, Instituted November 1811: Fourth Annual Report, from January 1st, 1815, to January 1st, 1816* (Bath: Richard Cruttwell, 1816), p. 11.
148. *State of the Bath City Infirmary*, p. 7.
149. *Improved Bath Guide*, p. 45; *Original Bath Guide* [1840], p. 98; *The Original Bath Guide* (Bath: William Lewis, 1876), pp. 77.
150. Lloyd, *United Hospital, Bath*, p. 8; *Bath Eye Infirmary*, p. 32.
151. *Letter to the President and Governors*, pp. 3–4.
152. *Collective Reports*, p. 93.
153. In 1744/45, for example, the *Bath Journal* carried reports relating to the General Hospital on 7 May, 29 October, 7 January, 25 February and 8 April; in 1760/61 there were reports on 5 May, 4 August, 3 November, 10 November, 9 February, 23 February and 20 April.
154. See footnote 84 above.
155. See, for example, *Bath Journal*, 10 May 1824; 15 March 1830.
156. *Bath Journal*, 12 September 1825; 5 December 1825; 1 February 1830; 12 April 1830; 3 May 1830; 5 July 1830.

PART FIVE
Status, Politics and Power

CHAPTER EIGHT

The Pursuit of Social Status

In Part Four of this book, we put forward a moral economy of Georgian medicine in which a tributary relationship between rich and poor was superseded by a proprietary one. The demise of paternalism embodied within this transition is consistent with Nicholas Rogers's view that by the end of the eighteenth century, 'Real civility, and by extension citizenship, rested fundamentally on middling, even middle-class, manners and morals'.[1] But as well as heralding a new ethical code, severing the link with property also enabled the emergence of a wider elite defined in terms of gentility which could be socially accumulated as well as genetically ascribed; like power, politeness was achieved through 'acquisition, production, [and] display ... rather than inheritance, formal title, and ancient lineage'.[2] In this part, we consider the socio-economic and political developments associated with the decline of civic virtue. Chapter 8 explores how the Bath Infirmary helped to expand the social élite by bringing together the aristocrats, gentry and middling men who co-operated in its finance and management, and by creating opportunities for them to exchange social status. Chapters 9 and 10 then examine the contribution of medical charity to the stability of the Georgian state, focusing on the mediation of political and religious divisions and the challenge to established authority posed by the lower orders.

Aristocrats and middling men

During the century after the Restoration, commercial prosperity transformed the social structure of Britain, rapidly expanding the middle orders to meet the business and professional, manufacturing and retailing needs of an affluent consumer society.[3] Jonathan Barry has extended the Stuart concept of the 'independent trading household' to this Hanoverian 'middling sort', arguing that their essential characteristic was economic self-reliance; not often on the payroll of others, he says, they defended their families against poverty by selling either 'the products of their hands' or 'the skills ... for which they had trained'.[4] This may be too all-inclusive a definition for the towns at the heart of the consumer revolution, whose middle strata began to identify themselves not just by escaping poverty but by using their surplus incomes to accrue gentility.[5] For a sector fragmented by wealth and occupation, religion and politics, this search for politeness offered a unifying cause,[6] but the urbane culture which initially resulted was not a distinctive bourgeois one, shaped without reference to the aristocracy and gentry. On the contrary, 'the fascination with gentility reinforced rather than undermined the cultural hegemony of the ... landed class',[7] and encouraged aspiring middling men to imitate their social values and behaviour. Consequently, it was the aristocracy which controlled admission to the enlarged élite by defining the accomplishments expected of the *nouveaux riches* not born to gentility. Moreover, even as the middling sort gained in power and influence from the later eighteenth century, their continued yearnings for politeness ensured that the social values of the aristocracy were not entirely supplanted. Rather, a process of convergence occurred in which the 'aristocratisation of the bourgeoisie combined with the eventual embourgeoisement of the aristocracy to redraw the dividing lines of society'.[8]

Historical accounts of how this integration took place have often emphasized the formative influence of material possessions for the developing middle class.[9] 'Whether commented on by natives or remarked on by foreigners', observes John Rule, 'the English middle ranks were usually first identified materially by the goods and services they purchased and by the status linked and revealed by that consumption'.[10] However, the pursuit of gentility involved relational as well as material ambitions. Such aspirations were admirably satisfied via the voluntary clubs and societies increasingly complementary to the civic and guild ceremonies inherited from the medieval town.[11] Not all these organizations involved those of middle rank, but the bourgeois economic and social predicament was ideally addressed in subscription schemes which applied the principle of the joint stock company to fashionable activities. Designed to improve accessibility by sharing the cost, these schemes allowed middling men and women to intermingle both among themselves and with the aristocrats and gentry who patronized the town.[12] The formula was especially compelling in the case of associated charities because they added the moral virtue of doing good to the economical quest for social kudos. The eighteenth-century voluntary hospital thrived on this mixture. Institutions sprang up not in industrializing regions where the health of the workforce was at risk as a result of mining and manufacturing, but in prosperous county towns which were social centres for the landed élite.[13] In this chapter, we examine the social rationale for the General Infirmary during the century when Bath evolved from a stylish resort into a popular residential location. First, the status assignations and occupational backgrounds of those who supported the institution are identified. Secondly, the economic, social and cultural networks which linked governors and subscribers are traced. Finally, these relationships are analysed with reference to the pursuit of social status, distinguishing between the use of the Hospital to seek public esteem and to fulfil social aspirations.

Who financed the Hospital?

The status assignations and occupational backgrounds of governors of the Bath Infirmary have to be tackled with care. In the first place, the benefactors from whom money was collected at the biannual charity services – a major source of income – were for the most part anonymous, only some late gifts being attached to known individuals. Even where the details of supporters were given, problems remain. Most (if not all) entries in the *Annual Reports* are legible, but the lists of governors and subscribers may not have been regularly updated, classifications did not always agree with the Minute Books, the duplication of Christian names and the use of initials makes differentiating between family members difficult, and neither ladies nor women titled Mrs or Miss are easily absorbed into a status hierarchy constructed around male assumptions. Compounding these mechanical problems is the mutability of status. In the 1718 edition of *The Present State of Great Britain and Ireland*, Guy Miège noted that 'the title of gentleman is commonly given in England to all that distinguish themselves from the common sort of people, by a good garb, genteel air, or good education, wealth, or learning'.[14] Therefore, while the position of aristocrats, baronets, knights and their 'honourable' relatives was comparatively straightforward, that of esquires and gentlemen was far more equivocal. Amanda Berry maintains that knowing whether hospital patrons styled themselves as esquire is impossible, and suggests that the title may have been conferred by the hospital authorities as a mark of deference.[15] However, 'linguistic fluidity'[16] cannot be reduced to status anarchy. That the Georgians continued to use the terms 'gentleman' and 'esquire' implies that they retained distinctive meanings. Charities flattering their benefactors too liberally risked offending those of higher rank. Yet, at the same time, there was an upward drift in assignations which generated expectations among the middling sort. In the early Georgian period, the appellation 'esquire' commonly signified a substantial country landowner, but the more affluent members of the professional and commercial classes were also 'grasping the very bottom rung of the titular ladder' and claiming the right to be addressed Mr or Gent.[17] As Penelope Corfield has elaborated:

> the concept of the 'gentleman' had already begun its famous social peregrination [by the 1720s], losing its oldest connotations of 'gentle' birth and 'idle' living, so that, in the later eighteenth century, individual vintners, tanners, scavengers, potters, theatre managers, and professors of Divinity could all claim the status, publicly and without irony.[18]

In discussing the social origins of those who financed and managed the Georgian Bath Infirmary, this 'social mutability'[19] must be kept constantly in mind.

Roy Porter has criticized the contention that voluntary hospitals owed most to the 'generosity of the middle classes', and argued that 'the big money came from the grandees', particularly in the early 'stages of seeding the infirmaries'.[20] Berry's work on 'the social structure of patronage' suggests that a 'particularist' reading of voluntary hospitals is appropriate. Across her three sample decades and three institutions, support from medical and military personnel was uniformly low. At the commercial centre of Bristol, however, 9.7 per cent of infirmary patrons were knights, esquires or gents, and almost 80 per cent were titled 'Mr, Mrs or Miss', whereas at the county towns of Exeter and Northampton a quarter fell into the first category and just under a half into the second. Yet despite this local variability, aristocratic support was minimal, with nobles constituting no more than 6 per cent of patrons.[21] The Bath Infirmary's experience of personal donors and annual subscribers confirms that the grandees were not major sponsors. Needless to say, the Hospital founded to make spa therapy available to poor strangers was inextricably bound up with the exclusive Company who holidayed at the resort. Furthermore, 'princely sums' were indeed donated by the landed élite, the royal family giving £700, and other aristocrats, baronets, knights and men of 'honourable' status almost £1 000, in the five years prior to opening. These groups continued to make substantial payments on an occasional basis: the Duke of Beaufort, for example, contributed £100 in 1742; Princess Caroline £100 in 1746; the Marquis of Stafford £100 in 1800; and the Duchess of Kent £25 in 1830.[22] But we must not over-generalize from such magnanimous gestures. Table 8.1 takes snapshots of personal donations at 15-year intervals between the opening of the annual subscription scheme in 1741 and 1830, charting the number, total value and average value of gifts received from different status groups. This type of income – though vital to the Hospital – was highly volatile and fluctuated in response to windfall payments, the mean ranging from almost £68 to under £14. Not all the spectacular contributions came from the upper echelons of the landed élite. Samuel Holden Esquire left a legacy of £2 000 in 1741/42 and Dr Bowen one of £1 800 in 1815/16, whilst Lawrence Williams Esquire bequested bank annuities worth £1 290 in 1770/71.[23] Furthermore, 'titled' benefactions – always small in number – only scored the highest average in 1800/01 when a gift from the Marquis of Stafford pushed up their share to 13 per cent; in the other sample years the grandees accounted for no more than 4 per cent of income from personal donations. Consequently, Table 8.1 contains scant evidence of aristocrats, baronets, knights and their ladies being fundamental to the financial security of the Bath Infirmary.

Annual subscribers generated only a small proportion of total receipts for the Bath Infirmary, but they form a bigger and more stable group with which to explore the status of financial supporters. No aristocrats, baronets, knights or ladies joined the scheme in its first year of operation and after 1741/42 their presence was no more than token.[24] Among the middling orders, who supplied the bulk of subscription income, four trends deserve comment (Table 8.2). Surgeons and apothecaries had 'invisible' qualifications and so they cannot be easily detected, but that few physicians subscribed is clear. Conversely, the presence of military officers after 1800 was noticeable and reflected Bath's popularity as a retirement centre for members of the armed forces.[25] The clergymen who themselves resided in the city, often recruited to meet the spiritual needs of the expanding population, also became more frequent subscribers, rising from nine in 1770/71 to 24 in 1830/31.[26] But most striking was the shifting position of esquires and gentlemen. In 1770/71, these two status groups were each supplying a third of annual subscriptions to the General Infirmary. By 1830, however, gentlemen subscribers had fallen dramatically, while esquires were flourishing. Simultaneously, the relationship between status and philanthropy was being reconfigured. In 1770/71, the social superiority of esquires was captured in their more generous contributions; not only was the average sum higher, but the modal payment was two guineas compared with one guinea for gentlemen. By 1830 status seniority was no longer expressed through a higher subscription, the majority of esquires dropping their payment to the standard guinea in a way that accorded with the notion of charity as a social nicety rather than an obligation of rank.[27]

Who managed the Hospital?

The status assignations of contributors suggests that it was not the grandees who kept the Bath Infirmary financially viable. Money was, of course, essential to the survival of the institution, but in an affluent society where surplus income was growing, a more stringent test of

Table 8.1 Bath General Hospital: the social status of personal donors, 1741–1830

	1741/42			*1755/56*		
Social status	*No. of donors*	*Total value of donations* £	*Average value of donations* £	*No. of donors*	*Total value of donations* £	*Average value of donations* £
Aristocrats	5	63.00	12.60	2	11.55	5.78
Baronets and knights	1	5.25	5.25	1	3.15	3.15
'Honourables'	—	—	—	—	—	—
Esquires	12	2 435.00	202.92	12	293.95	24.50
Gentlemen	4	26.25	6.56	3	7.35	2.45
Doctors	2	25.25	12.63	3	26.30	8.77
Clergy	2	8.85	4.23	3	11.55	3.85
Military officers	—	—	—	—	—	—
Ladies	2	10.50	5.25	1	21.00	21.00
Mrs/Miss	9	200.40	22.27	8	447.08	55.88
Unattributed	6	143.10	23.85	7	19.35	2.76
Total	43	2 917.60	67.85	40	841.28	21.03
	1770/71			*1785/86*		
Aristocrats	5	39.90	7.98	5	47.80	9.56
Baronets and knights	2	3.15	1.58	—	—	—
'Honourables'	1	1.05	1.05	2	1.30	0.65
Esquires	8	1 507.35	188.42	23	175.70	7.64
Gentlemen	5	58.50	11.70	8	96.30	12.04
Doctors	1	1.05	1.05	2	4.20	2.10
Clergy	2	10.50	5.25	9	28.35	3.15
Military officers	—	—	—	1	1.05	1.05
Ladies	—	—	—	4	54.20	13.55
Mrs/Miss	4	104.20	26.05	19	756.90	39.84
Unattributed	6	12.10	2.02	22	160.25	7.28
Total	34	1 737.80	51.11	95	1 326.05	13.96
	1800/01			*1815/16*		
Aristocrats	3	152.10	50.70	—	—	—
Baronets and knights	1	3.15	3.15	—	—	—
'Honourables'	—	—	—	—	—	—
Esquires	7	113.85	16.26	6	271.25	45.21

Table 8.1 continued

	1800/01			*1815/16*		
Social status	*No. of donors*	*Total value of donations* £	*Average value of donations* £	*No. of donors*	*Total value of donations* £	*Average value of donations* £
Gentlemen	9	67.85	7.54	2	1.53	0.77
Doctors	—	—	—	3	1 810.00	603.33
Clergy	5	202.10	40.42	1	50.00	50.00
Military officers	2	2.10	1.05	—	—	—
Ladies	2	2.10	1.05	—	—	—
Mrs/Miss	21	98.60	4.70	9	72.45	8.05
Unattributed	12	520.37	43.36	10	39.55	3.96
Total	62	1 162.22	18.75	31	2 244.78	72.41
	1830/31					
Aristocrats	3	32.10	10.7			
Baronets and knights	—	—	—			
'Honourables'	—	—	—			
Esquires	4	504.10	126.03			
Gentlemen	5	293.00	58.60			
Doctors	—	—	—			
Clergy	—	—	—			
Military officers	2	19.25	9.63			
Ladies	—	—	—			
Mrs/Miss	13	207.80	15.98			
Unattributed	11	29.10	2.65			
Total	38	1 085.35	28.56			

Notes:

1. Women donors have been placed in the aristocracy, baronetage or 'honourable' categories where their own titles permit. 'Ladies' of high rank who cannot be allocated in this way have been classified separately, as have all those called 'Mrs' or 'Miss'. The 'unattributed' grouping comprises donors for whom no status label was recorded.
2. There is some discrepancy between the totals for all personal donations given above and those in Table 3.4. The reason is that, although both sets of figures rely on the *Annual Reports*, this table uses the list of casual benefactions whereas Table 3.4 uses the annual accounts.

Source: *Annual Reports*.

Table 8.2 Bath General Hospital: the social status of annual subscribers, 1741–1830

	1741/42			*1755/56*		
Social status	*No. of subs*	*Total value of subs £*	*Average value of subs £*	*No. of subs*	*Total value of subs £*	*Average value of subs £*
Aristocrats	—	—	—	2	10.5	5.25
Baronets and knights	—	—	—	2	21.00	10.50
'Honourables'	—	—	—	3	15.75	5.25
Esquires	4	10.00	2.50	22	124.45	5.66
Gentlemen	10	6.25	0.65	39	58.53	1.50
Doctors	1	1.30	1.30	7	23.10	3.30
Clergy	4	2.95	0.74	6	13.50	2.25
Military officers	—	—	—	—	—	—
Ladies	—	—	—	—	—	—
Mrs/Miss	4	3.70	0.93	11	20.30	1.85
Unattributed	1	1.30	1.30	2	6.30	3.15
Total	24	25.50	1.06	94	293.43	3.12
	1770/71			*1785/86*		
Aristocrats	4	26.25	6.56	3	9.45	3.15
Baronets and knights	3	11.55	3.85	5	17.85	3.57
'Honourables'	1	5.25	5.25	3	10.50	3.50
Esquires	49	136.25	2.78	76	176.40	2.32
Gentlemen	45	58.75	1.31	44	55.65	1.26
Doctors	6	12.60	2.10	11	23.10	2.10
Clergy	9	12.60	1.40	22	29.40	1.34
Military officers	1	2.10	2.10	2	5.25	2.63
Ladies	1	5.25	5.25	5	13.75	2.75
Mrs/Miss	22	35.65	1.62	46	65.10	1.42
Unattributed	1	2.10	2.10	—	—	—
Total	142	308.35	2.17	217	406.45	1.87
	1800/01			*1815/16*		
Aristocrats	6	28.35	4.73	3	15.75	5.25
Baronets and knights	2	5.25	2.63	3	7.35	2.45
'Honourables'	—	—	—	1	2.10	2.10
Esquires	67	123.65	1.85	56	90.25	1.61

Table 8.2 concluded

	1800/01			*1815/16*		
Social status	*No. of subs*	*Total value of subs* £	*Average value of subs* £	*No. of subs*	*Total value of subs* £	*Average value of subs* £
Gentlemen	14	17.85	1.28	12	12.60	1.05
Doctors	5	8.40	1.68	2	3.15	1.58
Clergy	18	25.20	1.40	22	36.55	1.66
Military officers	1	1.05	1.05	3	7.35	2.45
Ladies	3	4.20	1.40	—	—	—
Mrs/Miss	45	62.85	1.40	50	68.05	1.36
Unattributed	—	—	—	5	10.50	2.10
Total	161	276.80	1.72	157	253.65	1.62
	1830/31					
Aristocrats	5	19.95	3.99			
Baronets and knights	4	8.40	2.10			
'Honourables'	—	—	—			
Esquires	66	90.95	1.38			
Gentlemen	10	13.65	1.37			
Doctors	2	3.15	1.58			
Clergy	24	43.05	1.79			
Military officers	11	17.50	1.59			
Ladies	2	4.05	2.03			
Mrs/Miss	49	66.35	1.35			
Unattributed	—	—	—			
Total	173	267.05	1.54			

Notes:

1. Women subscribers have been placed in the aristocracy, baronetage or 'honourable' categories where their own titles permit. 'Ladies' of high rank who cannot be allocated in this way have been classified separately, as have all those called 'Mrs' or 'Miss'. The 'unattributed' grouping comprises subscribers for whom no status label was recorded.
2. There is some discrepancy between the totals for annual subscriptions above and those given in Table 3.4. One reason is that although both sets of figures rely on the *Annual Reports*, this table uses the list of casual benefactions whereas Table 3.4 uses the annual accounts. More significant, however, is the omission here of corporate subscriptions, mainly from parishes but also medical institutions and local businesses.

Source: *Annual Reports*.

charitable commitment was the willingness to invest time in the management of hospital affairs and bear the opportunity costs that this involved. Therefore, administrative participation is subjected to a finer analysis than financial sponsorship, using quinquennial rather than 15-year samples. Although women comprised between a third and a half of all personal donors, and between 20 and 30 per cent of all annual subscribers (Tables 8.1 and 8.2), none of these female patrons were drawn into institutional management. But who among its male supporters carried the burden of administration, acting as governors and attending the general courts and weekly committees through which business was transacted? Whereas the majority of voluntary infirmaries tied membership of the governing body to financial sponsorship, at Bath automatic access was restricted to benefactors who had given a substantial sum of at least £40[28] and the remaining places were filled by election. The profile of the men thrown up by these joint processes to manage the Infirmary was both similar to, and different from, that of donors and subscribers (Table 8.3). At the top of the hierarchy, aristocrats, baronets, knights and men of 'honourable' status were more prominent as governors than contributors, and in 1739 they accounted for a quarter of the initial corporation. By the time the Hospital opened in 1742, there had been a net loss of six titled governors.[29] Sampling at five-year intervals reveals their representation declining further over the course of the long eighteenth century and by 1830 only one in ten governors were high-ranking members of the landed élite. With the middling sort, there was greater congruence between money and management. Physicians – not a major source of income – were likewise scarce among the governors. Conversely, the growing financial support of military men was reflected in increased presence on the governing body after 1820; while clergy governors almost doubled their representation to 20 per cent between 1775 and the close of the Georgian period. The transformation of the Mr into an esquire was also discernible. Mere gentlemen augmented their numbers in the middle decades of the century, but faded after 1770 and accounted for less than one per cent of governors by 1830. Simultaneously, esquires were strengthening their hold. Always by far the most abundant social category, their share had climbed from 40 to 50 per cent by 1770 and was approaching 60 per cent between 1800 and 1830, with a slight drop in the early 1820s.

Membership of the governing body signalled a formal affiliation with the Hospital, but the extent to which this nominal association was translated into active service varied according to status assignation. So who filled the offices of president and treasurer? And who attended general courts and weekly committees? The list of presidents reads like a roll call of the aristocracy. Six incumbents of this office up to 1830 were identifiable members of the royal family. Eight were spiritual lords. No fewer than 44 were aristocrats, while nine were baronets or knights (Appendix B). Among these titled presidents were distinguished military men such as the rear-admiral, Lord Rodney of nearby Rodney Stoke.[30] Others were aristocrats in waiting. The Right Honourable John Jefferys Pratt, for example, was MP for Bath when he was elected president in 1785, but he went on to inherit his father's title of Earl of Camden in 1794.[31] Local MPs of humbler origins also served, as did other men of lower status. However, their administrative or financial contribution had often been exceptional. The first president, Thomas Carew Esquire, an MP for Minehead, was responsible for shepherding the Act of Incorporation through Parliament;[32] the third president, the local businessman, Ralph Allen Esquire, had given 'the wrought stone for the erection of the building and £1,000 in money';[33] Francis Colston Esquire of Bristol was appointed in 1745, having the previous November donated £300 at a point of financial crisis;[34] and Charles Phillott Esquire was 'requested to accept the office of president' in 1822 after 43 years as a treasurer.[35]

The aristocratic majority was less diligent. In 1745, John Dalton dedicated his charity sermon to His Royal Highness the Prince of Wales, who 'first encouraged the Hospital with his bounty and now honours it with his protection as president'.[36] The office was bestowed on other nobles who were generous in their donations,[37] but the 'protection' that all presidents offered rarely went beyond keeping a distant fatherly eye on the institution. Though normally elected *in absentia*,[38] the Minute Books document only two candidates during the long eighteenth century who were unwilling to accept nomination: Dr Richard Frewin in 1750 and the Duke of Richmond in 1794.[39] In his letter of rejection, Dr Frewin mildly rebuked the governors for not being 'so kind as to have apprised me of your intention'. But neither this discourtesy, nor 'distain' for the Infirmary, was the reason for his refusal; he had turned down the 'honour ... with modesty, and I hope with decency, and prudence ... [because he] ... judged [himself] wholly unworthy of it' and believed that his replacement, Lord Viscount Palmerston, was a much better choice: a 'man of quality' with the 'interest and ability' to serve the institution well.[40] Dr Frewin's humility was perhaps a little contrived, for as a physician of high reputation, he was better qualified to be the president of an infirmary than to hold the Camden Chair of Ancient History at Oxford that he had accepted in 1729, only subsequently preparing himself for the post by purchasing large quantities of literature on the subject.[41] However, governors and incumbents of the presidency at Bath did not share Dr Frewin's rigorous conception of the duties. The text of a letter to the new president, dated 2 May 1744,

Table 8.3 Bath General Hospital: the social status of governors, 1739–1830

	Social status																			
	Aristocrats		*Baronets or knights*		*'Honourables'*		*Esquires*		*Gentlemen*		*Doctors*		*Clergymen*		*Military officers*		*Political appointment*		*Total*	
Year	*No.*	*%*	*No.*	*%*	*No.*	*%*	*No.*	*%*	*No.*	*%*	*No.*	*%*	*No.*	*%*	*No.*	*%*	*No.*	*%*	*No.*	*%*
1739/40	13	14.13	8	8.70	3	3.26	37	40.22	8	8.70	9	9.78	10	10.87	1	1.09	3	3.26	92	100.00
1750/51	14	13.21	3	2.83	2	1.89	46	43.40	17	16.04	12	11.32	8	7.55	1	0.94	3	2.83	106	100.00
1755/56	15	13.76	3	2.75	4	3.67	44	40.37	21	19.27	11	10.09	7	6.42	1	0.92	3	2.75	109	100.00
1760/61	11	10.38	6	5.66	4	3.77	45	42.45	19	17.93	9	8.49	9	8.49	—	—	3	2.83	106	100.00
1765/66	12	10.35	6	5.17	7	6.04	54	46.55	16	13.79	6	5.17	11	9.48	1	0.86	3	2.59	116	100.00
1770/71	17	13.28	7	5.47	3	2.34	66	51.56	19	14.84	5	3.91	8	6.25	—	—	3	2.34	128	100.00
1775/76	11	8.21	7	5.22	3	2.24	72	53.73	14	10.45	7	5.22	17	12.69	—	—	3	2.24	134	100.00
1780/81	10	6.85	9	6.16	3	2.06	79	54.11	16	10.96	8	5.48	17	11.64	1	0.69	3	2.06	146	100.00
1785/86	12	7.84	13	8.50	2	1.31	82	53.60	14	9.15	9	5.88	17	11.11	1	0.65	3	1.96	153	100.00
1790/91	9	5.29	9	5.29	1	0.59	95	55.88	14	8.24	10	5.88	27	15.88	2	1.18	3	1.77	170	100.00
1795/96	9	5.81	7	4.52	1	0.65	88	56.77	12	7.74	6	3.87	26	16.77	3	1.94	3	1.94	155	100.00
1800/01	12	8.00	6	4.00	1	0.67	89	59.33	4	2.67	7	4.67	26	17.33	2	1.33	3	2.00	150	100.00
1805/06	12	7.90	6	3.95	1	0.66	89	58.55	3	1.97	10	6.59	27	17.76	1	0.66	3	1.97	152	100.00
1810/11	13	8.33	7	4.49	1	0.64	93	59.62	1	0.64	9	5.77	28	17.95	1	0.64	3	1.92	156	100.00
1815/16	14	8.92	9	5.73	1	0.64	87	55.41	2	1.27	7	4.46	33	21.02	1	0.64	3	1.91	157	100.00
1820/21	11	7.43	9	6.08	1	0.68	75	50.68	1	0.68	8	5.41	38	25.68	2	1.35	3	2.03	148	100.00

1825/26	8	5.06	9	5.70	1	0.63	87	55.06	3	1.90	5	3.17	37	23.42	5	3.17	3	1.90	158	100.00
1830/31	7	4.76	9	6.12	—	—	85	57.82	1	0.68	5	3.40	32	21.77	5	3.40	3	2.04	147	100.00

Notes:

1. The social status of governors in 1739/40 has been compiled from the Hospital's Act of Incorporation. After 1749/50, a list of governors for the forthcoming financial year was published in the *Annual Report* eg. the names for 1750/51 represented the position on 1 May 1751.
2. All 'Doctors' were medical practitioners, with the exception of two Doctors of Law who were governors in 1739/40 and 1750/51 respectively. Doctors of Divinity (all of whom were ordained) have been classified as clergy.
3. The 'Clergy' category includes the Rector of Bath and the Bishop of Bath and Wells, who were *ex officio* appointments. Although clerics of all ranks are grouped under this heading, no more than three were bishops in any one sample year.
4. Political appointments comprised the Mayor and Justices of Bath who were *ex officio* governors.
5. The 'Total' column excludes governors for whom no social status is available: one in 1765/66, 1790/91 and 1795/96; two in 1750/51 and 1760/61; and three in 1820/21.
6. Percentages have been rounded up or down and so do not always total exactly 100.00.

Sources: 12 Geo. II, pp. 572–3; *Annual Reports*.

informed him of his unanimous election and asked him 'to appoint two proper persons' from the current weekly committee 'to represent you as deputies for carrying out the business of the House'.[42] Given this procedure, it was perhaps predictable that any administrative participation was exceptional. During his term of office in 1742/43, Ralph Allen did put in an appearance at 12 weekly committee meetings, and the presence of his brother, Philip, on 34 occasions suggests that he may have been regularly briefed. In the samples taken at five-year intervals, however, no other president attended a single weekly committee. Even general courts, which were the administrative high points of the Hospital year, were passed by, only Lord Bexley materializing to chair the meeting held on 31 January 1831. Essentially, therefore, presidents were eminent figureheads, recruited for their social prestige rather than to manage the institution.

The job of treasurer was potentially more onerous. Of the 18 men who filled the three posts available annually up to 1830, one was the Honourable Benjamin Bathurst, the first son of Earl Bathurst,[43] three were physicians and 13 were esquires, while Mr Charles Phillott ascended to the status of esquire in the early 1790s (Appendix C). The Minute Books suggest that most responsibility was devolved to one treasurer. Master of Ceremonies, Richard Nash, was energetic in transmitting donations to the Hospital[44] and his contemporary, William Oliver, was a similarly dedicated honorary physician and member of the weekly committee (Appendix G). In the early 1740s, however, it was the third treasurer, Francis Fauquier, who handled bills and legacies,[45] and started to make regular financial reports to the weekly committee.[46] Fauquier possessed a technical expertise which in 1756 enabled him to publish an influential *Essay on the Ways and Means of Raising Money for the Support of the Present War without Increasing the Public Debts*.[47] Benjamin Bathurst, his successor in 1745,[48] had no such special competence; indeed, in 1761 he became indebted to the Hospital to the tune of £180, having misappropriated the caution money for 60 patients. The money was duly repaid to Daniel Danvers,[49] who had been elected a treasurer in 1760[50] and took over prime responsibility for financial affairs until his death in 1779.[51] As well as regularly paying the tradesmen's bills and the servants' wages,[52] Danvers handled incidental tasks which ranged from dealing with executors[53] and selling stocks and shares[54] to taking legal proceedings against staff[55] and managing the Charmy Down estate.[56] Moreover, during the year of his death, he visited London 'to attest the nature and amount of the estates belonging to ... [the Hospital] before both Houses of Parliament' in what proved to be a successful attempt to escape from the restrictions of the Mortmain Act.[57] So closely was financial management identified with Daniel

Danvers that Hospital motions passed by the general court and the weekly committee referred to the treasurer in the singular without judging it necessary to name him.[58] Charles Phillott, who succeeded Danvers,[59] played an equally pivotal role during his long reign as a treasurer.[60] He was finally replaced by Edmund Anderdon in 1822,[61] who was likewise active in routine and *ad hoc* financial administration,[62] and also chaired the weekly committee until 1829.[63] Thereafter, much responsibility was transferred to Johnson Phillott. Anderdon was still checking the register's caution money account in 1831 – a procedure introduced in 1783, and implemented by the leading treasurer after 1792, following the discovery of fraudulent activities.[64] However, Phillott became chairman of the weekly committee, and also settled the bills arising from the refurbishment of the Hospital in the late 1820s.[65] The socio-economic background of these men who headed the financial team is significant. Edmund Anderdon was an apothecary (Appendix G), but Daniel Danvers and Charles and Johnson Phillott were all bankers[66] who, like Francis Fauquier, brought technical expertise to the finances of the Infirmary. In theory, abuse and corruption were prevented by the appointment of three treasurers who scrutinized each others' work.[67] In practice, the physicians and esquires who served as co-treasurers were sleeping colleagues, relying upon the integrity of a professionalizing group within the middling sort to deliver financial propriety.

A process of devolution was also evident in the general management of the Bath Infirmary. Whereas treasurers were skewed towards the status of esquire, however, those who participated in general courts and weekly committee were initially more socially diverse. General courts, poorly attended though not often inquorate throughout the Georgian period, were rarely graced with members of the aristocracy, baronetage or knightage (Appendix D). On 31 October 1770 Lord Londonderry chaired a general meeting, presumably at the invitation of the governors because he had no formal connection with the Hospital. Moreover, Lord Dupplin, Sir John Miller and Baron Dimsdale each attended one court in 1750/51, 1780/81 and 1790/91 respectively; while Sir Orford Gordon participated in one during 1825/26 and four held in 1830/31. But aristocrats and baronets like these were the exception. For the most part, courts were populated by the middling sort. Although physicians were more visible in the 1750s when the quota of honorary posts was temporarily doubled from three to six, they were never a major constituency and increasingly lost interest in administration after 1800. For clergy the trend, albeit variable, was in the opposite direction, their greater prevalence in the governing body feeding through to court attendance so that by 1830 they were second only to esquires, who accounted for half the governors participating in at least one general meeting. Esquires had not always been so dominant. When the court convened in May 1742, 40 governors held the status of esquire, yet just three were present, compared with ten of the 13 who carried the title Mr. The disproportionate attendance of Gents survived the rise and fall of their overall representation. In 1755/56, the sample year in which gentlemen's share of the governing body peaked at almost 20 per cent, they constituted more than 40 per cent of those appearing at one or more general meetings. Thirty years later, the proportions were 10 per cent and 30 per cent respectively. Only with the virtual disappearance of the assignation among the governors did evacuation of the court occur.

Appointment to the weekly committee was similarly structured. Honorary physicians and surgeons, together with key local clergy, were routinely recruited. Among the laity, however, managerial responsibility was more selectively distributed. Titled governors only infrequently found their way to the weekly committee, with the result that the middling sort were uppermost. During the earlier Georgian period, gentlemen were especially prominent. In 1755/56, for example, 19 members of the weekly committee were known as Mr and only three as esquire, but esquires outnumbered gentlemen by more than two to one on the governing body. Thirty years later, the relative chances of appointment remained uneven. Gentlemen had declined in absolute terms to 14, but they supplied seven members of the committee, compared with the 14 members drawn from 82 esquires (Appendix E and Table 8.3). Governors entitled Mr were not only more likely to be chosen; they were also more likely to attend. Though proximity to Bath was taken into consideration when picking the committee, overall attendance was poor and during each sample year a sizeable group failed to attend a single meeting. Fewer gentlemen than esquires were renegades; but of greater significance was the fact that more were present on at least ten occasions and hence made a regular contribution to running the Infirmary. With the departure of governors entitled Mr, esquires became the mainstay of hospital management, as physicians and surgeons withdrew their non-clinical involvement (Appendix F). In 1830, therefore, they were carrying the administrative burden of the institution, aided by a clutch of energetic clergy.

Moving from rates of appointment and attendance to the behaviour of individual governors reveals that the weekly committee was heavily dependent upon a faithful core of governors (Appendix G). Deputy president, Dr William Oliver, provides the most dramatic example, his presence at 49 weekly committees in 1742/43 outstripping the annual average for active physicians by 20. But other officers were also diligent, Mr Charles Phillott attending 39 meetings in 1785/86 and Edmund Anderdon Esquire 41 during 1815/16 – financial years when both were serving treasurers. Nor was regular attendance the monopoly of officers; for in 1770/71 the wine merchant, Mr Edward Parker, put in an appearance at 38 meetings. If the administrative core of which these men were distinguished parts is defined by participation in at least 20 weekly committees, we find that its membership shrank over the course of the long eighteenth century. In 1742/43, 15 governors met the criterion, but initial enthusiasm gave way to a reduced core of six to eight members until 1800/01 when just a solitary individual qualified. This collapse was brought about by the changing role of medical staff. Even after the paid apothecary had ceased to be a governor and the quotas for honorary appointments had returned to three, physicians and surgeons were typically towards the top of the attendance list and explained between a third and a quarter of all weekly committee attendances. Consequently, their abdication from the hospital administration created a temporary vacuum. In the longer term, however, recruitment came to reflect the professional values of the nineteenth-century city, as the clergymen appointed to serve Bath's expanding residential population began to assume the philanthropic duties which medical men had performed earlier in the Georgian period.

The location of the Bath Infirmary in a spa town and its dedication to poor strangers ensured that benefactors and governors were geographically far-flung. Consequently, it is difficult to move beyond an examination of status assignation to probe their socio-economic identities. In the case of the weekly committee, however, the bias towards nearby residents allows a more sophisticated analysis, using local histories, directories and newspapers, Corporation records and national biographical tools to search for the occupations of those whose employment is not disclosed by their title. Most difficult to identify conclusively are the country gentry: esquires like Edward Andrews of Mangotsfield in Gloucestershire, who attended five meetings in 1742/43; or John Lloyd of Ford, near Winscombe in Somerset, who attended 14 meetings in 1770/71 (Appendix G). However, distance meant that the governors participating in weekly committees were not just local but overwhelmingly urban. These men were markedly tilted towards the trades which catered for the visiting Company (Table 8.4). Apothecaries, for whom honorary posts were not an option, may have viewed being an active governor as an alternative source of professional status, especially given their subordinate position on the medical ladder. At a Georgian spa, however, dispensing medical wares was also a commercial service industry. Consequently, the apothecary – like the physician and surgeon – shared a common bond with the banker and lawyer, architect and

Table 8.4 Bath General Hospital: the occupational status of governors attending one or more weekly committees per annum, 1742–1830

Occupation	*1742/43* No.	*1755/56* No.	*1770/71* No.	*1785/86* No.
Physicians	5	6	3	4
Surgeons	1	6	4	3
Apothecaries	5	5	5	5
Clergymen	4	2	3	3
Lawyers	—	1	—	—
Businessmen: luxury products	5	3	2	2
Businessmen: non-luxury products	4	1	2	3
Other occupation	2	—	1	2
Visitor	3	2	2	1
Resident	1	—	—	—
Unknown	1	—	2	2
Total	31	26	24	25

	1800/01 No.	*1815/16* No.	*1830/31* No.
Physicians	3	1	2
Surgeons	2	1	3
Apothecaries	5	5	—
Clergymen	3	1	4
Lawyers	1	3	—
Businessmen: luxury products	1	1	2
Businessmen: non-luxury products	3	2	1
Other occupation	2	—	—
Visitor	—	—	—
Resident	3	1	6
Unknown	1	—	1
Total	24	15	19

Notes:

1. This table has been abstracted from Appendix G which lists the principal sources used. Identities there marked as uncertain have been classified. On the infrequent occasions where two occupations are given, priority has been accorded to medical employment.
2. The categories for physicians and surgeons include those holding honorary posts. In 1815/16, a truss-maker and surgical mechanist is accommodated with the surgeons.

3. The category for apothecaries includes the General Hospital's paid apothecary who was a governor in the 1740s and 1750s. A chemist and druggist has been absorbed in 1815/16.
4. The distinction between businessmen dealing in luxury and non-luxury products is difficult to draw. Examples of the former include a jeweller and toymaker, bookseller, dancing school master, portrait painter, wine merchant, lacemaker and tea dealer. Examples of the latter include Ralph Allen, the postal contractor and quarry owner, John Wood, the architect, a glazier, bankers, drapers, carriers and a grain merchant.
5. The category of other occupations includes the financial expert, Francis Fauquier, authors or poets, and the Masters of Ceremonies whose sources of income varied.
6. Visitors and residents are governors for whom no occupation has been traced. The former includes national politicians and dignitaries, and those living beyond the immediate vicinity of Bath; the latter are those with a local address.

painter, jeweller and lacemaker, wine merchant and bookseller whose activities were more obviously connected with the physical development of the city or the satisfaction of an appetite for non-essential consumption. This economic association of Hospital governors with the visiting Company helps to explain the loss of gentlemen from the governing body because, prospering with the resort, this élite among the commercial classes was socially mobile. Therefore, whereas the mid-century bookseller, James Leake, was known as Mr, his counterpart, Joseph Barrat – who in 1830 was the proprietor of a circulating library – enjoyed the distinction of esquire. Occupational continuity underpinned the changing contours of status assignation.

In asking who financed and managed the Georgian Bath Infirmary, we have identified a constituency of benefactors and governors which was socially mixed but hierarchically structured. Aristocrats and bishops, baronets and knights dominated the presidency throughout the long eighteenth century; but that pre-eminence was matched by neither financial nor administrative support. Titled donors made the occasional big-hearted gift, but their collective offerings both to casual income and to the subscription scheme were far outweighed by less elevated contributors. This middling sort also met most administrative needs. Aristocrats, baronets and knights, whose representation on the governing body sagged from a quarter to a tenth between 1739 and 1830, were conspicuous by their absence from general courts and weekly committees, leaving hospital management to doctors and clerics, gentlemen and esquires. The physicians and surgeons who carried a heavy administrative burden for much of the eighteenth century were largely motivated by the career rewards for their service. Professional status was likewise a consideration for the clergy who partially filled the gap opened up by the exit of medical men. Moreover, charity became increasingly instrumental as the Evangelical Revival generated denominational competition and pressure for religious reform.[68] But clerical involvement can also be attributed to the fusion of spiritual life with the socio-cultural commerce of the spa, especially since several ministers on the governing body were associated with the proprietary chapels set up to cater for visitors and residents (Appendix G). The diligence with which the commercial and professional classes attended meetings, and their preponderance at the general courts where nominations were made, suggests that they were not reluctant conscripts press-ganged by their social betters. For these occupational communities, running the Bath Hospital was integral to their economic and social networks. Tangible returns were delivered, some of which were financial. But, additionally, medical charity was a route to gentility, conferring social status upon those who committed money and time.

Economic and social networks

The most lively administrators of the General Hospital were caught up in a web of local economic and social relationships. Among the men who advanced the idea of an Infirmary, there were pre-existing commercial ties. The architect, John Wood, was patronized by Humphrey Thayer, who became treasurer of the fund in 1724. He also worked on behalf of Earl Bathurst, whose son, Benjamin, became an active governor. However, his best client was Ralph Allen: Wood operated as an enthusiastic London salesman for the Bath stone extracted from Allen's quarries and used this local material to build him the stately country house called Prior Park, which was completed in 1742.[69] Other governors were financially linked to Allen too: Samuel Purlewent was his attorney and steward; James Grist his apothecary, James Leake, a bookseller from whom he purchased, and John Chapman his domestic chaplain, while David Hartley, William Oliver and Robert Gusthart each served as his physician.[70] Later governors similarly had mutual economic interests; in particular, Daniel Danvers and members of the Phillott family, who were partners in a firm of Bristol bankers, went on to collaborate in setting up the Old Bath Bank which opened in 1768.[71] If the Infirmary tapped into relationships within the business community, it also contributed to the prosperity of the town. Throughout the Georgian period, the local economy revolved around a leisure industry that was greatly reliant upon the healing image of the springs. The General Hospital functioned as a medical showcase, its very presence investing water therapy with authority even if clinical trials were fitful and efficacy disputed. Therefore, although medical practitioners benefited most directly both from this demonstration effect – and from the access to fee-paying patients which honorary practice granted – the Infirmary also remitted a general commercial return because displaying the spa waters sold other goods too.

Complementing this generic economic glow was the profit to individual tradesmen and professionals from their business relationships with the Bath Hospital. In March 1742, Mr Samuel Howse was rewarded with a substantial order, 'having generously offered to supply ... all sorts of linen cloth at prime cost'. These special terms, and the ensuing sale of drapery items, may have facilitated the election of his son to a governorship in the 1750s.[72] But commercial concessions were also economically motivated. Already a governor when he donated two pieces of bathing linen in 1795,[73] the draper, Henry Edward Howse Esquire, was no doubt nurturing future custom both from the Infirmary itself and from colleagues on the governing body warmed by his benevolence. Good publicity was likewise an asset for those who dealt in luxury goods and services. Allen's donation of the stone for a charitable institution sited in a fashionable and expanding urban centre was a subtle but shrewd piece of advertising. John Wood – and the attorneys who handled legal briefs[74] – gave their assistance free of charge in reasonable expectation of a financial return from the enhancement of their professional reputations. And for the artist William Hoare, the Hospital doubled up as a gallery, housing his portrait of the treasurer, Daniel Danvers, and the scene of Dr Oliver and Mr Peirce examining patients, both of which he donated.[75] His commissions further reveal how governors may have gained indirectly from their alliance with the Hospital. Several patrons were presidents: Thomas Carew, Lord Chesterfield, Francis Colston, the Duke of Beaufort, Viscount Dupplin, William Pitt, Lord Clive, and Sir Lawrence Dundas. Other subjects were medical staff like Dr Oliver, Dr Hartley, Dr Charleton, Mr Peirce and Mr Wright, while a third group were governors. Hoare painted Richard Nash, Benjamin Bathurst, Robert Dingley, and Christopher Anstey,[76] and his pastels of Sir Robert Throckmorton's family still adorn the Tapestry Bedroom of their home at Coughton Court in Warwickshire.[77]

The social relationships which may have both facilitated such economic transactions and blossomed from them were of a familial and a socio-cultural kind. Although family names such as Chapman and Anderdon, Colbourne and Howse recurred among the active governors, it was the Phillotts who provided the most impressive instance of a dynastic network.[78] Joseph Phillott started the chain with his election as an honorary surgeon in 1767, a post which he held for over 50 years.

He was followed by his brother, Charles, who became a treasurer in 1779 and was honoured with the presidency for length of service in 1822.[79] Charles sustained the management of the Hospital during the difficult years of the Napoleonic Wars, ably assisted by a third brother, James, who was Archdeacon of Bath between 1800 and 1815. Finally, Charles's son, Johnson, like his father a partner in the family banking business, became a governor and treasurer, continuing the family tradition of active administration (Appendix G). As well as being the focus of a hereditary network, Charles Phillott was locked into the social relations of the Hospital by marriage because his wife was in all probability a daughter of Henry Wright, the long-standing surgeon and governor to whom Joseph Phillott had been apprenticed. Such marital associations between governors and honorary medical staff were not uncommon. William Oliver's daughter, Charlotte, was briefly married to the famous military physician, Sir John Pringle, before her premature death in 1753 at the age of 25.[80] Henry Harington's daughter married the Venerable Josiah Thomas, a respected Archdeacon of Bath;[81] while the second wife of Sir Benjamin Hobhouse, president in 1813, was a sister of Dr Caleb Hillier Parry.[82] Lay members of the governing body were also conjugally connected. Among early governors from outside the city, Frazer Honywood was married to Abraham Atkyn's daughter[83] and William Wollaston to Francis Fauquier's sister.[84] Later in the century, Peter Legh's daughter married Anthony James Keck[85] and Sir Matthew White Ridley married Sarah Colbourne, daughter of Benjamin Colbourne, a long-serving treasurer of the Hospital.[86] Local alliances were also cemented. Philip Allen's second wife was a sister of the Bath MP, Mr Philip Bennet;[87] Daniel Danvers' daughter married Samuel Howse, a local wine merchant who was probably descended from Samuel Howse, the draper;[88] and William Hoare's daughter, Mary, married a relative of the first Henry Hoare of Stourhead, the founder governor whose family perpetuated his interest in the Hospital by remaining on the governing body throughout the long eighteenth century.[89] Kinship ties were not confined to marriage. Sir Francis Knollys was a grandson of Humphrey Thayer;[90] Master of Ceremonies, William Wade, was a nephew of the military hero, George Wade, who was president of the Hospital in 1741;[91] Sir John Trevelyan was the nephew and heir of Sir Walter Blackett;[92] and the Honourable Philip Pusey was a half-brother of the Earl of Radnor.[93] Finally, the Reverend Martin Stafford Smith married Ralph Allen's niece, and lived at Prior Park, after the death of her first husband, William Warburton.[94]

Whatever the bond, these familial relationships occurred within the wider social and cultural networks in which members of the General Infirmary's governing body circulated. A number had esoteric interests.

Edward Harley, second Earl of Oxford and one of the initial corporation, surrounded himself with 'the more distinguished poets and men of letters', and 'had a passion for building and landscape gardening, and for collecting books, manuscripts, pictures, medals, and miscellaneous curiosities'.[95] Henry Hoare II was a patron of painting and sculpture, and created a classical landscape garden in the grounds of his Wiltshire country seat.[96] And John Julius Angerstein – known as the 'Father of Lloyd's' because he was responsible for transferring its business from the Coffee House to the Royal Exchange in 1774 – owned a large artistic collection which became the kernel of the National Gallery.[97] Within the early Georgian city, Ralph Allen was at the nerve centre of such cultural activities: a mandarin whose patronage encompassed men of local and national significance. Richard Nash apparently organized social amusements at Prior Park, although he was not a favourite.[98] But Allen was most renowned for the 'discriminate patronage of a brilliant group of men',[99] including among his coterie of eminent visitors politicians and religious leaders, artists and writers. Allen was a great friend of George Wade, and Pitt the Elder, both of whom represented Bath in Parliament and served as presidents of the General Infirmary.[100] Furthermore, his influence with Pitt is said to have oiled the appointment to the see of Gloucester of William Warburton, his niece's husband, who preached on behalf of the Hospital in 1742 and later became a governor. Warburton himself was originally introduced to the circle by Alexander Pope,[101] one of a string of literary protégés, and Prior Park was the setting for Gainsborough's study of the actor, theatre manager, playwright and Hospital governor, David Garrick.[102] However, William Hoare was the artist to benefit most from Allen's patronage, his lucrative practice owing much to the open door at Prior Park which granted access to many of the distinguished subjects whom he portrayed.[103]

For his admirers, Allen's cultivation of these political, religious, literary and artistic figures created an oasis of cultural refinement in Bath. Where previously there had been 'intrigue, libertinism, and vulgar gossip', he enabled 'society' or genuine 'social intercourse' – 'the confidential intermingling of persons to cultivate the "exercise of those graces which adorn the sociable life"'.[104] This nineteenth-century interpretation over-embellishes Allen's contribution as part of a mission to discredit Richard Nash, the Master of Ceremonies. None the less, the entourage at Prior Park was a cultural icon for the middling sort which, for those sufficiently familiar with Allen to receive an invitation, was a fountain of social prestige. Although this privilege was not exclusive to supporters of the General Infirmary, Allen's commitment to the institution and the density of participation by governors induced hopeful recruits to volunteer. By the time Allen died in 1764, Bath was entering a new phase in which the expansion of the resort began to trigger more structured social and cultural arrangements. Of course, informal relationships continued. Dr Caleb Hillier Parry enjoyed a lifelong friendship with the Bathurst family and became 'very intimate' with one of his famous patients, Lord Rodney,[105] who was president of the General Infirmary in 1783. Similarly, the local historian, the Reverend Richard Warner, was helped in his parish duties by the Reverend Thomas Falconer, a friend who like Warner was a governor of the Hospital in the 1820s.[106] Informal networks also survived. Sir John Miller was involved in the 'poetic academy' – frequented by fellow governor and poet, Christopher Anstey – which his wife organized at their Batheaston home until her death in 1781.[107] Moreover, Sir Richard Colt Hoare's 'Stourhead Circle' regularly brought together men with antiquarian interests, including his contemporary on the governing body, the Reverend Joseph Hunter.[108] Nevertheless, in Bath itself, the cultural enlightenment in which Allen had prided himself was increasingly sought through more structured forms. The expanding population of residents and visitors provided a ready market for open lectures and exhibitions.[109] For greater exclusivity, however, aspiring middling men turned to organized societies with a limited membership.

Like the honorary physicians, lay governors of the Bath Infirmary became engaged in these formal mechanisms of cultural refinement. There was a close association with the Bath and West Society. In 1777, Master of Ceremonies, William Brereton, and the banker and apothecary, William Street, attended the inaugural meeting; Sir Benjamin Hobhouse was its president between 1805 and 1817;[110] and in the mid-1820s, a half of the 23 vice-presidents, together with the sub-treasurer and secretary, were governors of the Hospital. This Bath and West Society had no fewer than 18 personnel in common with the first Bath Philosophical Society which was operative between 1779 and 1787. Despite its brief to discuss 'the arts and sciences, natural history, the history of nations or any branch of polite literature', the agenda of the Philosophical Society was predominantly scientific and a majority of its members – all of whom were elected by ballot to fill a fixed quota of 25 places – had a professional or amateur interest in this field of enquiry.[111] Therefore, although seven members of the Society were governors of the General Hospital in 1780 or 1785, three were physicians – two of whom were current or future honorary staff.[112] After two attempts at resuscitation, the Philosophical Society was finally reborn as the Literary and Scientific Institution in 1825. The governor, Sir John Palmer Acland, was one of the party who had submitted appropriate plans and acted as provisional tenants during the building programme, under the chairmanship of the Marquis of Lansdowne who became president of the General Infirmary in 1829.[113] In addition, at least one other governor, the Reverend Joseph Hunter, was a founder member and seven members of the first seventeen-man committee were also on the Hospital's governing body.[114] Unfortunately, full membership lists for the Institution, and for the Literary Club and the Harmonic Society also originating in the late eighteenth century, have not survived. From the evidence available, however, cultural organizations for the propagation of science appear to have been for a *cognoscente* who possessed sufficient expertise, in sharp contrast to the open, associated model of cultural activity popular from the post-Restoration period. Philanthropy, on the other hand, as much an Enlightenment accomplishment as learning in the arts or sciences, offered easier access to a lattice of socio-cultural relationships which was dependent upon only the payment of a small subscription and not a test of competence.

Despite this relative inclusiveness, however, charitable networks in Bath did exhibit signs of closure, both in their interlocking membership and in their social composition. In 1722, Henry Hoare I, a long-term campaigner for charity education in London and an active founder member of the Society for Promoting Christian Knowledge, laid the foundation-stone for a Blue-Coat School in Bath.[115] Charles Phillott, the later Georgian treasurer of the General Infirmary, was also a friend of philanthropic education so devoted that, in the words of a contemporary, he condescended 'to sit down to teach a poor shoe black the letters on the alphabet'.[116] When local participation after the charity explosion of the 1790s is pieced together more systematically from the *Improved Bath Guide* for 1812, Charles Phillott stands out as a star (Table 8.5). Over and above his responsibilities at the Bath Hospital and the Blue-Coat School, he was treasurer of the Society for the Suppression of Vagrants and the Bath Auxiliary Bible Society, a trustee of the Servants' Fund and a guardian of the House of Protection, who also 'ably supported' the Reverend Richard Warner in his 'humane exertions' to set up the Penitentiary.[117] But Charles Phillott was not the only governor to have his finger in several charitable pies. Officers were not named for every organization listed in the *Guide* and for a number only the incumbents of principal posts were specified. Even given this partial information, however, 23 members of the governing body as it stood in 1815 were identified as having an involvement in one additional charity, three in two, two in three, one in four, and one – Charles Phillott – in five. Furthermore, the 'freeze frame' of 1812 overlooks both past and future commitments. The Reverend John Sibley and William Anderdon had actively promoted the foundation of the Bath Casualty Hospital in 1788; Charles Phillott had been treasurer of the City Infirmary and Dispensary during the early 1790s; between 1808 and 1815, Lieutenant-General Sir William Cockburn

Table 8.5 Charitable participation by governors of the General Hospital in later Georgian Bath

Governor (1815)	*City Infirmary and Dispensary*	*House of Protection*	*Penitentiary*	*Society for the Suppression of Vagrants*	*Society for the Relief of Persons Imprisoned for Small Debts*	*Bath SPCK*	*Bath Auxiliary Bible Society*	*National Benevolent Institution*	*Blue Coat Charity School*	*Servants Fund*
George Edward Allen Esq.										Trustee
William Anderdon Esq.									Trustee	
Marquis of Bath							Vice-president			
Bishop of Bath and Wells						President				
Marquis of Camden							President			
William Clark Esq.					Auditor		Ctee			
Charles Crook Esq.									Trustee	
William Dickinson Esq. MP								General Ctee		
William Falconer MD							Ctee			
Wyndham Goodden Esq.					Auditor					
John Horton Esq.									Trustee	
Henry Edward Howse Esq.							Ctee			
Revd Robert Jacomb				Secretary						
Sir Walter James Bart.								General Ctee		
William Gore Langton Esq. MP	President						Vice-president	General Ctee		
Duke of Leeds								General Ctee		

T.B. Lethbridge Esq. MP								General Ctee		
Paul Cobb Methuen Esq.								General Ctee		
Caleb Hillier Parry MD								Local Ctee		
Earl of Pembroke								General Ctee		
Charles Phillott Esq.		Treasurer Guardian		Treasurer			Treasurer		Trustee	Trustee
Ven. Archdeacon James Phillott				Vice-president		Vice-president			Treasurer	
Revd John Richards		Guardian		Sub-treasurer						
Revd John Sibley									Trustee	
Revd Martin Stafford Smith									Trustee	
W.J.W. Taylor Esq.								Local Ctee		
R.G. Temple Esq.							Ctee			
Sir John Trevelyan Bart.					Vice-president					
Revd Richard Warner	Chaplain		Chaplain							
John Wiltshire Esq.				Vice-president			Ctee	Local Ctee		Trustee

Notes:
1. For a number of charities included in the *Guide*, no details of governors, etc. were given. In other cases, the information was partial.
2. Doctors are only included where they were not functioning as honorary medical staff.
3. There were two William Clarks on the governing body of the General Hospital in 1815, a father and a son.

Sources: *The Improved Bath Guide*, pp. 49–82; *Annual Report*, 1815/16.

chaired the committee of the Bath Society for the Suppression of Common Vagrants and Impostors; George Allen and Paul Methuen were serving the local Eye Infirmary in 1815, in the company of seven other governors; and Sir Orford Gordon chaired the annual general meeting of the Bath Penitentiary in 1825.[118] There was also intersection with the Bath United Hospital. Not only was almost half of its sixteen-man committee in 1831/32 drawn from the governing body of the General Infirmary, but it was the most active members who were recruited. Thus, M.T. Langton, William Basnet and Captain W.J. Lye, all of whom participated in more than 30 weekly meetings at the General Hospital in 1830/31, attended respectively 90, 74 and 38 sessions of the United Hospital's weekly committee between June 1827 and June 1829. Joseph Barrat and B.L. Lye, less frequent but still regular in their attendance at the General Infirmary, were more committed to the United Hospital, being present at 90 and 63 meetings respectively.[119]

The positioning of these energetic governors at the centre of a series of networks suggests that – to paraphrase Shani d'Cruze – they were acting as charity 'brokers', knitting together the middling sort through philanthropy and handling the sensitive interface with the traditional élite. Several factors affected the performance of this role: relevant professional expertise, commercial interests which were close to the social functioning of the resort, and leisure time to devote to good works. Overshadowing all these influences, however, was the social status which attached to the middling men who governed the Bath Infirmary and predisposed them to become urban cultural leaders.[120] This social status likewise earmarked those who were not brokers for positions of trust within philanthropic organizations – hence the appointment of esquires William Clark and Wyndham Goodden to audit the accounts of the Society for the Relief of Persons Imprisoned for Small Debts (Table 8.5). Governors who were aristocrats, baronets or knights, politicians or leading churchmen tended to occupy honorific posts when they became involved with other charities. In the case of the Bath Eye Infirmary, for example, the president and half of the 14 vice-presidents were on the governing body of the General Infirmary in 1815 and only two of these eight men were not aristocrats, baronets, knights or Members of Parliament. Conversely, just one member of the workaday committee was also a Bath Hospital governor, although at least three later acquired this distinction.

The concentration of governors among the vice-presidents of the Eye Infirmary, and their widespread penetration of charitable networks in the later Georgian city, intimates that the Bath Hospital was a socially exclusive institution. An analysis of annual subscribers at the City Infirmary and Dispensary, the Casualty Hospital, the Eye Infirmary, and the Penitentiary and Lock Hospital confirms this impression (Table 8.6). All five charities attracted only a sprinkling of titled subscribers. Doctors were also a modest contingent, the proportion at the Eye Infirmary reflecting the small subscriber body rather than large absolute numbers. Clergymen, on the other hand, were populous at the Penitentiary and Lock Hospital, perhaps won over by its overt agenda of moral reform, while the General Infirmary was slow to tap military officers and had fewer gentlemen subscribers. More complex is the situation of esquires, equally prevalent at both the General and the Eye Infirmaries. It is possible that, being newly founded and focusing on a fashionable speciality, the Eye Hospital enjoyed similar prestige to the long-established General Hospital. Complicating this interpretation, however, is the variation in women who were classified as Mrs or Miss and so defied allocation to the male categories which accommodated most of their male relatives. At the General Infirmary, 28 per cent of female subscribers fell into this grouping, slightly fewer than at the Casualty Hospital, the Penitentiary and the City Infirmary but insufficiently out of line to overthrow the clear status differential which set it apart from these organizations. At the Eye Hospital, on the other hand, only 14 per cent of subscribers were titled Mrs or Miss and, consequently, there were fewer unattributed women to swell the ranks of middling men. Thus if we assume that subscribers of both sexes were recruited from broadly similar socio-economic backgrounds, it is likely that the General Infirmary was better endowed than the Eye Infirmary with annual contributors who were esquires or the female relatives of esquires.

This deduction, together with the relative shortage of gentlemen among the annual subscribers, suggests that the social profile of the Bath Hospital was inclined towards the upper echelons of the middling sort.[121] Such exclusivity perpetuated itself, deterring donors from modest backgrounds. But it was also underpinned by the changing moral economy of medicine. The paternalist ethos of the General Infirmary may have discouraged subscriptions from middling men of lower social status who were committed to scientific philanthropy. Titled governors and esquires did not snub the new charities; they acknowledged the turning tide by filling honorific posts. However, their higher social position and their bonds with the landed élite preserved a residual belief in traditional obligations. Therefore, a degree of closure was achieved, not by direct but by indirect means. In theory, associated philanthropy was an open system; in practice, its networks kept alive the socio-moral heritages of different charities and betrayed the socio-economic origins of their benefactors.

During the span of the long eighteenth century, the cultural life of Bath was transformed as the informality of the early Georgian period

Table 8.6 The social status of charity subscribers in later Georgian Bath

Social status	*General Hospital subscribers 1800/01*		*City Infirmary and Dispensary subscribers 1792–94*		*Casualty Hospital subscribers and benefactors 1793*		*Eye Infirmary subscribers 1815*		*Penitentiary and Lock Hospital subscribers June 1816–December 1818*		*General Hospital subscribers 1830/31*	
	No.	%	No.	%	No.	%	No.	%	No.	%	No.	%
Aristocrats	6	3.73	3	1.62	5	2.16	1	1.11	10	2.46	5	2.89
Baronets and knights	2	1.24	4	2.16	1	0.43	3	3.33	10	2.46	4	2.31
'Honourables'	—	—	2	1.08	1	0.43	—	—	3	0.74	—	—
Esquires	67	41.61	57	30.81	50	21.65	37	41.11	109	26.85	66	38.15
Gentlemen	14	8.70	28	15.14	52	22.51	14	15.56	58	14.29	10	5.78
Doctors	5	3.11	3	1.62	6	2.60	6	6.67	4	0.99	2	1.16
Clergy	18	11.18	13	7.03	14	6.06	10	11.11	28	6.90	24	13.87
Military officers	1	0.62	8	4.32	5	2.16	3	3.33	28	6.90	11	6.36
Ladies	3	1.86	6	3.24	4	1.73	2	2.22	14	3.45	2	1.16
Mrs/Miss	45	27.95	61	32.97	79	34.20	13	14.44	123	30.30	49	28.32
Unattributed	—	—	—	—	14	6.06	1	1.11	19	4.68	—	—
Total	161	100.00	185	100.00	231	100.00	90	100.00	406	100.00	173	100.00

Note: Percentages have been rounded up or down and so do not always total exactly 100.00.

Sources: *Annual Reports*, 1800/01, 1830/31; *State of the Bath City Infirmary and Dispensary ... from 1 October 1792 to January 1 1794*, pp. 9–15; *The Sixth Year's State of the Casualty Hospital in the City of Bath ... for the Year 1793*, pp. 5–13; *Bath Infirmary for the Cure of Diseases of the Eye ... Fourth Annual Report from January 1 1815 to January 1 1816*, pp. 13–15; *The Collective Reports of the Bath Penitentiary and Lock Hospital from 1816 to 1824*, pp. 173–98.

gave way to organized structures which included new medical charities. Yet despite this more competitive environment, the General Hospital retained the exclusivity derived from its early connection with the élite visiting Company. Though not financially or administratively dependent upon aristocrats, baronets and knights, the Infirmary was able to attract contributors from higher socio-economic backgrounds than its rivals and recruit governors who were prominent in local philanthropic networks. Therefore, it remained a potent source of social kudos, holding out the tantalizing prospect of status accumulation in return for support. But what were the constituents of this status? And how did the Infirmary purvey the commodity?

The fulfilment of social aspiration

The pursuit of social status involved both the acquisition of public esteem and the fulfilment of social aspiration. Public esteem was a quality which cut across social boundaries; like the bourgeois ethic of respectability that was to underscore the mid-Victorian consensus, it was flexibly defined to accommodate different social levels.[122] Patients of the Bath Infirmary were thus worthy of public esteem because, though poor, they were deserving. For the early Georgian aristocrats and middling men among their patrons, responding to this legitimate need was a paternalist duty, the public execution of which was critical to their standing in the community. The traditional élite had in the past secured this recognition through heroic acts of personal giving.[123] But the context was changing. In particular, the social distance between rich and poor was growing. The indiscriminate practice of charity was under attack. And while 'temporal peers and the landed classes maintained their share of the expanding national income ... other groups ... [were doing] significantly better and ... beginning to close the gap'.[124] Furthermore, once the paternalist ideal started to wither in the later eighteenth century, it was replaced by a moral sensibility which included decadent aristocratic lifestyles among the causes of Britain's malaise. Therefore, associated philanthropy did not only appeal to the rising professional and commercial classes anxious to meet their charitable duties from relatively modest resources. To an aristocracy that was gradually losing economic and ideological supremacy, it was also 'a highly effective means of asserting grandee cultural hegemony'[125] and demonstrating a continuing social responsibility in the new era of benevolence. Given its roots in paternalism, the voluntary hospital was well equipped to meet these needs for social status by installing the aristocracy and gentry in high-profile institutional positions, and using their patrician presence to catch the aspiring middle orders. Therefore, the division of labour which emerged at the early Georgian Bath Infirmary remained feasible throughout the long eighteenth century. United by a shared desire for the public esteem of doing good, middling men and aristocrats and gentry entered into an exchange relationship in which financial and administrative inputs were traded for social prestige.

The thesis that voluntary hospitals fulfilled social aspirations runs counter to the characterization of Georgian philanthropy as more discreet than the extravagant personal munificence of the Tudors and Stuarts. It is true that authors like Thomas Day lauded anonymous giving, 'that placid unambitious benevolence, which gliding on like a gentle stream, uncelebrated and unknown, delights to scatter blessings upon mankind in obscurity'.[126] Equally incontrovertible is the fact that the corporate schemes of the eighteenth century had 'to tap the broad base of middle-class wealth as well as the more spectacular accumulations of a few plutocrats with fortunes but no families on which to bestow them'. None the less, the behaviour of individual philanthropists suggests that they did not 'supress their egotism'.[127] Ralph Allen, christened the 'Man of Bath', was one of several quasi-mythological figures who were used to personify reclusive giving. However, correspondence from the literary figures whom he patronized indicates that in private life Allen was a man who enjoyed flattery. His approval, wrote Samuel Richardson replying with gratitude for critical comments on material from *Pamela*, was valued 'in any serious, pious or beneficent turn, [more] than that of hundreds; since such would be the approbation of a gentleman, the constant tenor of whose life distinguishes in him a rectitude of thinking and a benevolence of mind'.[128] No doubt such 'handsome praise' was spoken 'with some confidence that it would not offend'.[129]

The local satirist, Philip Thicknesse, perceived Allen's aptitude for public self-aggrandizement when he described Prior Park as 'A noble seat which sees all Bath and ... was built, probably, for all Bath to see'.[130] Allen also chose to be seen through his medical charity. A native of Cornwall, he presented the Devon and Exeter Hospital with his own portrait in 1759, having previously made a substantial benefaction and served as chairman of the governors.[131] His dealings with the Bath Infirmary were likewise no secret. Though some *Annual Reports* referred coyly to 'one [unnamed] generous benefactor [who] gave a great part of the materials',[132] Allen clinched his association early by accepting the presidency in 1742; and if thereafter he withdrew from the routine administration, his brother, Philip, was a regular presence.[133] In other words, Ralph Allen was not a silent or anonymous benefactor.

His co-operation in a collective programme of medical philanthropy may have been less dazzling than the single-handed endowment of a hospital by Thomas Guy or John Radcliffe, but the reputation for unobtrusive benevolence was fed by the oxygen of publicity.

The paradox of Ralph Allen – reticent yet courting fame – implies that discreet benevolence was a convenient disguise for the pursuit of social ambition. For middling men eager to boost their social rating, associated charities created the opportunity to mix with fellow supporters and to be associated publicly with them. In order to satisfy the demand for refined interaction, voluntary hospitals organized events which intermingled governors and subscribers from different social backgrounds. At the Bath Infirmary, the laying of the foundation-stone was accompanied by much jollification.

> above twenty of the trustees and contributors met at the Rummer Tavern, and proceeded from thence to the place appointed ... When the ceremony was over, the gentlemen returned to the Rummer, where His Majesty's health, that of the Prince and Princess of Wales, General Wade, and other absent benefactors were drank, and all the demonstration of joy possible shown on this occasion ... [134]

There were further attempts at merrymaking in the late 1750s and early 1760s, when the governors became briefly involved in a series of musical concerts and advertised special dinners after meetings of the general court. In general, however, the Hospital year was free of social conviviality, even charity services being unaccompanied by the anniversary celebrations that were customary elsewhere. Therefore, the openings for social climbing were largely confined to dates in the administrative calendar.

The early Georgian increase in gentlemen governors, and their relative willingness to attend the general court, join the weekly committee and participate regularly in its meetings, suggest that among this group at the margins of gentility hospital management was regarded as a route to social prestige. The significance of socialization with the aristocracy should not be exaggerated, since titled governors were thin on the ground even at general courts. Access to esquires, less than diligent but more in evidence at administrative gatherings (Appendices D and F), took on a chronological pattern. Monthly analysis of participation in the weekly committee, undertaken at five-year intervals between 1742 and 1830 (Figure 8.1),[135] throws up a complicated series of peaks and troughs which reflects how the governors' behaviour was shaped by a myriad of personal and collective circumstances. None the less, total attendance, attendance by esquires, and attendance by gentlemen (until they almost disappeared from the governing body after 1800) all

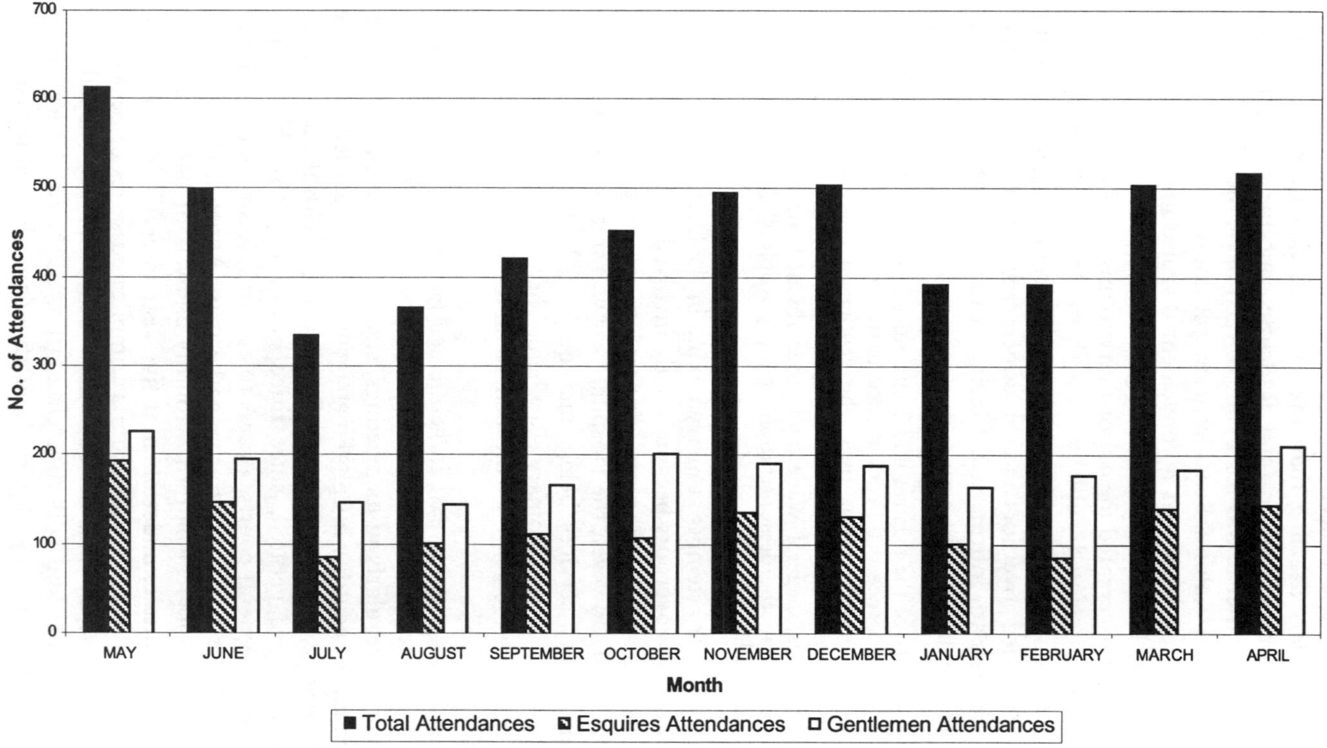

8.1 Bath General Hospital: the seasonal attendance of governors at weekly committees, 1742–1830 (five-year sample summary

Source: Minute Books.

exhibited a broad seasonal configuration, fluctuating in strength and in detail but still discernible at the end of the long eighteenth century. Essentially, numbers rose during the Spring Season, dropped off during mid-summer and rallied again for the Autumn Season with a final bulge at the end of the year. Whereas the December surge manifest the traditional linkage of Christmas, charity and hospitality,[136] the overlap with the two seasons points to a more specific niche within the social dynamics of the resort. Opening with the May general court, the Infirmary year was seasonally attuned and the weekly committees held during this month were among the best attended, their members perhaps activated by the fresh confirmation of appointment. But the administrative cycle aside, visitors to Bath also engaged in rites of passage which announced their arrival and drew them into the bustle of spa life.[137] For Hospital governors who were part of the peripatetic Company, the weekly committee was one such liminal mechanism – hence the rise in participation during the spring and autumn. Almost every early Georgian esquire who attended the committee was a member of the country gentry or upper bourgeoisie who transported themselves to Bath for the season (Appendix G). Their presence may have drawn in other governors, resident and itinerant, who also attended seasonally, keen to partake of the social status on offer. Furthermore, it also compensated the local gentlemen who endured the weekly administrative grind. Just as important for them, however, was the experience of meeting regularly as a social group because shouldering the governance of the Bath Infirmary, and meeting one another in the economic and social networks which criss-crossed the city, fostered a sense of common identity.

But did these associations transacted through the Hospital contribute to a metamorphosis of status? More specifically, did it transform Bath gentlemen into esquires? The retention of a smattering of gentlemen on the governing body, and their greater representation in the charities which mushroomed from the late eighteenth century, implies that the title of Mr continued to have significance within the status vocabulary. Though the assignations of individual supporters did progress over time,[138] the employment profile of active governors from the commercial classes was consistent throughout the Georgian period. Therefore, social mobility was not primarily responsible for the contraction of gentlemen on the governing body. What happened was an inflation of status titles which led to a reclassification of the élite trades and an ascent of the professional and commercial classes who ran the General Infirmary. Strengthened by flourishing occupations, bolstered by sporadic contact with more prestigious governors, and armed with a collective consciousness born of interaction with their peers, these gentlemen were able 'by a subtle mixture of individual assertion and social acceptance'[139] to negotiate entry into the category of esquire and hence acquire recognition as an élite within the urban middling sort. The rhythm of the resort sustained a seasonality in administrative participation, but by the late eighteenth century, there were few governors known as Mr and few visiting esquires at weekly committees. Although Bath itself remained more popular with visitors in the spring and autumn,[140] the esquires who now dominated the General Infirmary were predominantly middling men of local residence.

For the majority of governors and subscribers who were not active participants in hospital management, the transference of social status did not rely primarily upon cultivating sociability; rather the aspirations of the middle orders were addressed by publicizing their financial and administrative connections with the General Hospital. The allure of publicity as a means of social advancement was appreciated from the early days of the Infirmary. In the late 1730s, therefore, on the advice of their London banker, the trustees were careful to include even small sums so as not to offend modest contributors and wise enough to delay publication until 'the King was applied to and his benefaction received'.[141] Though the subsequent lists of donations – large and small – in local and national periodicals were partly designed to guarantee financial propriety, these bulletins and the separate coverage allotted to substantial gifts also served to advertise both the personal generosity of individual benefactors and the social status of the charitable with whom they were linked. Furthermore, when in 1783 the governors were able to rescind their decision to sell stock and cut the patient quota after the public responded magnificenty to a financial appeal, the names of those who had contributed to the emergency fund and the amounts which they had subscribed were attached to the explanation printed in the press and placed at the Pump Room, coffee houses and libraries.[142] Membership of the governing body was as much a source of social prestige as offering money. The names of principal officers were initially published in the local press,[143] and after 1748/49 a list of governors was appended to the printed *Annual Report*, with details of the celebrity president emblazoned across the top. From the early nineteenth century, aristocrats no longer took precedence over lesser mortals in the *Report*; for officers apart, the catalogue of governors now followed a strict alphabetical order.[144] But this minor concession to egalitarianism did not imply that the landed élite had been stripped of social prestige. Despite the status achievements of the middling sort, and any yearnings for parliamentary reform, gentility retained its aristocratic frame of reference and the governors of the Georgian Bath Infirmary continued to value coupling with their social superiors.

Although status by association was largely confined to being named as a governor or contributor amidst illustrious company, the capacity for self-advertisement was enhanced by a country-wide catchment area. Just as the city of Bath itself was 'the great hospital of the nation',[145] so the General Infirmary opened its doors to patients from beyond the immediate locality. In practice, the majority came from adjacent counties, as did annual subscriptions from parishes.[146] Throughout the long eighteenth century, however, publicity emphasized the geographical range of the institution. In the 'Short Account' attached to William Warburton's charity sermon of 1742, for example, readers were informed that public notices had been sent to all three kingdoms, giving details of the terms of admission and inviting applications.[147] Nineteenth-century publicity was still carrying the same message. As *The Improved Bath Guide* explained in 1812, the Bath Hospital was 'not merely a local charity, confined to the poor of a particular district, but extends its beneficient arms to receive indiscriminately all those whom poverty and disease have rendered proper objects of its benevolence'. It followed that the Infirmary was 'entitled to the patronage and charitable assistance of all the strangers that resort to this place'.[148]

The extent to which patrons from afar responded to these calls is difficult to establish. The *Bath Journal* did announce visitors arriving in the city, but these lists are not a reliable means of identifying 'outside' supporters because in all probability they were partial and biased towards the more élite members of the Company. When in the 1760s the *Annual Reports* indicated home locations, they revealed a strong non-Bath element with governors from London and the South East as well as the local region (Appendix I). The men who supported the Hospital throughout the Georgian period confirm this mix. Some had West Country interests. Both the Duke of Kingston who was president in 1757, and the Duke of Chandos whose son – the Marquis of Carnarvon – was president in 1759, were Bath landowners.[149] The early governor, Edward Southwell MP, lived at Kings Weston House near Bristol, the city which he represented in Parliament.[150] The Duke of Beaufort, a governor during the 1750s, occupied Badminton House in Gloucestershire;[151] and his relative by marriage, the mid-Georgian governor, Norborne Berkeley – subsequently Lord Botetourt – resided at Stoke Park in the Gloucestershire village of Stoke Gifford.[152] The late eighteenth-century governing body included Sir Caesar Hawkins, serjeant-surgeon to George II and George III, who had recently purchased the manor of Kelweston or Kelston near Bath; members of the Methuen family who owned land at Freshford south of the city, as well as their estate at Corsham Court in Wiltshire;[153] and Lord Francis Seymour who was not only Dean of Wells but also a son of the Duke of Somerset.[154] Complementing this regional contingent, however, were governors with few local roots: the aristocrats and baronets, leading clergymen, senior politicians, and military heroes who joined men of lesser rank and reputation as they thronged to Bath during the season. With such a geographically diverse collection of patients and patrons, the Bath Infirmary had a national profile; and, therefore, being designated an associate offered more than mere parochial recognition to the aspiring middle orders hungry for social status.

The esteem of mankind

Although social aspiration was critical to the dynamics of Georgian philanthropy, its appeal was strengthened by the 'esteem of mankind'[155] that was also a derivative of good works; as Robert Leyborne told the congregation before whom he preached on behalf of General Infirmary in 1753, the righteous benefactor had the praise, the esteem, the love, and the assistance of the sick poor 'to adorn his prosperity, and turn him from evil'.[156] Whereas the traditional élite regarded associated charity as a way of retaining the benevolent persona previously won through individual munificence, middling men from the professional and commercial classes saw it as a means of earning that reputation. For both groups, however, diverting money to charitable purposes helped to legitimate the possession of wealth. 'How well does that man deserve the prosperous fortune he has met with!' exclaimed Mrs Delaney, as she recounted how Ralph Allen had purchased a lodging-house to settle on the widow of a poor clergyman.[157] Visitors and residents embarrassed by the riches displayed at the fun city of Bath were particularly conscious of this escape hatch. But for those whose lives transgressed moral conventions, the rehabilitative properties of philanthropy were additionally attractive. Take the Hospital governor and bookseller, James Leake, who in the early 1740s, while regularly attending committee meetings to supervise the building programme, printed a pornographic book in which the female body was depicted as a 'Paradise of Pleasure, and a Garden of Delight'. Eleven editions, including one with illustrations, had been published by 1742, and Leake succeeded in attracting attention to the volume by producing a pamphlet critical of it.[158] We can only speculate that Leake's engagement in hospital administration, and the benefactions of those customers who consumed his pornography, were calculated to offset their moral misdemeanours. In the case of Master of Ceremonies, Richard Beau Nash, however, the restorative properties of charity are better evidenced.

The '*Arbiter Elegantiarum*' of early Georgian Bath, Richard Nash fashioned taste and etiquette at a formative stage of the spa's development. On its own, this concern with social niceties was enough to prompt accusations of superficiality, but Nash's sexual relationships were also colourful and in 1737 his good name was further tarnished by a gaming scandal; indeed, even his integrity as a custodian of public subscriptions for social events was called into question.[159] Yet for all these blemishes, the Beau was acknowledged as a great 'servant of the poor and the distressed', who made strenuous efforts on behalf of the General Infirmary. Though claims of diligent attendance at meetings are false, Nash was critical to the promotion campaign in London and functioned as an effective conduit for funds.[160] The 'choreography' of his funeral[161] celebrated these good works. The Corporation of Bath 'granted fifty pounds towards burying their sovereign with proper respect', Nash himself having died in dire financial straits. His biographer, Oliver Goldsmith, describes the procession in some detail:

> the charity girls two and two preceded, next the boys of the charity school singing a solemn ... hymn. Next marched the city music, and his own band sounding at proper intervals a dirge. Three clergyman immediately preceded the coffin, which was adorned with sable plumes, and the pall supported by the six senior aldermen. The masters of the assembly-rooms followed as chief mourners; the beadles of that hospital, which he had contributed so largely to endow, went next, and last of all, the poor patients themselves, the lame, the emaciated, and the feeble, followed their old benefactor to his grave, shedding unfeigned tears, and lamenting themselves in him.[162]

The coming together of political and cultural leaders with the beneficiaries of charity indicates its centrality both to the 'monarch of Bath' and to the city over which he ruled. For Nash, however, the pitiful image of the weeping disabled patients of the Hospital – albeit embroidered by artistic licence – cloaked the more disreputable aspects of his life and represented him as a respected philanthropist; as he himself had told the Duchess of Queensberry, 'Charity hides a multitude of sins'.[163]

Whether used to exonerate bad behaviour or to justify wealth, the public esteem derived from benevolence outlived the benefactor. Not only did obituaries record bequests and the offices that the deceased had held,[164] but charitable institutions functioned as memorials. This commemorative return was widely understood: Robert Nelson had argued in 1715 that the London hospitals were 'the standing monuments of the piety and munificence of our ancestors'; William Blizard urged at the close of the century that 'anniversary general meetings ... be considered as in commemoration of founders'.[165] The potential for remembrance found expression at Bath in the Reverend Mr Bayly's charity sermon of 1749, where he informed his congregation that hospitals remained 'the lasting monuments, not only of the taste and genius, but also of the piety and humanity of the founders'.[166] Supporters great and small were saluted by the continuity of the General Infirmary, while the exceptional contributions of Francis Colston, Richard Nash and Ralph Allen were marked by naming wards in their honour.[167] However, personal philanthropy was more publicly perpetuated in works of history, literature and art. Where historical studies listed governors, benefactors and subscribers, their charity was individually documented,[168] but with exceptional generosity came special commemorative rewards. Though Ralph Allen's personification of 'piety and charity' stemmed in part from his good works, his hospitality, his simple dress and manners,[169] the public projection of his personality as the model benevolent man was largely the outcome of its embodiment in the poetry and prose of those literary figures with whom he fraternized. In *The Epilogue to the Satires*, for example, Alexander Pope penned the lines: 'Let humble ALLEN, with an awkward shame,/Do good by stealth, and blush to find it fame.'[170] The fictional character, Squire Allworthy, in Henry Fielding's novel, *Tom Jones*, also hallowed the 'Man of Bath'. Having by a 'penetrating genius' raised 'a large fortune ... with the most perfect preservation of his integrity', the Squire discovered 'a taste superior to most' and showed

> a degree of goodness superior to all men, by acts of charity to objects, whose only recommendations were their merits, or their wants ... his private hospitality, and his public beneficence all denoted the mind from which they flowed, and were all intrinsically rich and noble, without tinsel, or external ostentation.[171]

Notwithstanding this literary paradigm, Allen's reputation for benevolence was most dependent upon his support for General Hospital. Following later editions of Defoe's *Tour*, guidebooks consistently cited him as a chief benefactor who, 'besides giving a very large sum of money', permitted 'the trustees ... to fetch from his stone-yard all the wall-stone, wrought free-stone, paving stone, and lime, that were necessary ... to complete the masons-work of the new edifice'.[172] Allen's investment in the Infirmary thus provided essential collateral, his gift of the materials connecting him to the very fabric of the building. As Bishop Warburton explained in a letter to Philip Doddridge written in February 1743, Allen was 'the greatest private character in any age of the world'. The Hospital was 'but a small part of his charities, and charity but a small part of his virtues'. But it was in the institution that his munificence was seen.[173]

Ralph Allen's artistic memorial at the Bath Infirmary was installed in 1757 with Warburton's presentation of a bust. The governors warmly welcomed the gift on the grounds that it would 'perpetuate a ... lively resemblance of ... [a] great benefactor'; though Allen was still living, they argued that 'it will remain an honour to have had so worthy a promoter, longer than marble will ever endure'.[174] Whereas Allen's bust was located behind the closed doors of the Hospital, the statue that immortalized Richard Nash's philanthropy was situated in the Pump Room at the social nucleus of the spa. Erected to mark his 'prudent management' of the town almost a decade before he died,[175] the statue depicts Nash carrying not a souvenir of his place in high society or a momento of his career at the tables, but a plan of the Infirmary.[176] Writing anonymously in the *Public Ledger* after Nash's death in 1761, William Oliver urged that the philanthropy which the statue so eloquently portrayed might now 'protect his memory'.[177] The publication of Goldsmith's sympathetic biography a year later ensured that Oliver's wish was granted. Though neither ignoring nor excusing Nash's failings, Goldsmith emphasized the virtue of his benevolence, which had to 'stand almost single against an hundred follies' and was 'large enough to outweigh them all'.[178] Literary images of the retiring Allen faded, but this biographical interpretation of the full-blooded Nash endured, isolating him as an energetic promoter of the General Hospital who, though ably supported by other trustees and governors, suggested 'the noble idea of its foundation' and brought the scheme to fruition.[179] Therefore, the Infirmary played an important part in drawing 'an impenetrable veil over his foibles'.[180] As a nineteenth-century commentator was later to advise:

> In reflecting on the numerous acts of levity which attach to the name of Beau Nash, let the recollection of his earnest advocacy of the interests of the General Hospital have its due weight, and let it soften the asperity of the critic, who would represent him as wholly occupied in folly and frivolity.[181]

The former gamester and socialite was at least partially reconstituted as a man of charity.

If Goldsmith established Nash's reputation, that of John Wood was the product of his own historical *Description of Bath*. On the agenda of this idiosyncratic book was Wood's view of how he had advanced the Infirmary project: an egotistical account, in which he credited himself with revitalizing the stagnant charity and modestly praised the 'magnificent' structure that was of his own design.[182] Allen's donation of the stone, on the other hand, was conveniently overlooked; and although Nash's fund-raising was mentioned, no judgement was passed. Wood's history, together with the biography of Nash, dominated the historiography of Bath for more than a century, later chroniclers recycling a familiar version of the Georgian past in which much hinged on the Master of Ceremonies and the architect.[183] By the end of the nineteenth century, however, an alternative reading was under construction. To the scrupulous bourgeoisie of later Victorian Britain, the nefarious

Nash was a less seductive figure. His sternest critic was the local writer, R.E.M. Peach, for whom he was a man of 'black morals': 'the great protoplasm of evil', whose influence on the city 'tended to evil rather than to good'. 'Gambling, immorality, and every species of blacklegism', continued Peach, were 'not rendered respectable because they may be concealed under a veil of pretence and hypocrisy'. Part of that 'pretence and hypocrisy' was the myth that Nash had contributed significantly to the foundation of the General Infirmary; for even the 'admirable projects' to which he had 'in his better days set his hand ... came to nought', despite the 'great forbearance and help of former colleagues'. Therefore, the Hospital 'lingered for years before it was brought to a successful issue', primarily by Wood now acting in concert with Allen.[184]

The quality which endeared Wood and Allen to the Victorians was their success as self-made men. When lack of money and a suitable site was frustrating plans for the Bath Hospital, argued Peach, it was Wood – a pupil at the Blue-Coat Charity School in the city – who 'came to the rescue, and by his energy, business aptitude, and judgment every difficulty was obviated'.[185] Allen's transposition from passive supplier of the stone to active promoter of the Infirmary was due in part to his impeccable moral credentials and to the revival of interest in the Georgian literature of which he was a feature. However, Peach was particularly impressed by Allen's entrepreneurial spirit. 'Our admiration is kindled', he wrote, 'as we follow the poor Post Office boy, with no advantages but those of a clear brain and a resolute and energetic temperament, skilfully and honorably surmounting great difficulties on his road to personal success'.[186] Conversely, William Oliver's profitable medical practice singled him out for less meritocratic acclaim because being from a landowning family and educated at Cambridge,[187] he was not archetypal of the 'from rags to riches' syndrome. Furthermore, the doctors who published studies of the Infirmary or the spa were prone to ignore his formative administrative contribution and simply note the appointment as an honorary physician.[188] Oliver's standing may have benefited from the establishment of physical medicine as a professional speciality during the first half of the twentieth century.[189] Certainly, it was just after the Second World War that he was accredited with founding the General Infirmary 'for those who could not afford to pay for treatment', never forgetting 'his duty as a doctor to heal the poor as well as the rich'.[190] But that resurrection was short-lived. Dr Roger Rolls's more recent work, which initially lists Oliver among the businessmen and speculators whose 'enthusiasm and generosity' led to the foundation of the Hospital, later notes his 'unfailing devotion' to its affairs.[191] In the post-war world of scientific medicine, however, neither lay administration nor old-fangled balneology cut much ice. Oliver's name lived on in the biscuit which he invented to accompany the waters, but he remains the unsung hero of the Bath Hospital. He had no biography or history to bid his case; and he lacked both Nash's flamboyance, and the material monuments of Allen's stone and Wood's building. As a result, his steady hand on the tiller during the crucial early years of the Infirmary has largely escaped the long-term public gaze.

Despite the vacillating interpretations of the founding fathers, histories and guidebooks have consistently narrated their connection with the Bath Infirmary and complimented them for their philanthropy. How pleasant it was, mused Jerom Murch in 1888, 'to think that our Triumvirs, Nash, Allen, and Wood, were not too much busied with the reception of the wealthy and fashionable to heed the sacred claims of those whose title was their sickness and their poverty'.[192] Modern guidebooks echo this parity.[193] Consequently, the tourists who tramp the streets of Bath today are still informed that Richard Nash, Ralph Allen and John Wood were the three good men who set up the General Hospital. The public esteem which their charity inspired during their lifetimes has been transmitted across the centuries.

In this chapter, we have explored the funding and administration of the Georgian Bath Infirmary in terms of the pursuit of social status. It has been postulated that although aristocrats, baronets and knights sought the 'esteem of mankind' from their association with the institution, their commitment to its finance and administration was dwarfed by the involvement of middling men, for whom medical philanthropy additionally quenched social aspiration. The patrician presence satisfied this thirst primarily through printed publicity because the grandees rarely attended the weekly committees and general courts at which less auspicious governors gathered. None the less, these occasions were critical to the lubrication of the middling sort, bringing together urban gentlemen and enabling them to mix with visiting country and metropolitan esquires during the Season. The resulting exchange of social status was no free-for-all. It was the more affluent members of Bath's professional and commercial classes – always dominant within the management structures of the General Hospital – who, by the late eighteenth century, had won sufficient kudos to be accorded the assignation of esquire. Their position at the top of the urban hierarchy now consolidated, these new esquires joined with the rural landowning classes to form a wider social élite defined by its gentility. But how far was this social cohesion matched by political and religious integration? And to what extent did the enlarged élite impose control over the lower orders? It is to these politics of medical charity that we turn in Chapters 9 and 10.

Notes

1. Rogers, 'Middling Sort', p. 180.
2. P.J. Corfield, 'Class by Name and Number in Eighteenth-Century Britain', *History*, 72 (1987), p. 61.
3. Borsay, *English Urban Renaissance*, pp. 204–10; Langford, *Polite and Commercial People*, pp. 67–8; Rule, *Albion's People*, pp. 74–5, 79, 81–2.
4. Jonathan Barry, 'Introduction', in J. Barry and C. Brooks (eds), *The Middling Sort of People: Culture, Society and Politics in England 1550–1800* (London: Macmillan, 1994), pp. 2–3. See also Shani D'Cruze, 'The Middling Sort in Eighteenth-Century Colchester: Independence, Social Relations and the Community Broker', in J. Barry and C. Brooks (eds), *The Middling Sort of People: Culture, Society and Politics in England 1550–1800* (London: Macmillan, 1994), pp. 181–2.
5. Porter, 'English Society', pp. 39–42.
6. Barry, 'Introduction', pp. 17–19; Barry, 'Bourgeois Collectivism?' pp. 89–90; L. Davison, T. Hitchcock, T. Keirn and R.B. Shoemaker (eds), *Stilling the Grumbling Hive*, 'Introduction', p. xxviii; Langford, *Polite and Commercial People*, p. 59.
7. Nicholas Rogers, 'Paul Langford's "Age of Improvement"', *Past and Present*, 130 (1991), p. 204.
8. Marjorie Morgan, *Manners, Morals and Class in England 1774–1858* (London: St Martin's Press, 1994), pp. 4–6. See also Borsay, *English Urban Renaissance*, pp. 317–18; Peter Earle, 'The Middling Sort in London', in J. Barry and C. Brooks (eds), *The Middling Sort of People: Culture, Society and Politics in England 1550–1800* (London: Macmillan, 1994), pp. 147–50; Langford, *Polite and Commercial People*, p. 4; Porter, 'English Society', pp. 39–42; Lawrence Stone and Jeanne C. Fawtier Stone, *An Open Elite?: England 1540–1880* (Oxford: Oxford University Press, 1986), pp. 290–95.
9. Langford, *Polite and Commercial People*, p. 121.
10. Rule, *Albion's People*, p. 85. Weber also defined status groups in terms of their '*consumption* of goods'. See Max Weber, 'Class, status and party', in Reinhard Bendix and Seymour Martin Lipset (eds), *Class, Status and Power: Social Stratification in Comparative Perspective* (London: Routledge and Kegan Paul, 1967), p. 27.
11. Clark, *Sociability*, pp. 13–14, 17–20.
12. Borsay, *English Urban Renaissance*, pp. 219–20, 251, 332–49.
13. Fissell, 'Physic of Charity', p. 90; Langford, *Polite and Commercial People*, p. 138; Porter, 'Gift Relation', pp. 160–61; Charles Webster, 'The Crisis of Hospitals during the Industrial Revolution', in E. Forbes (ed.), *Human Implications of Scientific Advance* (Edinburgh: Edinburgh University Press, 1978), pp. 214–15. A similar trend has been charted for dispensaries. See Pickstone, *Medicine and Industrial Society*, pp. 64–72.
14. Guy Miège, *The Present State of Great Britain and Ireland*, 4th edn (London: A. Bell, R. Smith and J. Round, 1718), p. 169.
15. Berry, 'Patronage', p. 41.
16. Corfield, 'Class', p. 39.
17. Borsay, *English Urban Renaissance*, p. 228.

18. Corfield, 'Class', p. 43.
19. Ibid., p. 60.
20. Porter, 'Gift Relation', pp. 158–60.
21. Berry, 'Patronage', pp. 40–45.
22. Benefactions of £50 and Upwards to 1883; *Annual Report*, 1800/01, 1830/31.
23. *Annual Report*, 1741/42; 1770/71; 1800/01.
24. The number of aristocrats, baronets and knights, 'honourable' and 'lady' subscribers was nine in 1770/71, and 11 in 1800/01 and 1830/31.
25. Fawcett and Bird, *Bath*, pp. 71–2.
26. Berry found that Anglican and Nonconformist clergy were more likely to support the Devon and Exeter Hospital than the Bristol Infirmary. See Berry, 'Patronage', pp. 49–50.
27. In 1770/71, 31 esquires but only eight gentlemen subscribed two guineas, and four esquires but 34 gentlemen subscribed one guinea. In 1830/31, 13 esquires and one gentleman subscribed two guineas, and 44 esquires and eight gentlemen subscribed one guinea. There was also a correlation between social position and subscription levels at the Northampton and Devon and Exeter Hospitals – though not at the Bristol Infirmary without a 'county' society. See Berry, 'Patronage', p. 74.
28. 12 Geo. II, p. 582.
29. Minute Book, 1 May 1740; 1 May 1741; 1 May 1742.
30. *DNB*, vol. 49, pp. 81–7.
31. *DNB*, vol. 46, pp. 290–92.
32. Letter Book, E. Brett to T. Carew, undated; T. Carew to W. Oliver, 10 April 1739. Sedgwick, *House of Commons*, vol. 1, p. 528.
33. Benefactions, p. 1.
34. Minute Book, 23 May 1744; 15 November 1744; 1 May 1745.
35. Minute Book, 1 May 1822.
36. Dalton, *Religious Use*, frontispiece.
37. The Duke of Kingston, for example, was appointed in 1757, having given £200 in the mid-1740s; while the Marquis of Stafford was in office when he gave his gift of £100 in 1800.
38. See, for example, Minute Book, 1 May 1742; 1 May 1755; 1 May 1770; 2 May 1785; 1 May 1800; 1 May 1815; 1 May 1830.
39. Minute Book, 1 May 1750; 1 May 1794; 7 May 1794; 21 May 1794.
40. Minute Book, 16 May 1750.
41. *DNB*, vol. 20, p. 275.
42. Letter Book, to the New President by order of the Court, 2 May 1744.
43. Sedgwick, *House of Commons*, vol. 1, p. 445.
44. According to one nineteenth-century historian of the Hospital, Nash 'obtained by his individual exertions' donations worth more than £2 000 'in the space of about six years'. See Falconer, *Mineral Water Hospital*, p. 31.
45. See, for example, Letter Book, F. Fauquier to W. Oliver, 29 May 1739; F. Fauquier to Mr A. Brooks, Attorney at Law in Kettering, 18 October 1743; Mr Brooke to F. Fauquier, 26 November 1743; F. Fauquier to Mr Serriere, 5 January 1744.
46. See, for example, Minute Book, 15 May 1744; 30 May 1744; 6 June 1744; 13 June 1744; 4 July 1744; 11 July 1744.
47. *DNB*, vol. 18, pp. 249–50.

48. Minute Book, 1 May 1745.
49. Minute Book, 21 October 1761; 9 January 1762.
50. Minute Book, 1 May 1760.
51. Minute Book, 20 October 1779.
52. See, for example, Minute Book, 30 May 1770; 28 November 1770.
53. Minute Book, 10 December 1766; 29 July 1767.
54. Minute Book, 1 October 1777.
55. Minute Book, 4 August 1773.
56. Minute Book, 18 March 1767; 30 September 1778.
57. Minute Book, 31 March 1779. 19 Geo. III, *An Act More Effectually to Enable the President and Governors of the Hospital or Infirmary at Bath, Established by an Act, Passed in the Twelfth Year of the Reign of ... King George the Second ... to Take or Acquire, and Hold, Any Lands, Tenements, or Hereditaments, or Any Interest in Lands, Tenements, or Hereditaments, and Any Money or Personal Property, to be Laid Out in Lands, Tenements, or Hereditaments, Pursuant to Any Will, or Otherwise, to the Amount Limited in the Said Act* (London, 1779).
58. Minute Book, 4 August 1773; 2 May 1774.
59. Minute Book, 10 November 1779.
60. See, for example, Minute Book, 3 March 1784; 28 October 1789; 25 November 1789; 24 October 1792; 1 May 1792; 27 August 1794; 24 February 1796; 2 May 1796; 31 July 1799; 28 May 1800; 29 October 1800; 30 October 1805; 13 November 1805; 17 October 1810; 6 February 1811; 15 November 1815; 14 February 1816; 7 February 1820.
61. Minute Book, 1 May 1822.
62. See, for example, Minute Book, 22 May 1822; 11 February 1824; 28 July 1824; 27 April 1825; 1 March 1826; 24 May 1826; 21 March 1827.
63. Minute Book, 13 May 1829.
64. Minute Book, 28 November 1792; 29 January 1800; 17 October 1810; 21 November 1821; 31 March 1831.
65. Minute Book, 6 May 1829; 18 November 1830; 27 January 1831.
66. Kirby, 'Mineral Water Hospital', p. 25; Thomas, 'Phillotts of Bath', p. 4.
67. Minute Book, 2 February 1738, 'Copy of a Letter to Mr Benjamin Hoare, Banker in Fleet Street, London'.
68. Corfield, *Power*, pp. 112–29.
69. *DNB*, vol. 1, p. 54; Boyce, *Benevolent Man*, p. 31; W.S. Dakers, *John Wood and His Times* (Bath: Mendip Press, 1954), pp. 12–13; Wood, *Bath*, p. 283.
70. *Full Vindication*, p. 13; Boyce, *Benevolent Man*, pp. 143, 264.
71. Kirby, 'Mineral Water Hospital', p. 25; Thomas, 'Phillotts of Bath', p. 1.
72. Minute Book, 11 March 1741; 23 January 1754; 1 May 1756; 5 November 1760.
73. Minute Book, 1 May 1790; 7 January 1795.
74. Minute Book, 10 February 1768; 11 October 1821.
75. Minute Book, 28 July 1762; 13 December 1780.
76. Evelyn Newby, 'The Hoares of Bath', *Bath History*, 1 (1986), p. 106; Evelyn Newby, *William Hoare of Bath* (Stroud: Alan Sutton and Bath Museums Service, 1990), pp. 26, 53.
77. *Annual Report*, 1760/61. Vincent Hemingway and Jeffrey Haworth,

Coughton Court and the Throckmortons (Norwich: Jarrold, 1993), p. 24.
78. Thomas, 'Phillotts of Bath', pp. 2, 4.
79. Minute Book, 10 November 1779; 1 May 1822.
80. *Bath Journal*, 31 December 1753; *DNB*, vol. 46, pp. 386–8.
81. Mainwaring, *Annals*, p. 217.
82. Kirby, 'Mineral Water Hospital', p. 103.
83. Namier and Brooke, *House of Commons*, vol. 2, p. 635.
84. Lewis Namier and John Brooke, *The House of Commons 1754–1790*, 3 vols (London: HMSO, 1964), vol. 3: *Members K-Y*, p. 563.
85. Ibid., pp. 1–2.
86. Ibid., pp. 353–4.
87. R.E.M. Peach, *The Life and Times of Ralph Allen* (London: D. Nutt, 1895), pp. 64–5.
88. *Bath Journal*, 28 August 1786. See note 72.
89. A.J. Turner, *Science and Music in Eighteenth-Century Bath* (Bath: University of Bath, 1977), p. 8; 12 Geo. vol. 2, p. 573.
90. Namier and Brooke, *House of Commons*, vol. 3, p. 14.
91. Susan Legouix Sloman, '"The immaculate Capt. Wade": "Arbiter Elegantiae"', *Gainsborough's House Review* (1993/94), p. 48.
92. Lewis and Namier, *House of Commons*, vol. 2, p. 96.
93. Michael Stenton, *Who's Who of British Members of Parliament: A Biographical Dictionary of the House of Commons*, 4 vols (Brighton: Harvester Press, 1976), vol. 1: *1832–1885*, p. 322.
94. Collinson, *Somerset*, pp. 146, 170.
95. *DNB*, vol. 24, pp. 394–5.
96. *Stourhead* (London: National Trust, 1990), pp. 42–8; Kenneth Woodbridge, *The Stourhead Landscape* (London: National Trust, 1971), pp. 8–14.
97. Royal Mineral Water Hospital, 'Notes on the Pictures'.
98. *Full Vindication*, p. 12; Boyce, *Benevolent Man*, pp. 8, 130, 142, 255; Walter H. Tregellas, *Cornish Worthies: Sketches of Some Eminent Cornish Men and Families* (London: Elliot Stock, 1884), p. 20.
99. Smith, *Bath*, pp. 66–7.
100. Peach, *Ralph Allen*, pp. 64–5; *DNB*, vol. 1, pp. 311–12; *DNB*, vol. 58, pp. 413–16.
101. *DNB*, vol. 1, pp. 311–12; *DNB*, vol. 59, pp. 305, 307; *Gentleman's Magazine*, 50 (September 1780), p. 409; *Annual Report*, 1760/61.
102. Boyce, *Benevolent Man*, pp. 230–31; Peach, *Ralph Allen*, p. 114; Tregellas, *Cornish Worthies*, pp. 9–10; *Annual Report*, 1785/86. Warburton also married Allen's niece.
103. Newby, 'Hoares of Bath', p. 110.
104. Peach, *Ralph Allen*, pp. 127–8.
105. Glaser, *Spirit of Enquiry*, pp. 5, 84.
106. Murch, *Biographical Sketches*, p. 127. *Annual Report*, 1820/21; 1825/26; 1830/31.
107. Namier and Brooke, *House of Commons*, vol. 3, pp. 138–9.
108. *A Brief Memoir of the Late Joseph Hunter FSA* (Lincoln's Inn Fields, London: printed for private distribution only by John Edward Taylor, 1861), p. 5; *DNB*, vol. 27, pp. 26–8; *Stourhead*, pp. 42–8; Woodbridge, *Stourhead Landscape*, pp. 8–14.

109. In 1786, for example, a Mr Donne was advertising lectures in the Lower Assembly Rooms in which scientific topics like geometry, astonomy and optics, electricity and magnetism would be 'clearly explained, on a proper apparatus, so as to be readily understood by ladies and gentlemen unacquainted with these subjects'. See *Bath Journal*, 16 January 1786. Scientific apparatus, geological specimens and works of art were also exhibited. See *Bath Journal*, 12 September 1825; 31 October 1825; 12 December 1825.
110. *DNB*, vol. 27, p. 46.
111. Members of the Bath Philosophical Society included Joseph Priestley; John Coakley Lettsom; the musician and astronomer, William Herschel; John Arden, a peripatetic lecturer on experimental science; Charles Blagden, who studied medicine at Edinburgh and acted as an assistant to Henry Cavendish; and the natural historians, Mathew Martin and John Walcott. See Williams and Stoddart, *Bath*, pp. 68–9, 103–8.
112. The honorary physicians were William Falconer and Caleb Hillier Parry; in addition, John Staker MD, who served the General Hospital between 1781 and 1784, belonged to the Philosophical Society. The five remaining members who were governors in 1780 or 1785 were Hon. Hugh Acland; Thomas Curtis Esq.; John Lloyd Esq.; the explorer, Constantine, Lord Mulgrave; and William Watson MD. See Williams and Stoddart, *Bath*, pp. 55–6, 68–9; *Annual Report*, 1780/81, 1785/86.
113. Mainwaring, *Annals*, pp. 247–8.
114. *Brief Memoir*, p. 5; *Bath Journal*, 24 January 1825; *Annual Report*, 1825/26.
115. Humble and Hansell, *Westminster Hospital*, p. 27; Peach, *Bath*, p. 139.
116. Thomas, 'Phillots of Bath', p. 4.
117. *Improved Bath Guide*, p. 58. See also Peach, *Bath*, p. 160.
118. Turner, *Charity*, p. 4; Kirkup, 'Bath Casualty Hospital', pp. 51, 53; *State of the Bath City Infirmary*, p. 8; *Bath Infirmary for the Cure of Diseases of the Eye*, p. 3; *Bath Journal*, 14 February 1825.
119. Royal United Hospital Minute Book, 24 January 1831; 6 June 1827–1 June 1829. Appendix G.
120. D'Cruze, 'Middling Sort', p. 182. See also Barry, 'Bourgeois Collectivism?' p. 101.
121. Evidence from elsewhere is in short supply, but we can extend the comparison to the Worcester Infirmary where in 1787 half the annual subscribers were gentlemen and only a fifth esquires. See Lane, *Worcester Infirmary*, p. 19, table 5.
122. Robert Gray, *The Aristocracy of Labour in Nineteenth-Century Britain c.1850–1914* (London: Macmillan, 1981), pp. 35–44.
123. Langford, *Polite and Commercial People*, p. 482.
124. Cannon, *Aristocratic Century*, pp. 130–31.
125. Porter, 'Gift Relation', p. 161.
126. *Select Miscellaneous Productions of Mrs Day and Thomas Day, Esq. in Verse and Prose* (London: T. Jones, 1805), pp. 89–90.
127. Langford, *Polite and Commercial People*, p. 482.
128. *Selected Letters of Samuel Richardson*, ed. John Carroll, (Oxford: Clarendon Press, 1964), p. 51.
129. Boyce, *Benevolent Man*, p. 120.
130. Thicknesse, *Bath Guide*, p. 76.

131. Adrian E. Hopkins (ed.), *Ralph Allen's Own Narrative 1720–1761*, Special Series No. 8 (no place of publication: Postal History Society, 1960), p. 11.
132. *Annual Report*, 1750/51.
133. Between joining the weekly committee in 1741 and his brother's death in 1764, Philip Allen atttended 369 meetings, his presence being most frequent in the 1740s.
134. *London Evening Post*, 11 July 1738.
135. For the five-yearly sample data, see Appendix H.
136. Lewis and Williams, *Private Charity*, pp. 120–21.
137. Borsay, *English Urban Renaissance*, pp. 271–2.
138. Charles Phillott was not the only gentleman governor to become an esquire. Among those so lifted in the quinquennial sample years were John Wood, Samuel Bush, Robert Dingley, John Donne, William Anderdon, Charles Crook, Harry Atwood, Samuel and Henry Edward Howse, and Henry and John Knight.
139. Corfield, *Power*, p. 12.
140. Barrett, 'Spas', p. 51; Hembry, *British Spas*, p. 58.
141. Letter Book, 14 March 1738, B. Hoare to F. Fauquier; Letter Folder, 13 May 1738, F. Fauquier to R. Allen.
142. Minute Book, 1 May 1783; 21 May 1783; 11 June 1783.
143. See, for example, *Bath Journal*, 7 May 1744; 4 May 1747; 4 May 1752; 7 May 1753; 6 May 1754; 5 May 1755; 3 May 1756; 9 May 1757; 5 May 1760; 4 May 1761.
144. See, for example, *Annual Report*, 1815/16; 1830/31.
145. Smollett, *Essay*, p. 70.
146. The geographical origins of patients are discussed in Chapter 9. The *Annual Report* for 1830/31 lists 118 parish subscribers, 39 of whom had paid for the year. Of the total, 46 were located in Somerset, 37 in Wiltshire and 14 in Gloucestershire.
147. [Bath General Infirmary], 'Short Account', in Warburton, *Sermon*, p. 27.
148. *Improved Bath Guide*, pp. 46–7. See also *Bath Chronicle*, 18 May 1797; Bath Chronicle, *Hot Water Hospital*, pp. 4, 16; *Original Bath Guide* [1840], pp. 98–9.
149. R.E.M. Peach, *Historic Houses in Bath and their Associations*, 2 vols (London: Simpkin, Marshall and Co., 1883), vol. 1, p. 54; Romney Sedgwick, *The House of Commons 1715–1754*, 2 vols (London: HMSO, 1970), vol. 2: *Members E–Y*, pp. 125–6.
150. Nicholas Kingsley, *The Country Houses of Gloucestershire*, 2 vols (Chichester: Phillimore, 1992), vol. 2: *1660–1830*, pp. 167–70; Sedgwick, *House of Commons*, vol. 2, pp. 431–2.
151. Kingsley, *Country Houses*, pp. 54–61.
152. Ibid., pp. 236–8.
153. Collinson, *Somerset*, pp. 125–6; Namier and Brooke, *House of Commons*, vol. 3, p. 134.
154. Collinson, *Somerset*, pp. xlix–l.
155. Thomas Secker, 'Sermon before the Lord Mayor, 1738', in T. Secker *Fourteen Sermons Preached on Several Occasions* (London: John Rivington, 1766), p. 65.
156. Leyborne, *Charity Conducive*, p. 34.
157. Tregellas, *Cornish Worthies*, p. 25.

158. Davis, 'Entertainments', p. 9; Davis and Bonsall, *Bath*, p. 42. In 1742/43, James Leake was present at 31 meetings of the weekly committee.
159. *Miscellaneous Works of Oliver Goldsmith*, pp. 527–31; Peach, *Ralph Allen*, pp. 217–24; Tyte, *Bath*, pp. 52–4; Fawcett and Bird, *Bath*, p. 51.
160. Bath Chronicle, *Hot Water Hospital*, p. 13; Falconer, *Mineral Water Hospital*, pp. 30–31. Between 1739/40 and 1752/53, Nash was present at only 64 weekly committee meetings; thereafter, he abandoned attendance altogether.
161. Sandra Cavallo, *Charity and Power in Early Modern Italy: Benefactors and their Motives in Turin 1541–1789* (Cambridge: Cambridge University Press, 1995), p. 135.
162. *Miscellaneous Works of Oliver Goldsmith*, p. 555.
163. Ibid., p. 542.
164. See, for example, Lewis and Williams, *Private Charity*, p. 19.
165. Nelson, *Address*, p. 199; Blizard, *Suggestions*, p. 94. In her study of Turin charities, Sandra Cavallo has identified this celebratory function from the later seventeenth century. See Cavallo, *Charity*, p. 134.
166. Bayly, *Sermon*, p. 20.
167. Minute Book, 27 April 1774; 21 January 1795.
168. See, for example, Wood, *Bath*, pp. 275–8, 299, 301–3; Collinson, *Somerset*, pp. 47–9; Warner, *Bath*, pp. 290–302.
169. *Letters from a Late Eminent Prelate to One of His Friends*, 2nd edn (London: T. Cadell and W. Davies, 1809), p. 508. See also Barbeau, *Life and Letters*, p. 248.
170. *Poems of Alexander Pope*, 8 vols (London: Methuen, 1939–67), vol. 4: *Imitations of Horace with An Epistle to Dr Arbuthnot and The Epilogue to the Satires*, ed. John Butt, 2nd edn (1953), p. 308.
171. Henry Fielding, *The History of Tom Jones*, ed. by R.P.C. Mutter (Harmondsworth: Penguin Books, 1966), p. 365.
172. Daniel Defoe, *A Tour Thro' the Whole Island of Great Britain*, 2 vols, 4th edn (London: 1748), pp. 297–8. See also *Bath and Bristol Guide*, p. 17; Bath Chronicle, *Hot Water Hospital*, p. 12; Collinson, *Somerset*, p. 170; Falconer, *Mineral Water Hospital*, pp. 28–9; Green, *Eighteenth-Century Architecture*, p. 106; *Improved Bath Guide*, p. 46; Ison, *Georgian Buildings*, p. 91; *Original Bath Guide* [1840], p. 99; Rolls, *Hospital of the Nation*, p. 22.
173. Tregellas, *Cornish Worthies*, p. 24.
174. Minute Book, 27 April 1757.
175. *Bath Journal*, 24 August 1752.
176. Murch, *Biographical Sketches*, p. 86; Peach, *Bath*, p. 80.
177. *Public Ledger*, 12 March 1761, p. 1.
178. *Miscellaneous Works of Oliver Goldsmith* , p. 542.
179. *Improved Bath Guide*, p. 45. See also Murch, *Biographical Sketches*, p. 86; *A Pictorial and Descriptive Guide to Bath* (London: Ward Lock, 1909), p. 52; Warner, *Bath*, p. 290.
180. 'The Life of Richard Nash, of Bath, Esq', *London Magazine*, November 1762, p. 630.
181. Bath Chronicle, *Hot Water Hospital*, p. 14. See also Falconer, *Mineral Water Hospital*, p. 33.
182. Wood, *Bath*, pp. 283, 291.

183. See, for example, Warner, *Bath*, p. 289; Falconer, *Mineral Water Hospital*, pp. 11, 30–33; Murch, *Biographical Sketches*, p. 355.
184. Peach, *Ralph Allen*, pp. xi, 218; Peach, *Bath*, p. 250.
185. Peach, *Ralph Allen*, p. 117.
186. Peach, *Ralph Allen*, p. viii. See also Lewis Melville, *Bath Under Beau Nash* (London: Eveleigh Nash, 1907), pp. 94, 98, 101.
187. *DNB*, vol. 42, pp. 153–5.
188. Falconer, *Mineral Water Hospital*, pp. 28–34; Freeman, *Thermal Baths*, p. 359; George D. Kersley, *The Three R's: Rheumatism, Rehabilitation, Research* (Bath: Ralph Allen Press, undated), pp. 27–8.
189. See, for example, Roger Cooter, *Surgery and Society in Peace and War: Orthopaedics and the Organization of Modern Medicine 1880–1948* (London: Macmillan, 1993), especially chs 6, 10 and 11; Rolls, *Hospital of the Nation*, chs 6, 7, 8 and 9.
190. Addison, *English Spas*, pp. 131–2. See also Ison, *Georgian Buildings*, p. 88; Smith, *Bath*, p. 65.
191. Rolls, *Hospital of the Nation*, pp. 14, 152.
192. Murch, 'Bath', p. 89. See also Mainwaring, *Annals*, pp. 328–9.
193. See, for example, *Bath: Official Guide Book 1986* (Bath: Bath City Council, 1986), p. 14.

CHAPTER NINE

The Integration of the Political Élite

In Chapter 8, we considered how the pursuit of social status at the Georgian Bath Infirmary contributed to the emergence of a broader social élite. This was achieved in two main ways: by enabling the passage of gentility from the landed to the commercial and professional classes, and by encouraging a sense of collective identity among the more prosperous urban gentlemen of the middling sort who assumed most responsibility for managing the institution. Though the civilized social world of which the Hospital governors were a part was not without friction, 'strong conventions of inter-personal behaviour' were put in place to ensure that 'unrestrained individual competition' did not degenerate into 'counter-productive levels of verbal and physical violence'. Consequently, civility became a 'flux that helped to weld together the new and old gentry'.[1] The memorial tablet to Richard Nash in Bath Abbey testifies to the contemporary pull of this social cohesion. Not only does the epitaph describe him as the 'umpire' of fashionable local society; but a cartouche bears the words 'Equa Pulsat Manu' – in translation, 'The Equality of a Handshake': a reference to Nash's desire to bring together the nobility and the middle orders, London and the provinces.[2] However, the calming properties of sociability were not enough to mend the political cracks which throughout the long eighteenth century afflicted the new élite; nor did they tackle the increasingly pressing problem of controlling the lower orders. Therefore, it is important to address the search for political stability in Georgian England and the role of the Bath Infirmary in such an endeavour. In this chapter, we examine the integration of the political élite. The focus falls first on the relationship between medical charity and the evolving fiscal-military state. Next the capacity of the General Hospital to appease religious divisions and political conflicts – symbolically as well as in practice – is assessed. And, finally, the institution is placed within the political environment of Bath, paying particular attention to its interface with the Corporation and its contribution to democracy. Chapter 10 will then examine the 'education' of the labouring classes.

Voluntarism and the state

Recent historiography has challenged the long established Whig orthodoxy that the Georgian state was 'decentralized', 'underfunded', 'amateurish' and 'weak'. This revisionist thesis takes as its starting point Britain's return to the power politics of continental Europe after a break of over 200 years.[3] Military and strategic prowess is judged an inadequate explanation. So, too, is the economic prosperity of the post-Restoration period, rooted in and dependent upon a relentless drive for commercial profit. Instead, much emphasis is placed on the mobilization of money and manpower for war, which between 1688 and 1714 led to the formation of a strong 'fiscal-military state' with high taxation, a national debt and an increasingly efficient system of public administration which included sophisticated mechanisms for transferring and servicing troops around the globe.[4] But if mighty at the external interface, eighteenth-century central government was more restrained in its internal relations because the disengagement of the Privy Council from domestic affairs after the Restoration was only partially offset by the redistribution of responsibilities to the cabinet, the Treasury and Parliament.[5] Therefore, policy on the home front became essentially a matter for local initiative rather than national direction. As a result, legislation was largely permissive; it was often sponsored by individual MPs; and its enforcement relied heavily upon an army of grass roots volunteers who served as JPs and overseers of the poor. Complementing these loose statutory frameworks, however, was a veritable array of philanthropic bodies whose enterprises complemented the domestic circumspection of the fiscal-military state.[6]

Despite their local origins, the charities which comprised the non-governmental sector were remarkably similar in their aims and practices. Where an umbrella organization existed – as in the case of the Society for Promoting Christian Knowledge – this consistency was aided by the circulation of guidelines to local branches.[7] Yet even when there was no such national structure, charities with comparable objectives set about their business in comparable ways. Consequently, though John Bellers failed in his bid for civilian state hospitals,[8] the voluntary infirmaries which grew up during the long eighteenth century were modelled on a template that was adapted to take account of particular circumstances. Communication played its part in shaping the common characteristics of the hospital movement. The national periodicals printed news of local schemes;[9] the provincial papers carried reports of proposals from outside their region;[10] and the institutions themselves exchanged information. Thus at Bath copies of a charity sermon, which included a survey of the Infirmary's current state of affairs, were swopped with the Northampton and London Hospitals,[11] and decisions of both a constitutional and a practical nature were taken with reference to experience elsewhere.[12] Such co-operation was facilitated by the involvement of governors with other charities. Henry Hoare I, one of the original proposers of the Bath Infirmary, had previously helped to found the Westminister Hospital.[13] Robert Dingley, the London merchant, was a chief instigator of the Magdalen Hospital.[14] Ralph Allen was associated with the Magdalen, St Bartholomew's and the Devon and Exeter Infirmary;[15] and a string of Bath governors supported the Foundling Hospital, among them Dingley and the artist, William Hoare.[16] Finally, the Gloucester Infirmary was instituted 'under the auspices of the late Lord Botetourt', who was also a Bath governor.[17] However, the unity of the voluntary hospital movement was based on more than overlapping membership and effective communication. These medical charities cohered because they implemented an evolving moral economy that was broadly in tune with the Georgian age: namely, the production of a fit and disciplined workforce through the regulated supply of medical care. Given this popular agenda, it was possible for a national network of infirmaries to be delivered slowly but surely by voluntary means. In eighteenth-century Britain, therefore, no clear demarcation existed between the public and the private spheres, and charities executed mercantilist policies which in other European nations were the exclusive preserve of the state.

The medico-moral agenda which the voluntary hospitals shared was critical to their role in defusing the 'partisan and sectarian antagonisms' which had racked the governing élite since the Restoration. Medical charity had the capacity to be a 'social balm' because of its affinity with the values of the Enlightenment. Whereas traditional philanthropy was directed towards educational and religious projects which inflamed the fractures of denomination and party, health care which sought to tame the poor in an institutional environment had a universal, humanitarian appeal and an empirical rationale which drew on the logic of the new sciences. Therefore, the voluntary hospital offered a neutral cause around which Anglican and Dissenter, Whig and Tory could consort.[18] But were the governors of the Bath Infirmary drawn from opposing groups? And how far did the institution assist in the search for stability and integration by healing religious divisions and appeasing political strife?

Healing religious divisions

After the supposed Puritan excesses of Cromwell's Commonwealth and the absolutist, pro-Catholic machinations of James II, the Revolutionary Settlement tried to create a balanced constitution in which church and state were complementary rather than rival autonomous forces. Though the non-jurors rejected this integration and refused to take an oath of loyalty to William and Mary, the early eighteenth century saw a gradual lowering of the religious temperature as the Occasional Conformity and Schism Acts were repealed and the Jacobite threat receded. In the Whig latitudinarians, governments had growing clerical support for William Warburton's new *Alliance Between Church and State*, in which the Anglican establishment abandoned its independent power in return for political protection.[19] But though Protestant Dissenters were granted a right of public worship which denied the Church of England a spiritual monopoly, they were excluded from national office. Attempts to remove the civil and political disabilities imposed on sectarian grounds were not successful until the Test and Corporation Acts were repealed in 1828 and Catholics were granted freedom of worship in 1829.[20] By the late 1780s, however, the context was changing. Following George III's rehabilitation of the Tories, latitudinarianism and the religious liberalism that was its accompaniment lost influence and was deflected towards more radical ecclesiastical and political reform.[21] At the same time, the Dissenters themselves were identifying with the democratic aspirations of the London Revolution Society, angered by Pitt's desertion and intoxicated by the endorsement of the Foxite Whigs. The repercussions were fierce. Opposition was not confined to the popular Church-and-King mobs. Nor was it limited to the High Church 'fringe' which had condemned the concessions of 1689. Unreservedly, the Anglican establishment denounced the demands as subversive. The French Revolution and the rise of popular radicalism from the 1790s strengthened this commitment to order in church and state. Sermons denigrated democracy and clergymen increasingly became magistrates. Religious and civil authority were one.[22]

Whereas the vast majority of landowners were at least nominally Anglican, Dissent was more common among the professional and commercial classes. For these middling men, and for the residuum of Recusant and Puritan gentry, religious liberty was not a right but a favour dependent upon the 'benevolent negligence' of a state which chose not to apply the letter of the law.[23] Throughout the long eighteeenth century, formal discrimination thus kept alive religious fissures within the expanded élite. Like other voluntary societies infirmaries offered a way of healing the wounds,[24] just as medicine became a 'secular priesthood' for would-be clerics whose careers were thwarted by religious restrictions.[25] Many institutions aimed to attract 'persons of every denomination' and so put into practice the Enlightenment virtue of toleration by bringing together different shades of theological opinion.[26] Although the Bishop of Bath and Wells and the Rector of Bath were *ex officio* governors, the General Infirmary was not an exclusive Anglican foundation[27] and shared the ecumenical objective.[28] Therefore, when the admission conditions were distributed to Church of England dioceses in 1742,

Dissenting meeting-houses were included among the locations to be targeted in London.[29] The cautious handling of the appointment of a hospital chaplain in 1770 – no doubt under the influence of the Evangelical Revival which had begun to penetrate the middling and upper orders – provides later and more sustained evidence of non-sectarianism. The governors were keen not to offend the religious sensibilities of contributors by raiding mainstream moneys. Therefore, they set up a separate subscription to raise a capital sum 'the income of which may produce a proper salary for a clergyman'. Moreover, after a candidate was finally elected by a packed general court of 43 governors in May 1775, the *Annual Reports* made clear that he was voluntarily supported.[30] The shortage of money, which delayed the original appointment and prompted an interim deduction from the charity collections, continued to haunt the scheme, but not until 1830 did the Infirmary shackle itself to the Established Church by claiming in law the power to nominate an Anglican chaplain and pay him from the general funds.[31]

An independently financed chaplaincy – which did not stop the neighbouring Bristol Infirmary from succombing to bitter sectarian conflict[32] – might have better negotiated religious differences at the General Hospital because Bath, a resort with long-standing Catholic sympathies[33] which thrived on bringing together the social élite, could ill afford to harbour denominational disputes. In any event, Jewish names were to be found among the first subscribers;[34] a bequest of £2 000 was made in 1741/42 by Samuel Holden, a wealthy director of the Bank of England who as chairman of the Dissenting Deputies Committee kept his colleagues 'politically quiet during the excise crisis';[35] and throughout the long eighteenth century, charity collections were regularly received both from local Dissenting congregations and from the Catholic mission at Bell-Tree House.[36] Religious minorities were also drawn into the administration of the Hospital. Mr Richard Marchant, a Bath banker of Quaker persuasion, was one of the five men who organized the first subscription in 1723,[37] while governors outside the pale of the Anglican communion included the Jewish MP and philanthropist, Lord Eardley (formerly Sir Sampson Gideon),[38] the Recusant honorary physician, Dr Richard Bostock,[39] and the Catholic baronet, Sir Robert Throckmorton, one of whose ancestors was executed in 1584 for plotting to invade England and place Mary, Queen of Scots, on the throne.[40]

If lay patrons were drawn from a variety of religious backgrounds, the theological politics of Georgian England were also articulated through the five clerics appointed to the presidency of the Bath Infirmary during the long eighteenth century: Dr Thomas Secker (1760), Archbishop of Canterbury;[41] Dr Charles Moss (1778), Bishop of Bath and Wells;[42] Dr Shute Barrington (1793), Bishop of Durham;[43] the Honourable Henry

Ryder (1816), Bishop of Gloucester;[44] and Dr G.H. Law (1825), Bishop of Bath and Wells.[45] Although Georgian bishops were not so disreputable as their fiercer critics alleged, nor were they all conscientious in their pastoral duties and generous in disposing of their wealth in the public interest.[46] Seen through the eyes of the late Victorian *Dictionary of National Biography*, however, those chosen to become president of the Bath Hospital were noted for their good works. Thomas Secker was a man of 'enlightenment and large-hearted charity' who had also studied medicine in his youth; Charles Moss 'warmly supported' Hannah More in her promotion of Christian education; Shute Barrington, who 'charitably aided' the needy, was president of both the Society for Bettering the Condition of the Poor and the School for the Indigent Blind when he died in 1826; G.H. Law was an 'active and practical bishop'; whilst Henry Ryder – an influential low churchman and the first evangelical to join the bench of bishops – not only helped to found a female penitentiary and schools for the education of the poor but also regularly participated in the teaching of children. This engagement with the new 'scientific' charities stridently committed to the moral reform of the lower orders reflected a growing political conservatism on the part of the Established Church which was also evident in changing attitudes to religious toleration. Despite his close connections with Bath society, William Warburton – engineer of the new relationship between church and state – never served the General Hospital as president, but the latitudinarian interest was represented by Dr Secker. Secker had no sympathy for the extreme, Hoadleian view that the church should be organized by the state because Christ had 'left behind Him no visible, humane authority ... no judges over the consciences or religion of His people'.[47] He was, however, 'a staunch supporter of the Hanoverian government' who came from a Dissenting family, had been educated at a Dissenting academy and 'maintained friendly relations with many leading Dissenters'. By the later eighteenth century, denominational boundaries were hardening. Bishop Barrington was 'a vigorous champion of the protestant establishment' who, believing that 'the corruptions of the Church of Rome were the principal causes of the French Revolution' excluded any political power from the concept of toleration which he applied to Catholics. Moreover, Bishop Law described himself as 'a friend of civil and religious liberty', yet 'strenuously opposed' repeal of the Test and Corporation Acts. No longer latitudinarian, these Anglican bishops resisted reform, aware that the integration of church and state made Catholic and Protestant Dissent an act of political defiance.

The later Georgian preoccupation with order which the spiritual lords displayed in their obstructive attitude to reform was manifest among lower clerics in an increased involvement with moulding the masses. Despite their *ex officio* status, the Bishop of Bath and Wells and the Rector of Bath attended few meetings of the General Infirmary.[48] However, clergymen did join the governing body in increasing numbers and assume more administrative responsibility. In 1825/26, their busiest sample year, they accounted for five of the 17 governors who attended at least one meeting of the weekly committee, and for a half of the 193 total attendances (Appendix G). Professional ambition, a coalescence of the spa's spiritual and socio-cultural life, and the Evangelical Revival may partly explain this activity, but the Hospital also provided a vehicle for moral reform and one that was open to non-Anglican ministers in the way that the magistracy was not. It may be for this reason that the local Presbyterian church supplied several active governors. The Reverend Dr Bennett Stevenson attended 27 meetings of the weekly committee during 1742/43; the Reverend Mr Frank over 20 in 1765/66, 1770/71 and 1775/76; and the Reverend Joseph Hunter 28 in 1825/26 and 22 in 1830/31. The Unitarian minister, the Reverend Thomas Broadhurst, was also present at 15 meetings in 1825/26 and 16 in 1830/31 (Appendix G). But the surge towards policing the lower orders overrode the denominational divisions within the social élite. Middling men from religious minorities who suffered civil and political disabilities because of their faiths did not generally identify a common grievance with the disenfranchised labouring classes over whose behaviour they ruled. Therefore, when Joseph Hunter preached on behalf of the General Hospital in 1810, he emphasized the advantages enjoyed by the poor.

> The most abject of those who fill the subordinate stations, and perform the menial offices in a Christian country, may look down in pity upon the lower orders of people in the several states of Greece, and in the city and adjoining territory of Rome. They were people with few, if any, political rights; they were even incapable of changing the master for whom they laboured; they had no opportunity of raising themselves by any extraordinary diligence or fidelity from this state of humiliating degradation ... Confined to the lowest rank of life, there many of them were born, and there they died. They married, but at the command of their masters: their offspring were his property ... Their servitude was of the hardest kind, their labour immense ... they were generally to be seen in chains; they were obliged to submit to every degrading purpose of their tyrant master ... [49]

The political message from Anglican and Nonconformist alike was clear: the poor in Britain should be grateful that they had been born into a Christian society where progress through effort was not denied by the bonds of slavery.

Georgian politics: faction and party

Though concurrence over the treatment of their social inferiors transcended religious denomination, the relationship between church and state was structured along political lines which were themselves contested. Therefore, we must ask to what extent the voluntary hospital appeased factional and party as well as sectarian conflict. The Revolution Settlement which gave Dissenters freedom of worship attempted to achieve a stable political constitution by balancing the monarchy against an aristocratic House of Lords and a elected House of Commons. For Tories with Stuart and hence Catholic sympathies, James II's departure was difficult to accept and by the early eighteenth century, the uneasy peace which followed the Glorious Revolution had collapsed into a 'rage of party' embracing economic as well as political and religious issues. Walpole's rise to power in 1721 was achieved by inflating the threat posed by a weak Jacobite plot. The effect was to outlaw the Tories from national politics and usher in a long Whig oligarchy. Opposition was hard to mount; and though the Tories retained support at constituency level and among the lesser clergy, they were marginalized in Parliament. Furthermore, despite sharing with malcontent 'Country' Whigs an abhorrence of how the 'Court' was corrupting economic and political life, the Tories did not endorse their wish to reduce religious restrictions. Consequently, the Country faction proved incapable of organizing a united campaign against the Court Whigs.[50]

After Walpole's fall in 1742 and the failure of a Broad-Bottom coalition of Whigs and Tories, Henry Pelham again managed to construct a durable ministry until his death in 1754. However, George III's rehabilitation of the Tories undermined the stability which had been the hallmark of early Hanoverian politics in the same manner that it weakened latitudinarianism. Administrations – headed by the Duke of Newcastle, the Earl of Bute, George Grenville, the Marquis of Rockingham and the Duke of Grafton – were all short-lived; and even Lord North in power after 1770 was unable to weather the storm of American independence, and the demands for electoral and economical changes invigorated by this loss and expressed by organizations like Christopher Wyvill's Association Movement. This reform campaign had its intellectual origins in the early Enlightenment, but whereas in Lockean theory men's natural rights were defended by civil liberties, radicals now demanded an extension of political liberties to secure a more democratic House of Commons and to improve the quality of government. Pitt the Younger's succession quelled the ministerial volatility which followed North's political demise, but parliamentary politics were beginning to respond to pressures from outside and shape themselves around the divisive issue of reform.

By the late 1780s Charles James Fox was regularly being described as leader of the opposition. Pitt in government saw his prime ministerial authority deriving from the monarch and not from a Commons majority. None the less, both parties acquired distinctive ideologies after 1794 when a majority of Whigs joined Pitt's coalition, leaving Fox with a hard core of dedicated reformers. The Napoleonic Wars put a temporary stop to political radicalism, tarring it with the brush of treachery. But with the middle ranks alienated from 1815 by a Corn Law which protected grain prices in the landowning interest, battle recommenced to forge a two-party system of parliamentary loyalty before the Reform Act enlarged the franchise in 1832.[51]

The conflict between Court and Country, Whig and Tory meant that the Georgian élite was torn along political no less than religious lines. Cultural pursuits were a means of mending these tears – not just early in the century when memories of the 'rage of party' were still fresh and the legacy of the Civil War and its aftermath more pervasive, but later too when demands for reform were jeopardizing domestic peace. Simultaneously, such activities increased the potential for conflict because the religious and political harmony promoted by cultural association enabled the rising middling sort to speak with a more united voice and challenge the preconceptions of the traditional élite.[52] Therefore, it is important to ask how far voluntary societies had an eirenic effect.

Addressing this question for the hospital movement, Adrian Wilson has compared eighteenth-century electoral contests in constituencies with and without an infirmary. In 'hospital boroughs', he found that whereas the incidence of contests prior to a foundation was 'effectively identical to the rate in "non-hospital boroughs"', afterwards the proportional number of contests fell by more than a third – albeit only temporarily for the duration of three general elections. For the counties, the eirenic factor operated in a more complex way. In the combined four general elections prior to foundation, 'contests in the "hospital counties" were about 66 per cent as frequent as in the "non-hospital counties"'; but the election '*immediately preceding* the moment of hospital foundation' was characterized by an 'incidence of contests ... slightly higher than the "control pattern"'. Foundations, however, were more than reactions to atypical conflict. Subsequently, contests became even less frequent, running at only about 36 per cent of the rate for 'non-hospital counties' in the combined three general elections after creation. In short, voluntary infirmaries in the counties both promoted and reflected political consensus; voluntary infirmaries in the boroughs only promoted it.[53]

The electoral history of Somerset and Bath offers inconclusive evidence as to whether the General Hospital defused political conflict. In the county, only the 1715 general election was contested up to 1790. In the borough, fewer elections were fought in the second half of the eighteenth century, but the foundation of the Hospital in 1739 did not interrrupt the unbroken string of contests until 1754 and although the general elections of 1761 and 1768 were uncontested, by-elections were fought in 1763 and 1766.[54] Yet Wilson himself recognizes that an absence of contested elections does not necessarily imply an absence of party disputes.[55] Furthermore, borough electorates varied enormously, and the towns which they represented fulfilled different economic and social functions which may have affected the political roles of voluntary hospitals. Therefore, it is important to move beyond electoral contests and explore the eirenic hypothesis in relation to political biography and the local community.

Identifying political affiliation

The role of Bath as an élite resort, and the place of the General Infirmary within the socio-cultural life of the city, ensure that many presidents and governors feature in the *Dictionary of National Biography*, or the History of Parliament series which contain meticulous portraits of MPs sitting between 1715 and 1790. These sources reveal that politicians from non-élite backgrounds were on the governing body of the Hospital. Thomas Coster, one of the founder members, owned a copper works in his Bristol constituency, and tin and copper mines in Cornwall.[56] Arthur Onslow, Speaker of the House of Commons and a mid-century governor, had family ties with the Levant Company.[57] Politicians on the late Georgian governing body also had connections with commerce. Sir Matthew White Ridley was heavily involved in trade in the North East; Benjamin Hobhouse was a banker and barrister; while Bath MP, John Palmer – the son of a local brewer, tallow chandler and theatre proprietor who in the 1750s had assisted the General Hospital – owed his personal prosperity to the development of mail-coach services.[58] But what were the factional and party affiliations of this governing body in which politicians from the landed élite were joined by MPs with industrial, commercial and professional interests? Table 9.1 profiles the Georgian presidents of the Hospital for whom political complexions have been traced, and indicates the year in which they served and the constituency (if any) which they held. Appendix J constructs a series of political vignettes, comprising governors of the Infirmary at fifteen-year intervals up to 1800 (when the History of Parliament volumes, essential for this examination of lesser known politicians, cease to yield the necessary information): 1739/42 towards the end of Walpole's administration; 1755/56 when the Duke of

Table 9.1 Bath General Hospital: the political affiliations of presidents, 1739–1830

Name	*Year*	*Constituency*	*Affiliation*
Thomas Carew Esq.	1739 and 1740	Minehead, 1739–47	Tory
Marshall George Wade	1741	Bath, 1722–48	Walpole administration
Ralph Allen Esq.	1742		Whig
Earl of Chesterfield	1744		Walpole opposition
Duke of Beaufort	1748		Tory
Duke of Bedford	1749		Whig
Lord Viscount Palmerston	1750		Pelham administration
Lord Dupplin	1751	Cambridge, 1741–58	Pelham administration
Duke of Devonshire	1752		Whig
Nathaniel Curzon Esq.	1753	Derbyshire, 1727–54	Tory
Marquis of Rockingham	1754		Whig
Sir John Ligonier	1755	Bath, 1748–63	
Rt. Hon. William Pitt	1758	Bath, 1757–66	Whig [Pitt-Newcastle administration]
Marquis of Carnarvon	1759	Winchester, 1754–61	Tory/Pitt-Newcastle opposition
Lord Henley	1761		Whig
Sir John Sebright	1763	Bath, 1763–74, 1775–80	Grenville administration
Earl of Lincoln	1765		Whig [nephew of Henry Pelham]
Duke of Beaufort	1766		Tory
Sir Lawrence Dundas	1769	Edinburgh, 1768–80	Grafton administration
John Smith Esq.	1771	Bath, 1766–85	North opposition
Henry Hoare Esq.	1776		Tory
Earl Spencer	1780		Whig
Earl Camden	1782		Whig
Lord Rodney	1783		North administration [up to 1782]
Abel Moysey Esq.	1784	Bath, 1774–90	Pitt opposition
Hon. John Jefferys Pratt	1785	Bath, 1780–94	Pitt administration
Earl of Mansfield	1787		Anti-Pitt Whig

Earl Nugent	1788		Independent
Lord Viscount Weymouth	1794	Bath, 1790–96	Pitt administration
Sir Richard Pepper Arden	1795	Bath, 1794–1801	Pitt administration
Duke of Northumberland	1796		Pitt opposition
Marquis of Stafford	1800		Whig
William Gore Langton Esq.	1801	Somerset, 1795–1807	Whig
William Dickinson Esq.	1802	Somerset, 1796–1806	Tory
Lord John Thynne	1804	Bath, 1796–1832	Tory
John Palmer Esq.	1805	Bath, 1801–08	
Thomas Buckler Lethbridge Esq.	1808	Somerset,1807–12	Tory
William Dickinson Esq.	1809	Somerset, 1807–12	Tory
Sir Benjamin Hobhouse	1813	Hindon, 1806–18	Tory[?]
Lieutenant-Colonel Charles Palmer	1815	Bath, 1808–26	Whig
Sir T. Shelley	1818	Seat unknown	
Earl of Brecknock [Rt. Hon. John Jeffreys Pratt]	1823		Tory
Earl of Liverpool	1824		Tory
Sir William Draper Best	1827	Bridport, 1812–[?]	Tory [Chief Justice of Common Pleas]
Marquis of Lansdowne	1829		Moderate Whig
Lord Bexley	1830		Tory

Notes:
1. Both the constituency and the affiliation relate to the period when the presidency was held.
2. A question mark indicates either that the political affiliation of the president, or his tenure of the constituency, is uncertain.

Principal Sources: 12 Geo. II, pp. 572–3; *Annual Reports*; *DNB*; Sedgwick, *The House of Commons 1715–1754*, vol. 1: *Introductory Survey, Constituencies and Members A–D*; Sedgwick, *The House of Commons 1715–1754*, vol. 2: *Members E–Y*; Namier and Brooke, *The House of Commons 1754–1790*, vol. 2: *Members A–J*; Namier and Brooke, *The House of Commons 1754–1790*, vol. 3: *Members K–Y*; Stenton, *Who's Who of British Members of Parliament*, vol. 1: *1832–1885*; *Bath Journal*; John Cannon, 'Bath Politics in the Eighteenth Century', *Proceedings of the Somersetshire Archaeological and Natural History Society*, **105** (1960–61); Sylvia McIntyre, 'Towns as Health and Pleasure Resorts: Bath, Scarborough and Weymouth, 1700–1815', (D.Phil. dissertation, University of Oxford, 1973); J.F. Meehan, *More Famous Houses of Bath and District* (Bath: B. and J.F. Meehan, 1906); Peach, *Ralph Allen*.

Newcastle was heading one of the unstable Whig ministries; 1770/71 as Lord North took over from the Duke of Grafton; 1785/86 during the first phase of Pitt the Younger's long administration; and 1800/01 after Pitt had been reinforced by the defection of conservative Whigs from Rockingham. Interpreting these tables calls for the utmost care. The vignettes are periodic 'stills' which ignore the dynamics of political life; they are based on lists of the governing body which may not have been frequently edited; they include long-serving individuals as well as new appointments; and, notwithstanding the rich sources, many remain unclassified, especially the local gentlemen and esquires who were so central to hospital management. But even where governors can be located with the biographical tools, attaching a reliable label is hazardous. For all its value, the *Dictionary of National Biography* is a product of late nineteenth-century Whig historiography which not only emphasized Whig/Tory divisions but also construed Georgian politics as confined to a narrow, self-interested élite. The History of Parliament project, though more recent, is also inclined towards this cynical view because, conceived by Sir Lewis Namier who also co-authored the volumes for 1754 to 1790, it displays his scepticism towards the influence of political ideas. And compounding all these problems are the difficulties of deciding affiliation at a particular juncture and amidst the shifting sands of Georgian politics.

The political manoeuvrings of men associated with the Bath Infirmary demonstrate the pitfalls which beset their classification. The Duke of Chandos, who as Marquis of Carnarvon was president of the Hospital in 1759, spoke for many eighteenth-century politicians when he declared that he 'abominated the distinction' between Whig and Tory.[59] In the absence of modern parties, politics revolved around personalities, with Walpole and the Whig magnates, North and Pitt the Younger taking the stage in turn. The result was a highly fluid political system. Confusion was the cause of some volatility as in 1737 when Sir William Wentworth – one of the original governors of the General Infirmary – supported an increase in the Prince of Wales's allowance, only to regret how he had cast his vote; according to Lady Isabella Finch, 'His brains ... [were] most puzzled on this affair'.[60] Calculation rather than ineptitude underpinned most decision-making. Politicians stood accused of selling themselves to the highest bidder. Lord Henley[61] and Earl Nugent[62] – presidents of the Bath Hospital in 1761/62 and 1788/89 respectively – each served a series of successive administrations during long parliamentary careers. Moreover, Lord Viscount Palmerston – president in 1750 – earned himself the disparaging title of 'Little Broadbottom Palmerston',[63] whilst Abel Moysey – a governor from the 1780s – was charged by the *English Chronicle* with undergoing 'a rapid metamorphosis in all his political sentiments', and switching his allegiance from the opposition to the government, after being appointed 'to the dignity of a Welsh judge'.[64]

Conviction as well as ignorance and opportunism contributed to the flux of Georgian politics. For the mandarins who held the reins of power, faction was a strong and destabilizing influence. Thus Lord Constantine Mulgrave – navy captain, former Admiralty spokesman in the House of Commons, and governor of the Bath Infirmary in 1785 and 1790 – was prevented from accepting a position in Pitt's new administration by his connection with Lord Sandwich who was committed to the Fox–North Coalition. Consequently, the appointment was delayed until Mulgrave was found a seat on the Duke of Newcastle's interest in 1784.[65] Granville Levison-Gower, who as the Marquis of Stafford became president of the Bath Hospital in 1800, twice resigned government posts during the unstable, later phase of the Whig oligarchy: in 1751 when he became attached to the 'Bloomsbury Gang' led by the Duke of Bedford and in 1765 when Rockingham took office. Having turned down an offer of the premiership after Shelburne fell in 1783, he became Lord President of the Council under Pitt and then Lord Privy Seal until he resigned in 1794 when the Duke of Portland joined the ministry. It is tempting to label Stafford as a reforming Whig, repulsed by the conservative colour that Pitt's administration acquired after the succession of Portland and his followers. By the time he took on the presidency of the Bath Hospital, however, Stafford had withdrawn from government,[66] and, consequently, there are dangers in assuming that he – and others appointed at the end of their careers – were still political figures of moment. Even if retirement did not induce a disdain of conflict, political disengagement may have reduced any capacity to activate factional or party rancour.

Amongst the MPs upon whom the grandees depended for parliamentary approval, a belief in independence was capable of producing fluid alignments. For governors of the Bath Hospital, this political posture was especially pronounced in the later eighteenth century. Though Robert Clive, Lord Clive of India, determined early in his parliamentary life to engage in 'No more struggles against the ministry', he demonstrated nevertheless a considerable autonomy and forged close links with the administration only at points of acute personal difficulty.[67] Samuel Eyre was more forthright, promising in his election address to be 'steady, uniform, and independent, not biased by interest, not attached to party'. Eyre's one recorded vote was with the opposition in 1767.[68] However, other MPs – like Paul Cobb Methuen, who spent only three years in the Commons during the early 1780s – did establish a reputation for independence.[69] Such men, who according to Namier were dominant in the

Lower House, had a predisposition to vote with the sitting government, but not all followed the example of Sir Edward Baynton who apparently supported every ministry under George III.[70] Their loyalty had to be won and retained.[71] Therefore, despite his admiration for Pitt the Younger, whom he described as 'the successor in name, virtue, talents, and situation' to the 'great and ever revered minister Chatham', Sir John Miller opposed the administration on the two occasions when his vote was recorded.[72] Sir Matthew White Ridley was similarly autonomous, for his parliamentary interventions in the 1780s had 'dealt with practical points, and especially with measures affecting the interests of his [Newcastle-upon-Tyne] constituents, rather than with wider questions of policy'.[73] The outcome of this independence was a complex series of voting patterns which perplexed even contemporaries. Take Sir Francis Knollys, an MP for Reading between 1761 and 1768. Outside Newcastle's whip when he entered Parliament, Knollys was originally defined as a 'Tory' in Bute's list of English and Welsh Members returned at the general election of 1761. Subsequently, however, the entry was deleted and replaced with the words 'Old Whig', Bute himself adding the rider that Knollys was 'rather a Walpolian'.[74] Categorization is no easier today, Georgian politicians not infrequently defying neat allocation to the headings Whig or Tory, government or opposition.

Appeasing political conflict

With these formidable problems of classification in mind, we can now chart the political affiliations of those who supported the Bath Infirmary and assess the extent to which it appeased political conflict. Table 9.1 suggests that if after 1800 Tories predominated among the presidents whose political loyalties have been traced, the Hospital at no stage during the Georgian period became the preserve of any one party or faction. Appendix J allows a more detailed look at political identities by using the biographies of presidents and governors to construct vignettes focusing on the effects of the Jacobite legacy, the tensions of the Whig oligarchy, and the revival of partisan politics. Bath had been a centre of 'royalist intrigue' since the Protectorate, a watering-place in the Tory West Country offering the ideal location for 'conspirators to gather under cover of seeking health or amusement'. By the time the General Hospital was founded in 1739, the Whig oligarchy was firmly entrenched, but Stuart sympathies remained strong in the city and Jacobitism, though a dying force, was briefly to resurge again in 1745 and 1751.[75] Both Whigs and Tories were represented in the first cohort of governors. On the Tory side was the first president of the Hospital who had been responsible for steering the Act of Incorporation through Parliament: namely, the Minehead MP, Thomas Carew Esquire, labelled by Horace Walpole 'a stout Jacobite'.[76] Among his political soulmates on the initial governing body were Sir William Wyndham and Thomas Strangeways Horner, both Tory MPs for Somerset. Horner had avoided arrest for his part in the 1715 Rebellion,[77] but Wyndham underwent several months of imprisonment, having given himself up as one of the leaders of the western uprising. Following Bolingbroke's advice, he kept his distance from later planned insurrections and seizing every chance 'to declare himself a strong Hanoverian', he had become the acknowledged 'head of those calling themselves Hanover Tories' by 1726. During the early 1730s, however, Wyndham did engage in discussions with the French about restoring the Stuarts,[78] his loyalty to the Hanoverian succession seemingly ambivalent. For the Whigs appointed to govern the Bath Infirmary in 1739, there was no such wavering. The Honourable Sir William Thompson, a former lawyer and parliamentarian, was famous for his role in the impeachment of the High Tory parson and Oxford don, Dr Henry Sacheverell, and of George Seton, the Jacobite Earl Wintoun.[79] George Wade and Ralph Allen, both presidents of the Hospital in the early 1740s, were more closely connected with the repression of Jacobitism in Bath itself. Though a local MP between 1722 and his death in 1748, Wade was 'much more' than a parliamentary representative; he was, in the words of a nineteenth-century historian, a 'fast friend' of the city, who 'lived in it and loved it, and identified himself with its ... institutions'. The origins of this intimacy lay in his dispatch to Bath with two regiments of dragoons during the 1715 Rebellion.[80] It was a tip-off from the young Ralph Allen – a 'staunch Hanoverian' who went on to finance a company of volunteers during the 1745 disturbances – which enabled Wade to detect the impending Jacobite plot.[81]

Although the Tory Party was reduced to a token parliamentary presence after the rise of Walpole, political conflict was succoured by the fractious ruling Whigs. On the governing body of the Bath Infirmary, there were both supporters and opponents of the Walpole administration. In 1732, George Wade had clashed with the malcontent Whig, William Pulteney, over army wages. Pulteney complained that British soldiers were far better paid than their continental counterparts; Wade, for the government, retorted that 'what [the German army] come short of ours in pay they do more than make up by plundering, oppressing and raising contributions upon the countries where they are quartered'.[82] The 'Country' or 'Patriot' critique of Walpole's administration, for which Pulteney – and the Hospital president of 1744/45, the Earl of Chesterfield – were prominent spokesmen, appealed beyond the Whig opposition to Tories like Sir William Wyndham who also accused the 'Court' of corruption. By the time the Hospital opened in 1742 Wyndham and Horner were dead, but a Tory voice was retained on the governing body through the moderate Thomas Prowse, who succeeded to Sir William's county seat,[83] and the more fanatical 'High-church zealot', Humphrey Sydenham.[84] In the immediate aftermath of Walpole's fall, Tories were embraced in the 'Broad-Bottom' administration. But the Whigs themselves were not united. Pulteney and Chesterfield, both instrumental in disposing of the 'Robinocracy', were no longer in sympathy once the job was done.[85]

During the remainder of the Whig oligarchy, different sections of the party continued to staff the governing body of the Bath Infirmary. Not all the recruits were factional. The Duke of Bedford, for example, appointed president in 1749, was renowned for his mediatory qualities, while, soon after holding the office in 1752/53, the Duke of Devonshire formed a short coalition with William Pitt the Elder, who found him an acceptable partner because he was 'uncontaminated ... by close association with the Pelhams'.[86] Pitt himself, however, was a man rarely away from the sharp end of political controversy. When chosen to fill the Hospital presidency in 1758, he had recently entered into a new coalition with Newcastle and won election as an MP for Bath. Pitt was most charismatic during his management of the Seven Years War (1756–63) before disagreements with George III and Bute forced his resignation in 1761. But if parliamentary tensions evaporated in this happy period, the same harmony was not apparent in his ministry of 1766/68. Elevated to the House of Lords, Pitt as the Earl of Chatham set out to replace conflict with conciliation; what he achieved was a universal animosity which pushed faction to its outer limits. In opposition against Lord North during the 1770s, Chatham dedicated himself to pursuing a more lenient approach to the government of America, asserting emphatically his belief that Britain had no right to tax the colonists. Though he no longer possessed the stature that he had enjoyed as William Pitt, his influential supporters included in their number the law lord, Earl Camden, and the Marquis of Rockingham, both of whom were governors of the General Hospital. Yet the three men were also divided amongst themselves. Camden was one of Chatham's closest associates. However, he chose to separate himself from Rockingham on issues where they were barely apart, and just before his death in 1778 publicly rejected the Rockingham Party's commitment to an immediate acknowledgement of American independence.[87] Conflict was courted to the last.

The hostility which Chatham's adversarial politics aroused was evident at his final appearance in the House of Lords when the judicial peer, Lord Mansfield, 'disgraced himself by exhibiting an ostentatious indifference'. Mansfield, a confidant of Lord North and his cabinet, had long been a rival. In 1787, however, his nomination to the presidency of the Bath Hospital brought him into the orbit of the late Chatham's friend, Lord Camden, who was still a governor. Mansfield and Camden themselves were protagonists. Whereas Camden was a Whig whose legal decisions in favour of John Wilkes during 1763 had won him great respect,[88] Mansfield was – in Macaulay's words – 'the father of modern toryism, of toryism modified to suit an order of things in which the House of Commons is the most powerful body of the state'. Consequently, the two law lords clashed violently over policies towards America, Camden maintaining that to tax colonists without a parliamentary voice was tantamount to robbery. Moreover, Mansfield's reputation was seriously damaged by Camden's criticism of his lacklustre performance during the 1770 debate on the exclusion of Wilkes from the Commons.[89]

In addition to the emnity between Lord Mansfield and Camden, the governing body of this period embraced local parliamentary representatives of different political persuasions: a situation in which Camden was also a player. Recorder of the city since 1759, he became concerned in the mid-1770s that both city MPs were supporters of Lord North and thus not of his own mind. When the ex-soldier and sitting Member, Sir John Sebright, announced his retirement in 1780, Camden took action and arranged for his own son, the Right Honourable John Jefferys Pratt, to stand. Duly elected, Pratt followed in his father's footsteps. Not only was he appointed a president and governor of the General Infirmary, but he also copied Camden's politics, voting against Lord North's administration and then backing Shelburne and Pitt. Re-elected, his fellow Bath MP, Abel Moysey – a justice and son of the Hospital physician of the same name – continued to support North and followed him into opposition with Fox.[90] In the early 1780s, therefore, just as in the 1740s, divergent political views were current among the governing body of the General Infirmary.

The rebirth of party in the closing decades of the eighteenth century began the restructuring of politics into the modern bi-polar system. The disruptive potential of this process, and the debate about reform at its core, was reflected in the cultural life of later Georgian Bath; for both the York Club and the Philosophical Society prided themselves in their political neutrality, and the latter specifically banned politics from its agenda, along with law, physic and divinity.[91] The political behaviour of Hospital governors also exhibited some resistance to partisanship, Sir John Trevelyan and Sir James Tylney Long joining the St Alban's Tavern group which aimed to bring together Fox and Pitt the Younger.[92] Their adherence to

Pitt after 1783 is suggestive of how party loyalties were to firm up. The long-standing governor and Somerset MP, William Gore Langton, who became president of the General Infirmary in 1801, was a 'steadfast' Whig and 'a strenuous supporter of the Reform of Parliament, the Roman Catholic Relief Act, and other measures of a liberal tendency'.[93] By the 1820s, the presidency of the Bath Hospital was being held by politicians who were clearly either Whigs or Tories. In 1824/25, for example, the incumbent was the Earl of Liverpool, Tory prime minister from 1812 to 1827.[94] The Chief Justice of the Common Pleas, Sir William Draper Best, was appointed in 1827. A Whig when he entered Parliament in 1802, he changed his politics and did service in Liverpool's ministry. Whereas Draper Best was 'a vehement supporter of the tory party, and strenuously opposed the Reform Bill' after his elevation to the House of Lords,[95] the Marquis of Lansdowne – who took up the Hospital presidency in 1829 – was an equally committed Whig. Chancellor of the Exchequer in the Ministry of All the Talents which was formed after Pitt's death in 1806, Lansdowne became a leading Opposition figure, promoting with enthusiasm the campaign for religious freedom and political reform. Furthermore, when the Whigs finally gained power in 1830 after a long spell in the wilderness, he was of sufficient importance to be offered the Treasury and the Foreign Office, though he actually chose the post of President of the Council.[96] Lansdowne's successor at the Bath Infirmary was also a man of high reputation. Lord Bexley, formerly Nicholas Vansittart, had been Chancellor of the Exchequer in Liverpool's administration. Upon retirement in 1823, he took an energetic part in the work of various religious and charitable societies, and also served as a director of the Greenwich Hospital.[97]

In many respects, Lord Bexley encapsulates the philanthropic environment of the early nineteenth century. An Anglican High Tory,[98] he represented a last ditch stand for paternalism. His enemy was the new moral economy of the market-place – increasingly welcomed by liberal Tories as well as Whigs – which destroyed reciprocity between rich and poor, and hence imperilled social and political order. At Bath, this mentality was enunciated in the scientific charities which sprung up from the 1780s. But the paternalism embodied within the General Hospital also retained a residual appeal, particularly among the urban élite and the landowning classes who visited the city. This lingering attachment to traditional obligations may account for the bias towards Tory presidents from the turn of the century. Furthermore, it also suggests that the financial prosperity which hit the Infirmary after Waterloo was not simply the product of a healthy economy released from the dead weight of war, but a local reaction against the *laissez-faire* strategy for poverty which was to dictate the reform of poor relief in 1834.

Unlike other provincial foundations, the Bath Infirmary made no direct reference in its original 'Plan and Elevation' to appeasing conflict between 'gentlemen of every party'. None the less, the pen portraits of those associated with the institution indicate that it did not become tied to particular political interests in the way that London medical charities developed partisan profiles.[99] Since the biographies are far from complete, the balance between different factions and parties cannot be discerned. What is evident is that throughout the long eighteenth century presidents and governors were recruited from politicians who were 'for' and 'against' the current administration. We can read from these mixed political affiliations a peacemaking role. The admission of Tories as well as Whigs to the first governing body can be seen as a gesture of reconciliation towards the largely historical wounds of Jacobitism. The absorption of Whigs from different factions can be seen as an attempt to counteract ruptures in the ruling oligarchy. The inclusion of radicals and conservatives can be seen as an effort to defuse the contentious reform debate. However, this ability to field political divergence demonstrates no inevitable eirenic effect.

There are two reasons. First, the governors belonged to pre-existing political networks just as they were enmeshed in economic and social relationships. Consequently, if some were foes, others were on the same wavelength. Political projects were shared as in 1745 when Humphrey Sydenham seconded Thomas Carew's motion for annual Parliaments[100] or in 1757 when the Earl of Chesterfield was instrumental in forming the administration which combined William Pitt the Elder with the Duke of Newcastle.[101] Political patronage similarly forged ties. In the case of Sir Richard Pepper Arden, president in 1795/96, the entwinement was pervasive, his success as a lawyer and politician being much attributed to 'the friendship of Pitt [the Younger], without whose patronage his career would have been far more arduous'.[102] But influence was also applied specifically to the electoral process. Rear-Admiral George Anson, later created a baron, owed his seat for Hedon in 1744 to the Earl of Bath.[103] Moreover, Ralph Allen used his interests on the Bath Corporation to secure the election of George Wade, Robert Henley, Sir John Ligonier and the Elder Pitt[104] – all of whom served as presidents of the General Infirmary. Allen's involvement in the election of local MPs is instructive, given that allegedly he never 'troubled himself to discuss party politics' and indisputedly extended hospitality to men like the Tory poet, Alexander Pope, and the Whig novelist, Henry Fielding.[105] It suggests that socio-cultural networks were capable of overriding political conflict. The apparent ideological neutrality of the Bath artist and Hospital governor, William Hoare, implies that commercial relationships too were impervious where fixed political opinions ran the risk of offending clients.[106] Thus, the political networks centred on the General Infirmary may have taken a back seat to the economic and socio-cultural returns of medical charity which in a spa town such as Bath were at an especially high premium.

To this qualification must be added a second factor: the limited potential for political integration through personal contact when attendance at Hospital meetings was so patchy. As a result of their regular encounters at the Hospital and at other venues in the city, the local élite of professional and commercial men may have started to develop the kind of independent political identity which was acknowledged in 1832 when the Great Reform Act enfranchized the urban middle classes. However, presidents and governors antagonistic to change were unlikely to have been converted by the ambitions of men with whom they mixed so infrequently, and scant attendance likewise rendered improbable any conciliation between factional or party opponents at a national level. Yet however minimal the eirenic factor, the governors who attended general courts were prepared to pick men at the heart of high politics with diametrically opposed views and these politicians were willing to be coupled publicly with an institution which also hosted their rivals. Therefore, we can deduce that the General Infirmary did function at a symbolic level. During an age in which the flames of political dissent were never extinguished, it carried the reassuring message that the governing élite was able to co-operate over the charitable provision of medical care for 'the honour and happiness of this country'.[107]

Local political institutions

Though the Bath electorate was narrowly confined to the oligarchic Corporation of 30 members, it was for much of the eighteenth century 'justly famed for its integrity, independence and zeal for the public good'.[108] Nation-wide, the paternalist ethos limited as well as legitimated the authority of the governing élite, and created obligations to the whole community as well as to the electorate. However, the political culture of Georgian England cannot be reduced to sparring for seats in a chamber dominated by the thin, landowning élite. On the contrary, the established framework of local government was joined during the course of the eighteenth century by a series of complementary vehicles for political communication which included voluntary societies as well as interest groups, petitioning and the press. These mechanisms, together with economic prosperity and socio-cultural organizations, helped to shape a more coherent middling sort and to compensate for the narrow parliamentary franchise by making central government more open to their influence.[109] But there were also ramifications for local politics, as the new agencies created opportunities for political integration while at the same time confronting existing structures of power. It follows that the eirenic hypothesis for voluntary hospitals has to be tested locally as well as nationally. Therefore, we now consider how the Bath Infirmary interacted with local political institutions and assess the extent to which it fostered democratic rights.

There has been a tendency to emphasize the 'synergistic' effects of interlocking town and county in a medical institution which served the region.[110] In the case of the General Hospital, governors and patients from the West Country were indeed numerous, and Members of Parliament for Somerset were appointed to the governing body along with those for the city (Appendix J). However, Bath was not the county capital, the region boasted other infirmaries at Bristol (1737), Exeter (1741) and Gloucester (1755),[111] and the Bath Infirmary's association with the waters bound it more closely to the resort rather than to its hinterland. Despite this identification with the town, civic pride was not universal, for while supporters saw the Infirmary as 'an ornament to this city',[112] opponents argued that it aggravated the affliction of vagrancy. Therefore, whereas civic authorities elsewhere made land or funds available,[113] the Bath Corporation drew up a petition against the Hospital Bill to be presented to Parliament if necessary, and succeeded in denying patients access to all but the Hot Bath.[114] The complex admissions/discharge procedure was designed to allay the fears of mendicity which gripped the Corporation. As we have seen, intending patients had to put forward descriptions of their symptoms, drawn up by a physician or 'skilful person' in the neighbourhood and attested by the local minister and churchwardens; the Infirmary then appraised each application and summoned suitable cases in sequence as vacancies arose, despatching the poor law certificates to overseers in the parish of St Peter and St Paul when patients arrived. Arrangements for release were equally stringent. Settlement rights were not acquired through residence at the Hospital and the Act stated categorically that patients were to be transported 30 miles from Bath in the direction of their home parish, the cost of the journey being met from their caution money. The penalty for subsequently loitering or begging within five miles of the town was a period of up to three months' hard labour in a house of correction. Additionally, the Act strengthened general powers to stamp out vagrancy in Bath and its suburbs of Widcombe and Walcot, imposing a maximum sentence of 12 months' hard labour.[115]

The Infirmary made strenuous efforts to publicize its entry procedures and before opening in May 1742 printed 12 000 advertisements explaining the 'admission and dismission of patients'.[116] As early as July 1742, however, the weekly committee was resolving 'to meet the Corporation of Bath at the Town Hall ... to consult of proper methods to clear the town of vagrants'.[117] Vagrancy remained a bone of contention. Between May and July of 1745, the governors regularly condemned in the *Bath Journal* those 'several persons [who] have lately reported to Bath, under pretence that they were to be admitted to the General Hospital', warning that 'no application will be received, unless the person be at his usual place of abode'.[118] By 1747 they were adopting an explicitly defensive tack. The Infirmary was beyond reproach; its governors 'do now and always will, strictly observe the directions of their Act of Parliament ... relating to the admission of patients'. It was the public who were at fault; they had ignored 'our former advertisements' and, therefore, they were to blame for 'all the evils which any poor persons shall suffer by coming to Bath irregularly'.[119] But these exhortations apparently proved insufficient to satisfy the Corporation, which weighed in during the Spring of the following year. 'Notwithstanding the repeated advertisements, and positive directions of the General Hospital at Bath, forbidding all patients to approach the city without proper credentials ... there are great numbers who daringly intrude, in a most impudent manner, under pretence of being recommended by their friends who are lodgers there.' Upon detection, they would be treated as incorrigible vagrants.[120]

After 1750 relations between the Hospital and the Corporation were less sullied by a preoccupation with vagrancy. The problem itself did not disappear. Late eighteenth-century poor law records show frequent payments for the return migrants to their home parishes;[121] the city spawned an early example of the national movement for bettering the poor when a local Society for the Suppression of Common Vagrants was founded in 1805;[122] and the abuse of out-patient papers from the United Hospital was so serious in the late 1820s that the governors published a press notice alerting benefactors to the evils of begging.[123] But though the General Hospital failed to stem the tide of beggars who journeyed to Bath for the waters,[124] and was powerless to assist the indigenous poor who multiplied with the number of visitors and residents, it was able to moderate the charge of causing vagrancy by practising continued vigilance towards street poverty. From the late 1740s, the conditions for admission were included in the *Annual Report* and details were published in both national[125] and local periodicals, the *Bath Journal* carrying advertisements at regular intervals until the late eighteenth century.[126] These regulations were amended in the light of experience. Military personnel were not a major constituency of patients.[127] However, in 1746 – no doubt in the aftermath of the

Jacobite Rebellion – the governors agreed to admit soldiers without parish certificates if their commanding officers signified a willingness to receive them back into the corps whatever their state of health when discharged from the Hospital. A similar stipulation was subsequently extended to governors of the Chelsea and Greenwich Hospitals before their pensioners were admitted.[128] Difficulties with Scottish and Irish applications prompted the requirement in 1756 that where there was no legal settlement in England or Wales a 'creditable person' approved by the weekly committee should not only specify the home parish but also promise to accept the discharged patient and arrange for conveyance to his or her place of abode.[129] These principles were implemented when cases were processed. Mary Hereford from the Foundling Hospital and George Wildash from Charterhouse were both minuted for admission only on condition that two governors from their parent institutions endorsed the undertaking which applied to other extra-parochial patients.[130] The settlement rule for parochial applicants was also enforced. Therefore, the request of John Davis's sponsor that justices in Monmouthshire be allowed to attest his certificate was turned down because although he had lived in Chepstow for 14 weeks, he was a parishioner of Woolaston in Gloucestershire.[131] This commitment to establishing responsibility for patients was essential if they were not to swell the population of beggars after discharge. When former inmates like James Merchant were found loitering, staff were told to apprehend them and bring them before the mayor.[132] But the Hospital's late eighteenth-century rules also enshrined an order of 1750 which instructed the house visitors to direct 'two of the chairmen ... every day to take up vagrants'.[133] Neither past patients nor the poor in seach of relief without authorization were to substantiate the accusation that the General Infirmary bred vagrancy.

Despite this concern about begging, the Minute Books contain no mention of dealings with the Poor Law authorities and governors of the General Hospital rarely dispensed public relief, their high occupational status setting them apart from the vintners and cabinet makers, barbers and plasterers who undertook this task. In the parish of Bath Abbey, for example, not a single overseer belonged to the governing body in the sample years up to 1830, and only three attended meetings at which accounts were received – all in the first two decades after foundation.[134] Furthermore, none of the six Bath parishes in the late 1820s had overseers who were governors.[135] With no more than four shared members in 1800, there was also little penetration of the Improvement Commission established to pave, clean, light and regulate the parish of Walcot.[136] However, the 54 Commissioners who oversaw the improvement of the Pump Room area included at least eight governors.[137] This was due to the involvement of the City Corporation, whose members were increasingly associated with the General Infirmary. For much of the Georgian period, the social exclusiveness of the visiting Company caused offence to some local tradespeople. From the 1760s the Corporation, through which their interests were vocalized, embarked upon a strategy to retain control as the spreading town's centre of gravity shifted northwards away from its old core; rival assemblies were even held in the resplendent Guildhall, completed in 1777.[138] Over time resistance to the Company weakened, as residents recognized the commercial advantages of the resort trade and visitors increasingly settled in the town. On the Corporation, this gradual reconciliation was reflected in the rising representation of medical practitioners, and governors of the General Hospital many of whose professional activities also thrived on the spa. In 1740 six of the 30 members were apothecaries; by 1800 seven apothecaries were joined by no fewer than ten physicians and surgeons.[139] The influx from the Infirmary's governing body was just as dramatic. Although overtures were directed towards the local political establishment by making the mayor and the two justices of Bath *ex officio* governors,[140] neither they nor the town clerk frequented the weekly committee on a regular basis unless they were already seasoned attenders (Appendix G). Sampling at fifteen-year intervals between 1755 and 1830 shows that governors who were on the Corporation comprised at least a quarter of those supporting one or more meetings of the committee. However, it was common membership which increased most significantly. In 1740, only two of the governing body besides the mayor and justices were councilmen; by 1800, the number was 12; after the Napoleonic Wars, it was in excess of 20.[141]

The absorption of governors into the Corporation poses questions about the political role of the Infirmary in relation to local parliamentary contests and the interface between residents and visitors. Relatively few general elections were fought in Georgian Bath. In 1741, only two governors – Ralph Allen and Samuel Bush – were councilmen and they both rejected the Tory, John Codrington, in favour of George Wade and Philip Bennett who backed Walpole's administration.[142] Examination of two further three-horse races demonstrates that the governing body accommodated differences of opinion within the Corporation just as it did national political conflict (Table 9.2). At the first election on 6 April 1784, William Pitt the Younger secured a parliamentary majority in the aftermath of his appointment as prime minister in the previous December. Pitt himself was nominated for one of the Bath seats, and although he was elected for Cambridge University three days before the poll, the Corporation decided to express their concurrence with his principles by retaining him in the ballot.[143] The 14 votes that he received meant only a slim defeat by one of the other candidates: John Jeffreys Pratt collected 27 votes, but Abel Moysey a mere 17. The 15 governors of the Hospital enfranchized as councilmen had preferences similar to the Corporation as a whole, 14 voting for Pratt, nine for Moysey and seven for Pitt. Pratt supported Pitt's ministry and Moysey opposed it. However, the endorsement of a mixed ticket comprising Pratt and Moysey by 15 councilmen – of whom eight were governors – suggests that balancing interests was an important criterion for the late eighteenth-century Bath electorate.

Our second contested election on 1 July 1830 brought Lord Grey to the premiership on the eve of the Great Reform Act. By the 1790s, the Pratt family had gained control over one Bath seat and the Thynnes (headed by the Marquis of Bath from Longleat in Wiltshire) over the other, but their supremacy did not go unopposed and after John Jeffreys Pratt, now Lord Camden, dropped Major-General Charles Palmer for his son, the Earl of Brecknock, in 1826, one councilman exclaimed that he 'could never submit that this city should become the close property of two peers'.[144] A Whig who was popular with the Bath public, Palmer initially lost to Brecknock but beat him by two votes in 1830 and rejoined the Tory, Lord John Thynne, as the second MP. Both Palmer and Thynne were backed by 15 members of the full Corporation, and by 11 of the 21 governors of the Hospital who were enfranchised in the city. But political divisions were sharpening. Only nine councilmen, six of them governors, voted for the winning Palmer/Thynne package, whereas an unequivocal 'party' position was taken up by 19 electors, 14 of them governors. Most but not all of this allegiance was to the Tory camp. Therefore, although men from across the political spectrum were still embraced, the late Georgian Corporation was predisposed towards the paternalist ethos for which the General Infirmary, and the more illustrious political figures among its patrons, stood. Conversely, Bath was to return a radical MP in 1832. The old Corporation was at variance with the new electorate.

In addition to reflecting parliamentary politics, the Bath Hospital was crucial to relations between residents and visitors. The convergence of governors and councilmen does not necessarily imply that the Infirmary was a force for political integration, not least because the most active members of the governing body made their livings from economic activities which thrived on the spa. When in 1819 John Parish attacked its extravagant treatment of 'foreign invalids' in a bid to improve funding for the Penitentiary and Lock Hospital, he openly accused the Corporation of reversing 'the *good old adage*, that "Charity should begin at home"'; since 1742, he complained, 'the Worshipful Body have had preached from their pulpits ... "that of all charities which we have to

Table 9.2 Bath General Hospital: the voting behaviour of governors who were members of the Bath Corporation at general elections in 1784 and 1830

(a) 6 April 1784

Governors	*Candidates*		
	Abel Moysey Esq.	*Hon. John Jeffreys Pratt*	*Rt Hon. William Pitt*
Mr William Anderdon	X	X	
Mr Harry Atwood	X	X	
Francis Bennett Esq.		X	X
Mr George Chapman		X	X
Leonard Coward Esq.		X	X
Simon Crook Esq.	X	X	
Dr Henry Harington	X	X	
Mr Edmund Hutchinson	X	X	
Abel Moysey Esq.	X	X	
Mr Charles Phillott		X	X
Mr Joseph Phillott	X		X
Mr Thomas Rundell		X	X
Dr William Watson		X	X
Walter Wiltshire Esq.	X	X	
Henry Wright Esq.	X	X	
No. of votes from governors	9	14	7
No. of votes from all councilmen	17	27	14

(b) 1 July 1830

Governors	*Candidates*		
	Rt Hon. Lord John Thynne	*Major-General Charles Palmer*	*Rt Hon. Earl of Brecknock*
George Edward Allen Esq.			X
Edmund Anderdon Esq.			X
Thomas Croxall Cam Esq.	X	X	
William Clark Esq.	X	X	

Table 9.2 concluded

(b) 1 July 1830 continued

Governors	*Candidates*		
	Rt Hon. Lord John Thynne	*Major-General Charles Palmer*	*Rt Hon. Earl of Brecknock*
Robert Clarke Esq.	X	X	
Thomas Clutterbuck Esq.		X	
Charles Crook Esq.	X	X	
Dr John Ford Davis			X
Sir George Smith Gibbes	X	X	
John F. Gunning Esq.	X		X
George Kitson Esq.		X	X
Peter Marriott Esq.	X	X	
George Norman Esq.		X	
Charles Phillott Esq.			X
Johnson Phillott Esq.			X
Joseph Phillott Esq.	X		X
Eleazer Pickwick Esq.	X		X
James Sloper Esq.		X	
Joseph Hume Spry Esq.		X	
William Tudor Esq.	X		X
G.H. Tugwell Esq.	X		
No. of votes from governors	11	11	10
No. of votes from all councilmen	15	15	13

Note: One member of the Corporation was absent at each election.

Sources: Bath Corporation Minute Books; Bath General Hospital *Annual Reports*.

look to, the *first* is – that charity which begins *abroad*"'.[145] Despite this onslaught, the Corporation did not finally deprive the General Infirmary of one of its pair of annual sermons until the Bath United Hospital opened in the late 1820s. Far from indicating civic support, however, the allocation of two annual charity services may have indicated an isolation within the local community if church and chapel collections, targeting the Company, were regarded as the suitable way to fund an institution which catered for the visiting poor. This interpretation is consistent with the apparently limited collaboration between the two bodies. In 1743, a piece of land was leased from the Corporation as a burial ground. Thirty years later, the civic authorities were thanked 'for their charitable supply of water to this House'; and in 1779 gratitude was again expressed for the readiness with which councilmen instructed their MPs to forward the Hospital's petition for exemption from the Mortmain Act.[146] It is possible that these last two incidents, when the Corporation was locked in battle with the fashionable upper town, were bids to cultivate an institution located within its territory yet bonded to the Company. After the initial clash over vagrancy, however, there is little documented involvement in the Infirmary's affairs.

Although parallel membership may have obviated the need for formal communication, the reserve of the Corporation was also symptomatic of local ambivalence towards the institution. Set apart by its historical association with the visiting Company and its desire to help poor strangers, the General Hospital was resented for detracting attention from the local sick poor. So argued the broadsheet which in the 1790s proposed enhancing the Pauper Scheme into a City Infirmary and Dispensary. 'While the benevolent contributions of the wealthy are chiefly conferred on an Hospital ... which ... excludes the inhabitants of Bath itself, there does not perhaps exist any other city of the same opulence, in which the afflicted poor suffer such misery and want.' The subscribers hoped

> for the benevolent contributions of the resident inhabitants, and of the families who have property in the neighbourhood ... [but] they likewise flatter themselves that the Company resorting to Bath, who already see a well-endowed Hospital for the reception of strangers from all parts of the kingdom, will, in return for the benefits solely appropriated to the poor of their respective districts, contribute to relieve the afflicted within Bath itself, who, without the aid of this institution, have not even the means of employing the waters so bountifully bestowed by providence on their native city.

With such support, it would be possible 'to rescue Bath from the reproach of being the only city of its population and wealth in this country, which has neglected to provide an asylum for its own sick poor'.[147] The creation of the City Infirmary and Dispensary did not quell the hostility felt by critics of the General Hospital.[148] The Corporation manifested its concern for the resident poor in financial support for local medical charities: £50 to the Bath City Infirmary and Dispensary in 1811; £50 to the Penitentiary and Lock Hospital in 1816; £300 to the Casualty Hospital in 1820; and a further £700 in 1823 when its merger with the City Infirmary and Dispensary was put in motion.[149]

The General Hospital was given no such assistance, despite its periodic cash crises. Therefore, the fact that many governors were now councilmen brought no change to the long-standing hands-off policy. Mindful of the controversy which surrounded charity for 'foreigners', the Corporation defined civic obligation in terms of provision for the indigenous poor, ever swelling to serve a growing resident population.

Medical charity and democracy

For Charles Lucas – the Irish radical who played a key role in the mid-century sulphur controversy – the Bath Corporation exemplified the political flaws of the Establishment. But if local government was in the hands of an exclusive élite, to what extent did Georgian society nurture more democratic forms of participation which complemented existing structures of power? Kathleen Wilson has argued that while voluntary hospitals confirmed and redistributed 'social authority and power', their 'internal structures' and the values which they espoused also challenged 'the customs and imperatives of patrician society' and therefore fed 'the radical critique of the eighteenth-century state'. Even before the campaign for economical and political reform got under way in the 1760s, voluntary infirmaries were making a stand against the corruption of clientage by setting up open and efficient administrative procedures. They were also generally responsive to the decline of the paternalism traditionally associated with patrician landowners, and developed out-patient facilities and corporate subscription schemes deemed more conducive to independence on the part of the poor. But, above all, since 'there were [normally] no rules or requirements that allocated greater power to men of wealth and position', the vast majority of voluntary hospitals were subscriber democracies in which for the price of a small contribution the middling sort joined with their social superiors to manage the institution.[150] The United Hospital in Bath conformed to this political paradigm. Thus when Dr James Muttlebury resigned from his post as an honorary physician in June 1828, a total of four candidates were willing to fill the vacancy. The governors enquired initially of the remaining physicians whether there were objections to any of the names being placed on the ballot paper. But for one of their number this arrangement was unsatisfactory. Therefore, at the instigation of Dr Edward Barlow – prominent in the national campaign to reform the medical profession and also physician to the General Infirmary – the candidates were asked to provide 'testimonials of qualification'. Dr Barlow was foiled in his attempt to secure votes for 'subscribers of one pound' on the grounds that the committee had 'no power to alter the rules already made'. None the less, the Guildhall was hired to accommodate the large body of subscribers who attended the special general meeting at which the election was held and tellers were appointed to ensure that the votes for each candidate were properly counted.[151]

The democratic conventions which Edward Barlow sought to extend at the United Hospital were absent from both the constitution and the procedures of the General Infirmary. In the first place, only benefactions of at least £40 attracted the distinction of governor, so that annual subscribers and donors of less substantial lump sums who wished to exercise democratic rights were dependent upon being chosen by the governing body.[152] There is little to suggest that the two routes to governorship were socially polarized. The early *Annual Reports* do not specify those governors who met the financial qualification, but not all the big gifts came from aristocrats and men recruited by election were drawn from a variety of status groups. Between 1739 and 1742, for example, there were 16 appointments which included an aristocrat and a clergyman, three doctors, five esquires and six gentlemen.[153] The identification of £40 governors in *Annual Reports* from the late eighteenth century indicates that as inflation eroded the real value of the threshold, the 'purchase' of seats on the governing body grew: in 1785/86 one in five governors qualified in this way, by 1830/31 one in three. However, this egalitarian influence did not override the confinement of automatic political rights to benefactors of £40, which ensured that the governmental structure of the Bath Hospital was an oligarchic rather than a democratic one.

The General Infirmary was oligarchic in its operation as well as in its constitution. Not only did medical recommendation virtually exclude the lay sponsorship of patients, but the majority of governors played little part in the administration of the institution. This abdication extended to the opportunities for patronage that were available. The importance of elections in shaping the governing body was reflected in the higher than average attendance at the May general court when vacancies were usually filled. Participation likewise rallied when senior paid staff were appointed. The election of a matron typically drew at least ten governors[154] and the election of an apothecary at least 20.[155] The post of register had greater pulling power, attracting several attendances of more than 30.[156] However, it was the choice of honorary medical staff which afforded the best opportunity for patronage. Without detailed accounts of individual elections, unambiguous trends are not easily discernible (Table 9.3). In general, only between 10 and 20 per cent of the governing body materialized to cast their votes. Of course, engagement was curtailed by the geographical distribution of governors recruited from the visiting Company. But Minute Book

Table 9.3 Bath General Hospital: the number of governors present at the election of honorary medical staff, 1740–1830

Position	*Date*	*Name(s)*	*No. present*
Physician	1 May 1740	Edward Harrington	15
		William Oliver	
		Alex Rayner	
	15 May 1744	Richard Bostock	24
		Thomas Brewster	
		David Hartley	
	1 May 1747	Abel Moysey	18
		William Woodford	
	2 November 1748	John Summers*	13
	2 June 1757	Rice Charleton	27
	20 May 1761	Robert Gusthart*	20
	6 September 1780	Henry Harington*	17
	10 January 1781	Daniel Lysons*	23
	16 May 1781	John Staker*	22
	12 May 1784	William Falconer	33
	30 October 1799	Caleb Hillier Parry*	43
	9 April 1800	James Holman	51
	28 December 1804	George Smith Gibbes	51
	23 April 1817	John Ford Davis*	26
	4 February 1818	Charles Parry*	13
	3 March 1819	Edward Barlow*	18
	17 July 1822	James Muttlebury*	17
	28 July 1830	John Bampfylde Daniell	22
Surgeon	1 May 1740	Jeremiah Peirce	15
	24 June 1742	Archibald Cleland	22
		John Donne	
		Thomas Palmer	
		Henry Wright	
	15 August 1744	Philip Ditcher	14
	15 November 1744	Giles Jones	22
	3 June 1767	Joseph Phillott	45
	31 January 1781	Harry Atwood*	17
	12 February 1794	Morgan Nicholls*	14
	21 May 1806	William Tudor*	34
	2 April 1817	George Kitson	48
	17 May 1820	J.G. Elkington*	18
	15 August 1821	W. Terry*	18
	9 May 1827	Richard F. George	60

Notes:
1. All honorary medical staff were appointed by general courts.
2. Where an individual is marked with an asterisk, the Minute Book records that he was elected unanimously.

Source: Minute Books.

entries give no indication that posts were openly contested and not infrequently the few who were present reached decisions which were recorded as unanimous. Just how much significance should be attached to this term is unclear because its omission may be no more than a clerical oversight. At four of the five appointments with a turnout of over 40 the decision was not described as unanimous, but not all such elections generated large numbers and so we cannot equate a high participation rate with electoral conflict. A chronological pattern is similarly elusive. Although an unprecedented 60 governors attended when Richard Francis George was appointed to his surgeon's post in 1827, a mere 22 were present at the election of the physician, John Bampfylde Daniell, three years later.

The failure of the Bath Infirmary to embrace wholeheartedly the principles of political reform is not surprising. By the late 1820s, there were signs of politicization among the governors who dealt with routine administration as the more professional system of record-keeping was used to arbitrate the outcome of disputed meetings. These governors probably held the county franchise, but only seven of the 26 proposing or seconding motions or amendments after the procedure was minuted from February 1829 were councilmen.[157] Throughout the long eighteenth century, experience of hospital management may have helped such men to increase their representation on the Corporation[158] and thus join the political élite of Bath which elected MPs for the borough. Therefore, the General Infirmary consolidated traditional structures of authority, leaving middling men of lower social status, excluded from the governing body by its oligarchic constitution, to learn the lessons of democracy from local charities whose management was open to modest subscribers.

In examining the search for political integration among patrons of the General Hospital, we have detected forces pulling in different directions. At the local level, an institution dedicated to spa therapy for poor strangers remained a focal point for antipathy towards visitors, despite the adaptation of social and political relationships to the spa economy. Furthermore, the exclusivity of the early Company was preserved in the constitution of the Infirmary which was supportive of the *status quo* and failed to mollify contributors without a franchise who turned to charity in order to exercise democratic rights. The campaign for electoral reform which convulsed later Georgian Britain, and the political and religious factions which had previously split the élite, were more readily mediated through the capacity of the Hospital to bring together men of divergent views and hence symbolize unity. Irrespective of politics or religion, however, governors were bound together by a shared commitment to police the sick poor. The moral economy which underpinned this regulation underwent a transformation during the course of the long eighteenth century as, even at the Bath Infirmary with its Tory sympathies, the mutual obligations of paternalism were depleted by a *laissez-faire* model of charity which assumed that the labouring classes were essentially degenerate. It is the implementation of these values that we address in the next chapter, paying particular attention to the disciplining of patients and servants, and its implications for political stability.

Notes

1. Borsay, *English Urban Renaissance*, pp. 278, 318.
2. W. George Ford (ed.), *Some Notes for Visitors* (Bath: Abbey Church of St Peter and St Paul, November 1982), pp. 25, 57. See also Fawcett and Bird, *Bath*, p. 47.
3. Lawrence Stone, 'Introduction', in L. Stone (ed.), *An Imperial State at War: Britain from 1689 to 1815* (London: Routledge, 1994), pp. 1–2.
4. John Brewer, *The Sinews of Power: War, Money and the English State 1688–1783* (London: Unwin Hyman, 1989), pp. xiii–xviii; Stone, 'Introduction', pp. 1–9.
5. Joanna Innes, 'The Domestic Face of the Military-Fiscal State', in L. Stone (ed.), *An Imperial State at War: Britain from 1689 to 1815* (London: Routledge, 1994), pp. 97–108.
6. Andrew, *Philanthropy and Police*, pp. 98, 202; Davison et al. (eds), *Stilling the Grumbling Hive*, 'Introduction', pp. xv–xvi, xxix–xxx; Langford, *Polite and Commercial People*, pp. 485–6, 493–8; Langford, *Public Life*, p. 494–5.
7. Hitchcock, 'English Workhouse', pp. 114, 224–32, 257.
8. Bellers, 'Essay', pp. 181–3. It is significant that there was state medical care for soldiers and sailors; the military hospitals at Chelsea and Greenwich opened in the late seventeenth century, those at Gosport and Plymouth in the mid-eighteenth century. See Innes, 'Domestic Face', pp. 110–11; Rodger, *Wooden World*, p. 110.
9. The *Gentleman's Magazine*, for instance, published regular items on the hospital movement. See **1** (1731), p. 172; **11** (1741), 441, 474–7, 497; **20** (1750), pp. 184, 282, 426, 522; **40** (1770), pp. 94, 277, 341; **61** (1791), p. 175; **100** (1830), p. 556.
10. On 14 January 1751, for example, the *Bath Journal* appended the proposal for a hospital in Exeter to its announcement that a subscription was being opened to build an infirmary for the local sick poor.
11. Minute Book, 28 May 1746; 25 June 1746.
12. No upper limit was imposed upon the appointment of governors because this was the practice followed by general hospitals in the capital. See Letter Book, E. Brett to T. Carew, undated. On occasions consultation even preceded the simple purchase of domestic equipment. See Letter Folder, J. Hollinter to F. Fauquier, 13 November 1740. Minute Book, 21 January 1742; 29 July 1752.

13. Humble and Hansell, *Westminster Hospital*, p. 5; Wood, *Bath*, p. 275.
14. Owen, *English Philanthropy*, p. 57.
15. Boyce, *Benevolent Man*, pp. 41, 77, 186, 237, 263.
16. Newby, *William Hoare*, pp. 8, 33.
17. Thomas Fosbrooke, *An Original History of the City of Gloucester*, introduced by Peter Ripley, first pub. 1819 (Dursley: Alan Sutton, 1976), p. 219.
18. Porter, *Disease*, p. 35. See also Hunter, *Science and Society*, pp. 26–9; Porter, 'Gift Relation', p. 153; Speck, *Stability and Strife*, Part 2; Wilson, 'Urban culture', p. 177.
19. Cragg, *Church*, p. 61; Gascoigne, 'Anglican Latitudinarianism', pp. 23–4.
20. Gilbert, *Religion*, pp. 8–12; Langford, *Polite and Commercial People*, pp. 39, 41–4, 258–9.
21. Gascoigne, 'Anglican Latitudinarianism', pp. 33–8. See also Dickinson, *Liberty*, p. 202.
22. Andrew, 'On Reading Charity Sermons', pp. 588–91; Cragg, *Church*, pp. 172–3; Hempton, *Methodism*, pp. 56–7; Robert Hole, *Pulpits, Politics and Public Order in England 1760–1832* (Cambridge: Cambridge University Press, 1989), pp. 250–54; Innes, 'Politics and Morals', pp. 67–8; Vidler, *Church*, pp. 33–4.
23. Langford, *Polite and Commercial People*, pp. 73–4, 292–3. See also Hempton, *Methodism*, pp. 30–31.
24. Barry, 'Bourgeois Collectivism?', p. 109; Langford, *Polite and Commercial People*, p. 74.
25. William Birken, 'The Dissenting Tradition in English Medicine of the Seventeenth and Eighteenth Centuries', *Medical History*, **39** (1995), pp. 197–215.
26. McLoughlin, *Liverpool Infirmary*, p. 18. See also Lawrence, *Medicine*, pp. 20–21; Porter, 'Gift Relation', pp. 153–5.
27. 12 Geo. II, pp. 572–2. Kersley and Cosh, *Royal National Hospital*, p. 24.
28. [Bath General Infirmary], 'Short Account', in Dalton, *Religious Use*, p. 23.
29. Minute Book, 11 March 1742. See also Russell, *Exeter Hospitals*, p. 27.
30. Minute Book, 1 May 1770. *Annual Report*, 1780/81; 1785/86; 1790/91; 1795/96; 1800/01.
31. Minute Book, 2 May 1774; 1 May 1775; 9 May 1775; 18 May 1775; 1 May 1780; 1 May 1820. 11 Geo. IV, p. 18.
32. Smith, *Bristol Royal Infirmary*, pp. 35–9.
33. J. Anthony Williams (ed.), *Post-Reformation Catholicism in Bath*, 2 vols (no place of publication: Catholic Record Society, 1975), vol. 1, pp. 42–85.
34. Malcolm Brown and Judith Samuel, 'The Jews of Bath', *Bath History*, **1** (1986), p. 151.
35. Sedgwick, *The House of Commons*, vol. 2, pp. 144–5. *Annual Report*, 1741/42.
36. *Annual Report*, 1742/43; 1755/56; 1770/71; 1785/86; 1800/01; 1815/16; 1830/31. See also J. Anthony Williams, *Bath and Rome: The Living Link: Catholicism in Bath from 1559 to the Present Day* (Bath: Seabright's Bookshop, 1963), pp. 33–4.

37. Wood, *Bath*, p. 278; Boyce, *Benevolent Man*, p. 145.
38. Namier and Brooke, *House of Commons*, vol. 2, pp. 498–9.
39. Rolls, *Hospital of the Nation*, p. 159.
40. *Annual Report*, 1770/71; 1785/86. Hemingway and Haworth, *Coughton Court*, p. 5.
41. *DNB*, vol. 51, pp. 170–73.
42. *DNB*, vol. 39, pp. 181–2.
43. *DNB*, vol. 3, p. 294.
44. *DNB*, vol. 50, pp. 45–7.
45. *DNB*, vol. 32, pp. 227–8.
46. Cragg, *Church*, p. 124; Vidler, *Church*, 135.
47. *The Works of Benjamin Hoadly*, 3 vols (London: W. Bowyer and J. Nichols, 1773), vol. 2, p. 404.
48. The Bishop of Bath and Wells was present at no general courts during the quinquennial sample years; the Rector of Bath was present at one or more in just over half of these sample years, none of them after 1810/11 (Appendix G).
49. Hunter, *Ameliorated Condition*, pp. 12, 14–15.
50. For a more detailed discussion of early eighteenth-century politics, see Linda Colley, *In Defiance of Oligarchy: The Tory Party 1714–1760* (Cambridge: Cambridge University Press, 1982), especially chs 4 and 5; Dickinson, *Liberty*, Part 2; Geoffrey Holmes, *The Making of a Great Power: Late Stuart and Early Georgian Britain 1660–1722* (London: Longman, 1993), Part 2; Geoffrey Holmes and Daniel Szechi, *The Age of Oligarchy: Pre-Industrial Britain 1722–1783* (London: Longman, 1993), Part 1; Langford, *Polite and Commercial People*, chs 2 and 5.
51. For fuller accounts of later Georgian politics, see Dickinson, *Liberty*, Part 3; Dickinson, 'Radicals and Reformers', pp. 123–4; Holmes and Szechi, *Age of Oligarchy*, Part 3; Langford, *Polite and Commercial People*, chs 8 and 11; Frank O'Gorman, *The Emergence of the British Two-Party System 1760–1832* (London: Edward Arnold, 1982); D.G. Wright, *Popular Radicalism: The Working Class Experience 1780–1880* (London: Longman, 1988), chs 1–4.
52. Leonore Davidoff and Catherine Hall, *Family Fortunes: Men and Women of the English Middle Class 1780–1830* (Chicago: University of Chicago Press, 1987), p. 419; R.J. Morris, 'Voluntary Societies and British Urban Elites, 1780–1850: An Analysis', in P. Borsay (ed.), *The Eighteenth-Century Town: A Reader in English Urban History 1688–1820* (London: Longman, 1990), p. 356.
53. Adrian Wilson, 'Conflict, Consensus and Charity: Politics and the Provincial Voluntary Hospitals in the Eighteenth Century', *English Historical Review*, **111** (1996), pp. 609–14.
54. Sedgwick, *House of Commons*, vol. 1, pp. 514–15; Namier and Brooke, *House of Commons*, vol. 1, pp. 116–17.
55. Wilson, 'Conflict', pp. 606–7.
56. Sedgwick, *House of Commons*, vol. 1, p. 583.
57. Ian R. Christie, *British 'Non-Elite' MPs 1715–1820* (Oxford: Clarendon Press, 1995), p. 20.
58. Ibid., pp. 70, 81, 90.
59. Namier and Brooke, *House of Commons*, vol. 2, pp. 125–7.
60. Sedgwick, *House of Commons*, vol. 2, p. 529.

61. *DNB*, vol. 25, pp. 417–19; Sedgwick, *House of Commons*, vol. 2, pp. 127; Namier and Brooke, *House of Commons*, vol. 2, p. 605.
62. *DNB*, vol. 41, pp. 269–71; Sedgwick, *House of Commons*, vol. 2, pp. 302–3; Namier and Brooke, *House of Commons*, vol. 3, pp. 218–22.
63. Sedgwick, *House of Commons*, vol. 2, pp. 464–5.
64. Namier and Brooke, *House of Commons*, vol. 3, p. 179.
65. Ibid., pp. 277–8.
66. *DNB*, vol. 33, pp. 148–9. Among the other presidents who were appointed in retirement were Lieutenant-General Popham (1819) and Sir James Mansfield, a former solicitor-general and chief justice of the common pleas (1814). See *DNB*, vol. 36, pp. 91–2; Namier and Brooke, *House of Commons*, vol. 3, pp. 109–10, 308.
67. Namier and Brooke, *House of Commons*, vol. 2, pp. 225–8.
68. Ibid., p. 410.
69. Namier and Brooke, *House of Commons*, vol. 3, p. 134.
70. Namier and Brooke, *House of Commons*, vol. 2, pp. 69–70.
71. Holmes and Szechi, *Age of Oligarchy*, pp. 281–2.
72. Namier and Brooke, *House of Commons*, vol. 3, pp. 138–9.
73. Ibid., pp. 353–4.
74. Ibid., pp. 14–15.
75. McIntyre, 'Towns', p. 80. See also Fawcett and Bird, *Bath*, p. 47; Hembry, *English Spa*, pp. 113–14, 133.
76. Sedgwick, *House of Commons*, vol. 1, pp. 528–9.
77. Sedgwick, *House of Commons,* vol. 2, p. 150.
78. Ibid., pp. 562–4.
79. *DNB*, vol. 56, pp. 226–7; Sedgwick, *House of Commons*, vol. 2, pp. 467–8.
80. Peach, *Ralph Allen*, p. 155; *DNB*, vol. 58, pp. 413–16; Sedgwick, *House of Commons,* vol. 2, pp. 501–2.
81. Peach, *Bath*, p. 248; Peach, *Ralph Allen*, pp. xii, 154–7.
82. Sedgwick, *House of Commons*, vol. 2, p. 501.
83. Ibid., p. 371.
84. Ibid., pp. 459–60.
85. Langford, *Polite and Commercial People*, p. 207; *DNB*, vol. 54, pp. 25–37.
86. Langford, *Polite and Commercial People*, pp. 27, 232.
87. *DNB*, vol. 45, pp. 354–67; Namier and Brooke, *House of Commons*, vol. 3, pp. 290–99; John Cannon, 'Bath Politics in the Eighteenth Century', *Somerset Archaeological and Natural History Society Proceedings*, **105** (1960–61), p. 93.
88. Namier and Brooke, *House of Commons*, vol. 3, pp. 322–4. See also *DNB*, XLVI, pp. 285–8.
89. *DNB*, vol. 39, pp. 409–15; *DNB*, vol. 46, pp. 285–8.
90. Cannon, 'Bath Politics', pp. 100–102. See also *DNB*, vol. 46, pp. 290–92; Namier and Brooke, *House of Commons*, vol. 3, pp. 179, 324, 419.
91. Peach, *Bath*, p. 176; Williams and Stoddart, *Bath*, p. 68.
92. Namier and Brooke, *House of Commons*, vol. 3, pp. 52–3, 563–4.
93. J.F. Meehan, *More Famous Houses of Bath and District* (Bath: B. and J.F. Meehan, 1906), pp. 110–11.
94. *DNB*, vol. 29, pp. 311–15.

95. *DNB*, vol. 4, pp. 420–21.
96. *DNB*, vol. 45, pp. 127–31.
97. *DNB*, vol. 58, pp. 140–44.
98. Hilton, *Age of Atonement*, p. 227.
99. *Gentleman's Magazine*, 11 (1741), p. 497. See also Brockbank, *Royal Infirmary, Manchester*, p. 6; Croxson, 'Economic Analysis', pp. 77–83; Croxson, 'Public and Private Faces', pp. 142–9; Frizelle and Martin, *Leicester Royal Infirmary*, pp. 27–8; Porter, 'Gift Relation', pp. 154–5; Wilson, 'Conflict', pp. 603–5.
100. Sedgwick, *House of Commons*, vol. 2, pp. 459–60.
101. *DNB*, vol. 54, pp. 30–31.
102. *DNB*, vol. 2, pp. 74–5.
103. Sedgwick, *House of Commons*, vol. 2, p. 415.
104. Sedgwick, *House of Commons*, vol. 1, pp. 313–14; Sedgwick, *House of Commons*, vol. 2, pp. 127, 501; Namier and Brooke, *House of Commons*, vol. 1, p. 366; McIntyre, 'Towns', pp. 85–8.
105. Peach, *Bath*, p. 248. See also Kingsley, *Country Houses*, pp. 100–101; McLynn, *Crime*, p. 144.
106. Newby, *William Hoare*, p. 7.
107. Frizelle and Martin, *Leicester Royal Infirmary*, pp. 23–4. See also Bevan, *Salop Infirmary*, p. 12.
108. William Pitt the Elder to the Corporation, 12 April 1761, Chatham MSS, quoted in Cannon, 'Bath Politics', p. 87. See also Christie, *British 'Non-Elite' MPs*, p. 197.
109. See, for example, Cannon, *Aristocratic Century*, ch. 4; John Cannon, *Samuel Johnson and the Politics of Hanoverian England* (Oxford: Clarendon Press, 1994), pp. 269–87; H.T. Dickinson, *The Politics of the People in Eighteenth-Century Britain* (London: Macmillan, 1995), chs 1–3; Frank O'Gorman, *Voters, Patrons and Parties: The Unreformed Electoral System of Hanoverian England 1734–1832* (Oxford: Clarendon Press, 1989), pp. 227, 234, 384–7; Rogers, 'Middling Sort'.
110. Wilson, 'Conflict', pp. 2–3. See also Porter, 'Gift Relation', p. 155; Hume, *Newcastle Infirmary*, p. 5; Leader, *Sheffield General Infirmary*, pp. 6–7; Rook, Carlton and Cannon, *Addenbrooke's Hospital*, p. 80; Steer, *West Sussex Hospital*, p. 19.
111. Woodward, *To Do the Sick No Harm*, p. 147.
112. Leyborne, *Charity Conducive*, p. 16.
113. See, for example, Bevan, *Salop Infirmary*, pp. 7–8; Copeman, *Norfolk and Norwich Hospital*, p. 1; Hume, *Newcastle Infirmary*, p. 7; Jacob, *General Hospital*, p. 12.
114. Bath Corporation Minute Book, 12 March 1739. Letter Book, R. Nash to E. Brett, undated. See also McIntyre, 'Bath', p. 238; McIntyre, 'Towns', p. 99.
115. 12 Geo. II, pp. 575–8. Minute Book, 16 February 1738, 'Plan and Elevation'.
116. Minute Book, 4 March 1742.
117. Minute Book, 22 July 1742.
118. See, for example, *Bath Journal*, 22 May 1745; 15 July 1745.
119. *Bath Journal*, 18 May 1747.
120. See, for example, *Bath Journal*, 13 March 1749; 3 April 1749.
121. Baly, 'Care of the Sick Poor', p. 2.

122. Andrew, *Philanthropy and Police*, p 174; Turner, *Charity*, pp. 1–2.
123. Bath United Hospital Minute Book, 23 February 1829; 5 July 1830.
124. This was an objective of the 1723 proposal. See Wood, *Bath*, pp. 279, 282.
125. See, for example, *Gentleman's Magazine*, 17 (June 1747,) p. 270.
126. See, for example, *Bath Journal*, 8 June 1747; 3 November 1755; 19 March 1770; 30 January 1786.
127. Only 40 of the 1 619 entries in the Casebook for 1750 to 1758 were identified as soldiers. See Table 10.4.
128. Minute Book, 1 May 1746; *Annual Report*, 1747/48, 1780/81.
129. Minute Book, 19 May 1756.
130. Minute Book, 13 November 1799; 15 September 1802.
131. Letter Folder, W. Jane to the Register, no date; Register to W. Jane, 10 March 1785.
132. Minute Book, 21 October 1807.
133. Minute Book, 15 June 1750. Rules.
134. Bath Abbey Overseers Accounts, 1729–41, 1741–50, 1750–58, 1770–74, 1783–86, 1815–36. No Accounts covering 1800/01 survive.
135. *Keene's Bath Directory*, (Bath: John and James Keene, 1829), pp. 57–8.
136. *Robbins' Bath Directory*, (Bath: G. Robbins, 1800), p. 134.
137. Neale, *Bath*, pp. 255–7.
138. Fawcett and Bird, *Bath*, pp. 48–9, 61–2; Hembry, *British Spas*, p. 66.
139. McIntyre, 'Bath', p. 224.
140. 12 Geo. II, p. 573.
141. Bath Corporation Minute Book, 1740–1830. 12 Geo. II, pp. 572–3. *Annual Report* and Minute Book, 1755/56; 1770/71; 1785/86; 1800/01; 1815/16; 1830/31. At Bristol and Northampton during the 1790s, a majority of councillors also supported the local infirmary. See Berry, 'Patronage', p. 49.
142. Bath Corporation Minute Book, 15 May 1741.
143. Cannon, 'Bath Politics', p. 103.
144. Ibid., p. 105.
145. *Report of a Committee ... to Examine a Statement Circulated by Mr. Parish*, pp. 3, 14.
146. Minute Book, 9 February 1739; 6 July 1743; 20 July 1743; 26 May 1773; 18 November 1779; 27 January 1779. Bath Corporation Minute Book, 15 January 1779.
147. *Bath City Infirmary*, pp. 1–2.
148. See, for example,Warner, *Bath*, p. 304.
149. Bath Corporation Minute Book, 12 February 1811; 23 July 1816; 24 January 1820; 7 February 1823. Local poor law authorities, whose paupers were excluded from the General Hospital, paid annual subscriptions to the Casualty Hospital, the Bath City Dispensary, and the Bath Penitentiary and Lock Hospital. See Bath Abbey Vestry Minutes, 2 May 1819.
150. Wilson, 'Urban Culture', pp. 167, 170, 172–6.
151. Bath United Hospital Minute Book, 19 June 1828; 23 June 1828; 30 June 1828; 7 July 1828; 8 July 1828. Loudon, *Medical Care*, pp. 147–51.
152. 12 Geo. II, p. 582.
153. Minute Book, 20 October 1739; 1 May 1740; 1 May 1741; 1 May 1742.

154. See Minute Book, 24 December 1741; 31 October 1770; 15 April 1772; 14 April 1773; 13 April 1774; 15 November 1777; 24 June 1778; 22 June 1785; 1 February 1815; 15 November 1826.
155. See Minute Book, 2 May 1743; 2 May 1757; 23 February 1763; 19 May 1784; 7 October 1829.
156. See Minute Book, 13 October 1779; 25 May 1796; 6 March 1805; 12 February 1812; 15 February 1826.
157. Minute Book, 25 February 1829 to 28 April 1831. Bath Corporation Minute Book, 27 September 1830.
158. See also Wilson, 'Urban Culture', p. 177.

CHAPTER TEN

The Education of the Lower Orders

In Chapter 9, we considered the extent to which the Georgian Bath Infirmary fostered the development of an integrated political élite. Within the city itself, the Hospital preserved a residual animosity between the visiting Company and the local community, and retained an oligarchic constitution which failed to satisfy the democratic aspirations of the many middling men who were disenfranchised. Its contribution to closing the fault lines which had divided British society since the Civil War was equally limited because although presidents and governors were recruited from conflicting factions and parties, their rare attendance at meetings of the general court and weekly committee made the eirenic effect minimal. At the symbolic level, however, the Infirmary demonstrated the willingness of an expanding élite to sink their religious and political differences by coming together in a scheme to control the poor. In this chapter, we explore how the evolving moral economy which underpinned such unity was applied to those inhabiting the Bath Hospital. First, medicine will be placed within the context of Enlightenment materialism. Discussion will then move to the operation of these ideas in the architecture and design of the institution, and in the relations of confinement as they affected both the servant and the patient communities. The chapter will conclude with an examination of the actual and the figurative transaction of power in medical care.

Medicine, materialism and the Enlightenment

During the early modern period, neighbourhood segregation and a differentiation of cultural activities increasingly weakened the informal, personal contacts between rich and poor which had previously been used to implant authority.[1] The repertoire of formal techniques which were developed to replace these traditional methods included an institutionalized approach to poverty which dated back to the Elizabethan house of correction.[2] Though Foucault much exaggerated the 'great confinement' of marginal social groups which occurred in the later seventeenth century,[3] an interest in institutional provision fitted with the materialism of the English Enlightenment. Akihito Suzuki has taken historians to task for projecting 'the late Enlightenment marriage of Lockean philosophy and medicine on to the early Enlightenment'.[4] It is important to note the tightening interpretation of materialism, which reached its apotheosis in Bentham's famous Panopticon or penitentiary; for by the end of the eighteenth century utilitarian reformers, committed to the socializing potential of the pleasure principle, were insisting that since mind and body were one, routine and repetition imposed by 'the external force of authority would first become a habit and then gradually be transformed into a moral preference'.[5] But as Suzuki himself admits, early Georgian doctors 'championed belief in the malleability of the mind as confidently as the later materialist thinkers ... [and] preached that the moral and intellectual powers of man could be enhanced by the art of medicine, through taking care of the body, rather than through religious and spiritual means'.[6] Therefore, the spectacular proposals of the utilitarian era should not be allowed to overshadow the less advanced associationism of the early Enlightenment which offered an intellectual rationale for moral education throughout the Georgian period.

The voluntary infirmary played a central part in the application of medical materialism. Private patients suffering from the diseases of overconsumption were free to ignore homilies about moderation and seek advice elsewhere in the medical market-place.[7] In the hospital, however, doctors had a laboratory in which to practice the moral improvement of the poor, relieving their physical ailments whilst simultaneously restoring virtue and religion.[8] The early promoters of the voluntary infirmary recognized this regulatory function. In 1737, for example, the first annual report of the Winchester Hospital stressed that:

> great numbers of the poor will be insensibly reclaimed by the exact regularity of manners, which is maintained in an hospital as well as by the frequency of such reflections as are naturally suggested in the house of mourning ... For we can never hope to secure their affections, soften their passions, reform their manners, and possess them with a sense of their duty to God and their superiors so effectually as by this feeling way to instruction.

In short, sickness dismantled resistance to moral change.[9] Charity sermons, such as that delivered by Reverend Josiah Tucker on behalf of the Bristol Infirmary in the mid-1740s, reiterated the theme, describing hospitals 'as Schools of Christian Education for the adult Poor; and as a Means conducive towards a National Reformation in the common People'.[10] The trustees of the Bath Hospital went further in tackling the problem of order in early modern society and aimed to inculcate in patients practices which upon discharge might be learnt by the labouring classes at large. In the words of the original 'Plan and Elevation': 'it is to be hoped, that the success which may reasonably be expected from the regularity of these poor creatures, may induce others of better condition voluntarily to imitate them in the management of themselves, that they may receive the like benefits'.[11] But how did the General Infirmary set about educating its inmates in the ways of healthy, sober and godly living? And to what extent did it achieve its disciplinary goals?

The architecture of order

The moral reform of the poor at Bath exploited both the physical environment in which patients and servants were housed and the social relations in which they engaged. Constructed in the style of a classical mansion with five windows on each side of the door and a central pediment resting on four Ionic columns, the building exemplified the architectural austerity of many Georgian voluntary hospitals.[12] This simplicity may have expressed the frugality of the trustees, anxious not to waste their precious funds on inappropriate adornment. However, Palladianism had made pretention unfashionable by deprecating the heavy decoration of the Baroque and so plainness also embodied a social prestige into which supporters could tap.[13] Of greatest relevance to the education of the lower orders was the political significance of reproducing a classical country house in the town. First, the Infirmary itself recreated an image of the traditional authority of the rural élite which 'radiated outwards' over the surrounding landscape.[14] Indeed, its frontage echoed the almost palatial north side of Queen Square in Bath, completed by John Wood just before the hospital project: an elegant terrace of houses hiding behind a unified classical façade with a huge pediment. A second derivative from the architectural form of the Infirmary was an association with order. Whereas the irregularity of the previous 'Gothic' style was berated for its barbarity and chaos, classicalism was venerated for its proportion and symmetry; and since the purpose of these principles was to unite the separate parts of the structure into a coherent whole, the classical style became a potent symbol for social harmony.[15] In his study of how prisons fabricated virtue, Robin Evans has argued that until the late 1700s architecture performed no more than this emblematic function, representing the good society in a visible way but unacknowledged as a causal agent with the power to bring about moral reform. If less ruthlessly systematic than Bentham's later model institutions, however, these buildings did 'map the location of staff and inmates, guide their movements and mediate transactions between them'.[16] Therefore, we must understand the physical structure of the Bath Infirmary not just as a metaphor for authority but also as a tool for engineering personal and social change.

The thesis that architecture failed to move beyond mere representation until the final decades of the eighteenth century starts from a false dichotomy between symbol and action. In practice, it is unlikely that patients and servants who climbed the steps of the General Hospital were not intimidated by its imposing façade, reminiscent of the country houses occupied by the aristocracy and gentry. Governors too were affected by the symbolic paternalism, the urban middling sort winning increased authority from their stake in an institution which sought to replicate a power base of the landed classes. But if the reforming impulses of the Bath Infirmary began with its political imagery, they were continued through the organization of space. The Hospital consisted of three floors: a ground storey or basement 'appropriated for offices and lodging rooms for some of the servants'; a chamber or upper storey split into five wards; and a 'principal' or middle storey which was the medical and administrative nerve centre as well as the location of two wards.[17] The dispatch of servants to the bottom floor, partially below ground, signified their subordinate position within the institutional hierarchy. Moreover, by preserving the Palladian convention of a high middle storey – which in other voluntary infirmaries was often abandoned for floors of equal height – the Bath Hospital articulated the importance attached to the medical and managerial tasks carried out on this level and to the doctors, governors and paid staff who implemented them.[18] The floor plan reiterated these gradations of authority. We can piece together the layout of the principal storey by comparing the surviving 'Plan and Elevation' (Figure 10.1), printed 'for the sake of ornament, and to gain a point in the purchase of the land', with John Wood's description of the finished building, incorporating the changes which he made with the trustees' approval. In addition to reducing the number of wards from five to two, the later design shifted the matron's parlour and bedchamber from a situation overlooking the courtyard to the right-hand side of the entrance on the north front. The surgery displaced by this move was shunted into the spot previously occupied by the governors' board room, which was resituated to the south on the west front. Therefore, the Hospital opened with the apartments of the apothecary and the matron on either side of the vestibule, adjacent respectively to the rooms for the physicians and the surgeons.[19]

The availability of the senior paid officers relative to the honorary medical staff and the governors conformed to the classical canon of mansion design which positioned closest to the main entrance the hall and the saloon, least discriminatory in terms of admission. But whereas the exclusive residence was often structured around a series of interconnected rooms which controlled access to the more privileged spaces, circulation within the hospital was primarily via corridors which in the

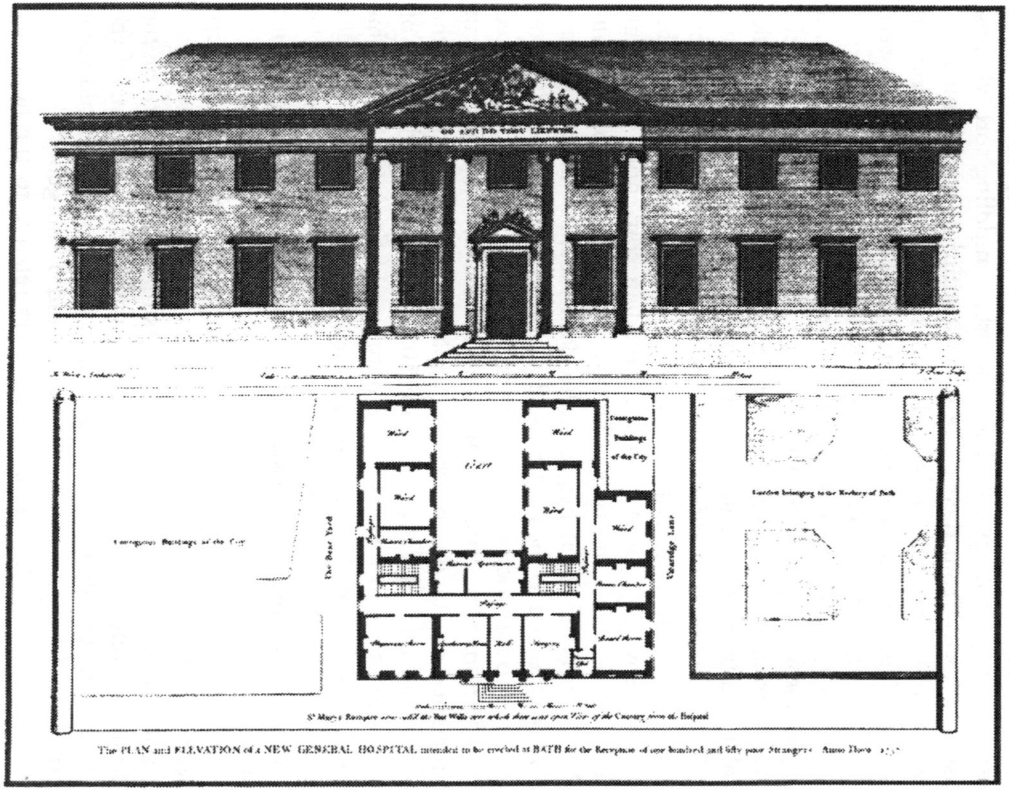

10.1 Bath General Hospital: plan and elevation, 1738. [The date on the illustration refers to the Julian calendar.]

country house were secondary routes for unseen use by servants. These passages had two effects. First, they defined firm boundaries around the different status groups that operated within the institution, sealing separate identities for patients and employees, physicians, surgeons and the governing body, which were not easily breached by informal negotiation. Secondly, having erected a spatial hierarchy, the corridor became the means by which interaction occurred between the discrete sectors, enabling the efficient movement through the building which was essential to the supervision of both inmates and paid staff.[20] It is unfortunate that no details survive of how the wards were arranged at the Bath Infirmary. However, the passages which run across the central block and down the two wings testify to the dominance of the arterial communication system. The apothecary and matron by the door were its gatekeepers, watching the traffic in patients and servants, goods and services. Surveillance extended to the courtyard at the centre of the Hospital which, being enclosed on three sides, ensured that the institutional eye pervaded even taking the air. During the course of the long eighteenth century, the General Infirmary underwent two major construction programmes: in the 1790s when the attic storey was added to accommodate more patients; and in the 1820s when major refurbishment of the interior raised ceilings and improved ventilation. Quite how these alterations affected the internal configuration of space is unclear, but the now top-heavy patrician, classical exterior continued to pronounce the authority of those who ruled the institution and the subordination of those in their charge.

The relations of confinement

Complementing the influence of the physical environment were the socio-political relations of hospital confinement. In his classic sociological study of *Asylums*, published in 1961, Erving Goffman argued that in the 'total institution' reward and punishment, together with 'processes of mortification' or humiliation, were used to teach the inmate the 'house rules' and to induce 'radical shifts in his *moral career*'.[21] The 'central feature' of the total institutions outlined by Goffman was the way in which they broke down the barriers normally separating work, sleep and play. As he explained:

> First, all aspects of life are conducted in the same place and under the same single authority. Second, each phase of the member's daily activity is carried on in the immediate company of a large batch of others, all of whom are treated alike and required to do the same thing together. Third, all phases of the day's activities are tightly

> scheduled, with one activity leading at a prearranged time into the next ... Finally, the various enforced activities are brought together into a single rational plan purportedly designed to fulfil the official aims of the institution.

Two consequences flowed from this 'rationalisation of everyday living'. Total institutions were closed in the sense that their inmates had 'restricted contact with the world outside the walls'; and the use of a 'bureaucratic organization' to meet the needs of 'whole blocks of people' produced a rigid staff–inmate split, with each group conceiving 'of the other in terms of narrow hostile stereotypes'.[22] Applying Goffman's ideas to a Georgian context has difficulties because relatively little is known 'about the patterns of life within the hospital, beyond what the rule books stipulate'.[23] However, we can use his concept of the total institution to launch a tentative exploration of how power was transacted at the Bath Hospital.

The governors' 'rational plan' was evident in the rules of the Infirmary, framed to confront the vices which, according to materialist thinking, underpinned both physical disease and moral turpitude. In the early set of regulations, published in John Wood's *Description of Bath*, both patients and the poor employed to supply nursing and housekeeping services were banned from consuming liquors and provisions illicitly smuggled into the Hospital. Swearing, abusive language and indecent behaviour, smoking and playing at cards and dice were also forbidden; and going out without permission, or staying away overnight, was proscribed. Further restrictions applied to patients. Clinical directives were to be obeyed. Strict sexual partitioning was also adopted, with men and women lodged in segregated wards to prevent improper liaison. And loitering in the city and entering alehouses when legitimately absent were outlawed.[24] The extant Rules from the later eighteenth century confirmed these initial regulations, but additionally embraced orders previously passed by the governors to improve behaviour at the baths: male and female patients were to visit on separate days; consuming alcohol or offering it to the bath guides was prohibited; and the head nurse was instructed 'to see decency and good order observed' when the women bathed.[25] After the briefs of paid officers were redrawn in 1774, the apothecary was required 'To attend the men patients to the bath', while the matron's responsibilities now included occasionally visiting the bath 'to see that a proper decorum is preserved' amongst the women patients.[26]

The apothecary and the matron were at the centre of the Hospital's disciplinary system; they were the 'Master and Mistress' of an paternalist, institutional household or family in which, unusually, the common subordination of servants and inmates was particularly underlined by their shared rules.[27] In the initial regulations, it was the matron who oversaw the behaviour of patients and servants; both groups were instructed to be 'submissive and obedient' to her, and the porter at the door was under orders to prevent any patient from leaving unless he was satisfied that she had given permission. Following the expansion of job descriptions in the 1770s, the matron was charged with lodging 'complaints with the house visitor, or committee, against any of the servants or patients who misbehave themselves'. However, the apothecary acquired her former duty 'to regulate the patients in their going out, and coming in'; and he was also mandated 'to see that proper order is kept up by the nurses, chairmen, and patients'.[28] The rules designed to implement the Hospital's reforming mission were systematically transmitted. Soon after the opening in 1742, tables of orders was hung in all the wards.[29] Notices were also displayed when new restrictions were imposed;[30] and in 1828 a subcommittee recommended that 'each patient on admission, and every other person concerned, should be furnished with a separate printed copy of ... [the] rules and instructions'.[31] But the voice of authority was imparted most forcefully in the ritual reading of the regulations required each week:[32] a symbolic performance which underlined the politics of control within the institution.

The secular constraints put in place to reform the moral fibre of patients and servants were reinforced by the cultivation of a religious ethic. Though 'improving' literature was donated by individual benefactors[33] and by organizations like the Auxiliary Bible Society and the SPCK,[34] prayer books and bibles were also purchased by the governors[35] and in 1819 they agreed to join a parochial library.[36] The imposition of religious observances was more significant. There was no dedicated chapel until the new block opened in 1861,[37] but on the Sabbath patients sufficiently mobile were 'allowed to go to their respective places of worship' and from 1750 the steward was also expected to say prayers in the wards.[38] Hardening attitudes to the poor enabled religion to tighten its grip within the more coercive, scientific approach to philanthropy. As early as 1760, a correspondent in the *Gentleman's Magazine* advocated replacing rotating clergymen with one chaplain so that 'public infirmaries ... might ... extend their salutary influence ... to the minds and morals of the patients'; would not 'a well chosen minister', it was asked, 'form a better judgement of the temper and disposition, weaknesses and wants of each patient, and the representations, admonitions, or comforts, suitable to their respective circumstances?'[39] In the mid-1770s, the apothecary to the Bath Hospital acquired the duty of reading 'prayers in the wards three times at least in every week when the officiating clergyman cannot conveniently attend'. Almost contemporaneously, however, a single chaplain was appointed.[40] Details of his duties have not survived, but in 1830 the weekly committee resolved that 'the rules and regulations relative to the conduct of the patients be read by the chaplain on the first Sunday of every month after divine service'.[41] Policing the poor received a religious seal of approval.

The servant community

Since supervision by the governors was largely confined to the intermittent calls of house visitors, the implementation of their rational plan was heavily dependent upon paid employees. Although servants were 'obliged to discover ... to the matron, on pain of expulsion' any violation of the Hospital rules,[42] their embodiment within the same regulatory code as patients suggests that there was no rigid staff–inmate split characteristic of the total institution. This impression is reinforced by the absence of a firm division of labour; for the Bath Infirmary – like other voluntary hospitals[43] – expected patients who were able to co-operate with servants in nursing, washing and ironing the linen, cleaning the wards and undertaking any other jobs required by the matron.[44] Such commonality arose from the paternalist ethos which the Infirmary applied to the recipients of its charity and extended to its staff. Rates of pay are difficult to compare with modern time series,[45] not just due to local and occupational variations but also because posts attracted a combination of 'board, washing and lodging' as well as a wage.[46] However, the governors' paternalism was clearly displayed in their benevolent attitude to employees. Workmen were absorbed into the festivities when the foundation-stone was laid in July 1738, their contribution acknowledged with the gift of a 'handsome present'.[47] Diligent staff were also rewarded with internal promotion;[48] wages were augmented for good conduct;[49] and gratuities were bestowed in return for exceptional loyalty and service.[50] Therefore, the 'meritorious' performance of the Hospital apothecary, Mr William Farnell, won him a salary increase and no fewer than three gratuities during a career which spanned over four decades.[51] The dedication which these sums honoured led the governors to install an assistant when Mr Farnell became too incapacitated to fulfil all his duties.[52] In so doing they continued a long-standing concern for the health and welfare of employees. As early as 1738, when a labourer was injured building the Hospital, the contractor was authorized 'to pay ... [him] during the course of his lameness one half of his weekly pay'.[53] Similar paternalist gestures followed. By defraying the brewer's 'expenses in the smallpox'[54] or by admitting to the wards three servants 'affected with the itch' through washing linen,[55] the governors were responding to conditions acquired during the course of employment. But when the brewer and baker was granted 'three months' leave of absence owing to his ill state of health',[56] or the steward was permitted 'to go into the country on his own affairs for a fortnight',[57] there was no obligation to compensate; indeed, George Whittaker, 'having given notice to quit', was even permitted to vacate his job for a month 'on account of the illness of an aged mother', if he found a substitute acceptable to the Hospital officers.[58] The commitment to staff well-being also applied to those no longer fit for employment. Nurse Tympany became a patient after being discharged from her post,[59] and valued employees 'incompetent from age' or 'bodily infirmity' were awarded gratuities to assist them in retirement, wages being converted into permanent pensions where assiduity was combined with long service.[60]

But did the workforce, protected by this web of paternalism, reciprocate with 'submission ... and civility and respect'?[61] The window into daily life opened by the House Visitors Books which remain for 1742 and 1743, and from 1754 to 1759 give little credence to the disorderly view of the Georgian infirmary, for during the seven years that these records cover only 15 incidents of a disciplinary nature were noted. Dismissal for misconduct, identifiable from the Minute Books, conveys the same impression (Appendix K). Apart from the steward and matron sacked for corruption in 1773, and the departure of a second matron five years later, it seems that senior paid officers performed their duties to the satisfaction of the governors. Among the domestic and technical staff, three cooks, three bakers and brewers, two maids and two laboratory staff were discharged. The nurses and chairmen committed more misdemeanours, their offences – where specified – involving dishonesty, alcohol and provisions, insolence and insubordination, and illicit absence. Nurses were dismissed for 'taking the money of the patients' and for misappropriating Hospital property. Nurse Hester Waters, accused of 'obstructing the charity of this House in advising a person not to put his benefaction into the Box but to give it to the porters',[62] was sacked two months later 'for being disguised in liqueur'. Nurse Hitchcock lost her job 'for permitting spiritous liqueurs to be drunk on her wards', whilst 'staying out beyond the time allowed' proved to be the downfall of Nurse White. Absconding was also a transgression of the chairmen. Not only did Samuel Rogers and John Stagg elope, but John Rudman, discharged 'for his misbehaviour in the House', had previously been reported to the house visitors for taking five hours to fetch oatmeal from Bathwick (on the perimeter of the city) and for 'going out without leave and not returning the same day'.[63] Overall, however, only 19 nurses and 17 chairmen were minuted as being dismissed for misconduct between 1742 and 1830. Consequently, their misdeeds were relatively isolated; they did not spell a breakdown of order amongst the employees closest to supervising patients.[64]

Although staff indiscipline was never endemic at the Bath Infirmary, the 'social anatagonisms' of the eighteenth century led to a perceived deterioration in master–servant relations[65] and may explain the accelerating rate of recorded dismissals apparent post-1800 (Appendix K). It also predisposed the later Georgian governors to address the calibre of those whom they employed at the Hospital. After 1775, chairmen, nurses and servants were forbidden to nominate deputies until the matron had received 'the approbation of the house visitors' and the decision had been ratified by the weekly committee.[66] In addition, a number of posts were filled 'on trial' from the turn of the century.[67] And in 1828 the general principle of annual gratuities for 'good conduct and attention to ... duty' was approved and subsequently implemented on the grounds that cash incentives 'would more certainly attain the desired effect than a fixed higher rate of payment'.[68] In the case of nurses, however, an exception was immediately made and their wages were raised from £8 to £10 per annum, and then to £12 combined with increments of £1 for satisfactory behaviour until their incomes reached £15 per annum.[69] The main motivation for this increase in basic salary was the need to recruit 'younger and more active nurses ... in the place of many of those, who from age, or bodily infirmities, are now incapable of well performing their necessary duties'. Within the next 12 months, no fewer than five nurses were discharged on these grounds and a sixth tendered her own resignation.[70] Furthermore, a rule was passed specifying that 'in the future the ages of the nurses to be appointed shall not be under 30 nor exceeding 40'.[71]

Yet despite this emphasis on physical efficiency, the reform of the nursing regime at the later Georgian Bath Infirmary was also laced with medical and moral concerns. The regulation that nurses 'behave with tenderness to the patients'[72] evinced the 'aspiration to create a caring environment',[73] but throughout the long eighteenth century responsibilities were focused on cleaning the wards and serving meals rather than ministering to more personal bodily or clinical needs.[74] In 1829, however, the ability 'to read writing' was made a formal precondition for employment as a nurse.[75] Although enforcement may have proved difficult, this criterion did show early recognition that as medicine adopted a more scientific methodology, doctors required an ancillary staff with sufficient education to follow more complex clinical instructions and to report significant changes in the patient's condition.[76] Imposing a reading test was thus the first step on the road to the professionalization of nursing. Nevertheless, the occupational competence of nurses was rarely challenged at the Georgian Bath Infirmary, most complaints revolving around moral behaviour and not the ill-usage of patients or the neglect of housekeeping tasks.[77] Therefore, given the contemporary perception of literacy as a sign of respectability, we can also see the requirement that nurses be able to read as an attempt to apply the moral values of the Evangelical Revival.[78] The exclusion of married women whose husbands resided in Bath[79] can also be construed in an Evangelical light, assuming that a residential post was regarded as incompatible with the sexual (and domestic) dues of marriage. But the moral agenda was most overt in the recommendation – linked to the payment of increments to staff in the late 1820s – that when patients appeared before the weekly committee prior to their discharge, they should be asked whether any of the servants had indulged in 'the frequent and secret custom of ... receiving bribes and gratuities'.[80]

The campaign to reform the servant body at Bath, which had preoccupied some hospitals since the 1780s and became widespread from the 1830s,[81] altered the relationship between governors, paid officers, servants and patients. In 1829, the matron lost a discretion that she had previously enjoyed when the weekly committee took on responsibility for the selection of nurses[82] and later made the appointment 'subject to ... proper testimonials of ... character'.[83] A greater degree of formality was also introduced to the disciplinary procedure. Complaints from the house visitors were followed up by the weekly committee from the early days of the Hospital.[84] In 1802, however, two chairmen called Daniel Martin and John Baker were summoned 'to answer a complaint preferred against them by Samuel Howse Esquire', one of the governors and possibly a house visitor, who was also asked to be present 'to substantiate his charge'.[85] The Minute Book records nothing of this encounter, but in 1828 a chairman by the name of Daniel Martin was again before the committee 'for very improper conduct in neglecting his duty' and on this occasion a dismissal notice was issued. The quasi-judicial approach was most developed in the case of Nurse Edwards who was discharged in 1830, along with a patient called David Meddings – he for bringing in provisions without the agreement of the physicians and surgeons, and she for permitting him to do so.[86] An appeal was lodged against the decision in which the nurse claimed that 'she was actually ignorant of the patient having infringed the rules of the Hospital'. It was successful. The weekly committee agreed to reinstate Edwards, having admonished her 'to be particular circumspect in her future conduct'.[87]

The procedural formalities which involved the governors more closely in the appointment and discipline of staff not only reduced the autonomy of the apothecary and the matron; they may have also undermined cohesion within the servant body. Evidence is thin on the ground. None the less, a capacity for collective action was demonstrated in 1778 when, after James Hawkins was given notice to quit as a chairman, five of his colleagues resigned in protest; 'having made a proper submission', they were reinstated the following week. Fifty years later, conversely, Nurse Morris was sacked for using 'improper language' because of 'a complaint having been made by Nurse Gregory'.[88] But if relations between servants were fragmenting, what was happening to their interface with patients? The common rules implied a degree of solidarity, and on occasions delinquent members of the two communities were partners in crime. In 1754, for example, a complaint was registered against a chairman for being 'absent from the Hospital and keeping James Phillips, a patient, with him till late at night'.[89] From the foundation, however, the duties of staff created potential for the kind of conflict which flared up in July 1747 when the porter clashed with the 'men in the King's Ward ... [who] insisted upon going out and were with difficulty restrained'.[90] Efforts to improve the quality of servants may have widened their gap from patients. However, steps were also deliberately taken to restrict interaction when in 1830 the honorary physicians and surgeons recommended a full-time assistant for the apothecary. Previously, male patients had been employed in the dispensary and the laboratory, but this was 'a practice which present attention to order and regularity throughout the establishment forbids'.[91] Such mixing was no longer judged conducive to a disciplined environment.

The patient community

The increasing social distance between patients and employees hints at the gradual emergence of a staff–inmate split typical of Goffman's total institution. For most of the long eighteenth century, however, there was no strict demarcation in place and so we must ask by what other means the governors attempted to enforce their moral agenda. Despite subjecting patients to the control of a single authority dedicated to the rehabilitation of both mind and body, the Bath Infirmary afforded their integrity a measure of protection as a result of its paternalist ethos. No doubt the lower orders arriving at the Hospital for the first time were disconcerted by their unfamiliar surroundings, but they were not exposed to the 'processes of mortification' which the total institution employed to dismantle the 'presenting culture' of its inmates. Therefore, although compelled to wear a medallion when temporarily vacating the premises,[92] patients' personal identity was not supressed by the issue of a uniform and their clothes were expected to be in a satisfactory state of repair. That the governors deplored the ragged condition in which inmates arrived at the Infirmary[93] suggests a belief in minimum standards. This was carried through to cleanliness and diet. Given the attention paid to hygiene and the practice of summoning patients only when a bed was free, it is unlikely that the premises were excessively dirty or overcrowded. Diet too was monitored, responsibility resting with the honorary physicians and surgeons. Patients required their permission before breaching the institutional regime by drinking tea or taking meals outside the Hospital, but food intake was also specified[94] and when, due to grain shortages during the Napoleonic Wars, the daily ration of bread was fixed at 14 ounces 'with a small addition of potatoes', the medical staff signed an undertaking that this was 'a sufficient quantity' for each patient.[95] In 1827, the quota of bread was still 14 ounces a day. In addition, there was a daily allowance of a pint and a half of beer, together with 'ten ounces of meat on Sunday, Tuesday, Thursday, and Saturday. And one ounce of cheese and one ounce of butter on Monday, Wednesday and Friday'. The governors made public the rations which they prescribed. Two years later, after the doctors had produced a revised table, copies were 'painted on ... boards and hung in the three passages of the Hospital'.[96] If cheap and tedious by twentieth-century standards, the meals which patients ate were reasonably nutritious and in all probability compared favourably with the diet of the labouring classes outside. Unlike the total institution, therefore, the Bath Infirmary did not pursue a policy of less eligibility which degraded its inmates by forcing them to tolerate filthy conditions and unpalatable food.

The allegiance to paternalism which encouraged minimum standards of provision also dictated that patients – like servants – be given a method of redress. When in 1743 Archibald Cleland was dismissed for sexual abuse during his surgical practice at the Hospital, the accusations were allegedly made to nurses and patients, with the apothecary serving as a conduit channelling the complaints to the weekly committee.[97] However, it was the house visitors whom the original rules required to 'receive the complaints of the patients, and servants, each of which they shall examine apart'; and this regulation was reaffirmed in the 1820s when a notice was fixed in every ward explaining the grievance procedure.[98] Under this supervisory system, the house visitors processed numerous requests for clothing to be purchased from the patients' caution money;[99] but it seems that few complaints were received.[100] When they were, the reaction was not always favourable. In 1830, for instance, no fewer than nine inmates were 'dismissed for misconduct in conspiring to find fault with the provisions', even though the simultaneous sacking of the cook suggests that their dissatisfaction may not have been unreasonable.[101] A week later the committee heard an appeal from two of the nine men.[102] The governors, persuaded that both had been drawn into the disturbance by the other rebels, agreed to readmit them. But whereas Nurse Edwards was reprimanded for her error of judgement, these disgraced patients secured their pardon by making 'a proper apology'.[103] The distinction may point to a subtle differentiation between staff and inmates. The paternalist ethos remained dominant. In their dealings with employees, however, the governors were beginning to develop a contractual relationship in which both parties had rights as well as duties. In their dealings with patients, on the other hand, there had been less erosion of traditional obligations. Paternalist charity did not encourage recipients to complain or donors to accept the legitimacy of their criticism.[104] Therefore, forgiveness was only forthcoming on the admission of guilt.

The governors sought to minimize lapses on the part of their charges by keeping their behaviour under close surveillance. The house visitors' inspections documented for the 1740s and 1750s reveal only 18 cases of 'irregularity'. These misdemeanours, used in conjunction with the reasons for dismissal specified in the Minute Books, indicate several areas of wrongdoing. Patients were pronounced guilty of speaking abusive or profane language,[105] of committing theft[106] and of making false allegations against others.[107] In 1789 indecency was at the centre of a wrongful claim when two patients were accused 'of a detestable crime, which upon the recent scrutiny appeared to be wholly destitute of foundation';[108] but sexual malpractice was also substantiated, as in 1795 when William Manwaring was expelled for 'indecencies of a nature too gross to be particularly mentioned'.[109] However, the misconduct referred to by far the most frequently involved drunkenness[110] and being 'absent without leave'.[111] Although patients may have become inebriated inside the Hospital, intoxication also went hand in hand with truancy.[112] Other institutions incarcerated their inmates in response to indiscipline outside the walls,[113] or even closed during the season to avoid upsetting fastidious visitors.[114] For patients of the General Infirmary, however, medical treatment at the Hot Bath necessitated regular trips into the city, and religious observances at local churches and chapels also continued. These excursions posed serious problems. The house visitors were not mandated to oversee extra-mural activities, but their extant Minute Books indicate that they did so. On 5 July 1742, patients at the Hot Bath were found to be well behaved and 'very well attended',[115] and when in 1757 a house visitor positioned himself to scrutinize patients who were well enough to attend Divine Service in the Abbey-Church, it was 'but doing them common justice, to say, that they behaved with great decency'.[116] But orderly behaviour was not always achieved. In the early 1740s, the house visitors registered complaints 'against some of the men patients for being without their linen and swimming naked in the Bath'.[117] An order passed by the governors in 1779, forbidding all patients 'to swim, dive or behave disorderly in the Bath on pain of immediate expulsion',[118] indicates that delinquency during bathing was an ongoing problem.

So too were illicit absences. Inmates left the Hospital without permission, in some cases 'lying out ... several nights'; those whose excursions were authorized did not always return on time;[119] and whilst away they were tempted into 'begging about the streets under false pretences'[120] or calling at inns and drinking pots of ale.[121] In the 1770s, and at 'the request of the committee appointed for setting the duty of the clergyman', the chairmen and officers were instructed to 'attend the patients to and from their respective places of worship'.[122] A decade later the governors determined to seek a complementary means of pursuing sobriety by printing handbills which warned publicans that if they offered hospitality to patients of the General Infirmary, an application would be made to the magistrates not to renew their licences.[123] These attempts to tighten external supervision were a response to changing circumstances. The redrawing of attitudes to poverty and the transition of Bath from a lively resort to a genteel residential town combined to reduce the tolerance of riotous behaviour and generate pressure for the greater confinement of patients within the Hospital. The new wing opened in 1861 included both an exercise yard and a chapel, thereby allowing inmates to take the air and attend a place of worship without leaving the institution. Moreover, from the perspective of 1857, the *Bath Chronicle* also interpreted the construction of baths on the premises in 1830 as a way of dispensing with the services of the chairmen 'whose conduct is represented as being extremely obnoxious'.[124] Therefore, though the level of closure associated with a total institution had not been reached, contact between the General Hospital and the city was reducing by the end of the Georgian period.

The ability of patients to abscond, together with the lack of a polarized staff to police them inside and outside the Infirmary, demonstrates that surveillance was not all-encompassing. None the less, sampling from the generally reliable patient statistics published in the *Annual Reports* shows that dissolution was by no means rampant (Table 10.1). The ultimate sanction of dismissal for irregularity was imposed upon only handful of inmates in any sample year; and after 1755 misconduct accounted for more than 1.5 per cent of annual discharges only during the Napoleonic Wars, when national insecurity heightened anxieties about the unruly poor. This is a proportion which compares favourably with the decadal averages for the Salop Infirmary, which were normally in the region of

Table 10.1 Bath General Hospital: patients discharged for irregularity, 1742–1830

Year	*No. discharged for irregularity*	*% discharged for irregularity*	*All discharges*
1742/43	2	2.67	75
1745/46	2	1.82	110
1750/51	—	—	233
1755/56	5	1.85	271
1760/61	2	1.01	199
1765/66	1	0.30	335
1770/71	3	1.09	275
1775/76	1	0.33	305
1780/81	5	1.49	335
1785/86	4	1.41	284
1790/91	—	—	313
1795/96	7	2.07	338
1800/01	3	1.08	278
1805/06	5	1.81	277
1810/11	5	1.87	268
1815/16	5	1.67	300
1820/21	2	0.58	344
1825/26	3	0.79	382
1830/31	3	0.79	381

Source: *Annual Reports*.

2.5 per cent between 1746 and 1836.[125] So why did patients acquiesce in the governors' programme of medico-moral rehabilitation?

Unlike the inmates of a total institution, the patients of the Bath Infirmary were not compulsorily detained. Between 1742/43 and 1759/60 no fewer than 188 (or 9 per cent) left at their own request,[126] and when the Hospital first opened, temporary leave of absence was also granted so that patients could 'go home for the air'.[127] This voluntary status was reflected in admission as well as discharge. Since Bath residents were excluded, all patients travelled from outside the city centre. Analysing the parishes of origin listed in the Admissions Register and the Casebook shows that recruitment had a regional thrust with over 40 per cent of entries between 1742 and 1758 coming from Somerset or the adjacent counties of Gloucestershire and Wiltshire (Table 10.2). Treatment outcomes published in the *Bath Journal* during the 1820s indicate a similar picture; for example, just over half of those discharged

Table 10.2 Bath General Hospital: the geographical origins of patients, 1742–58

Register, 1742–52			*Casebook, 1750–58*		
County	*No.*	*%*	*County*	*No.*	*%*
Somerset	296	18.02	Somerset	274	16.92
Gloucestershire	216	13.15	Gloucestershire	218	13.47
Wiltshire	213	12.96	Wiltshire	198	12.23
Devon	137	8.34	Devon	92	5.68
Middlesex	114	6.94	Middlesex	91	5.62
Dorset	73	4.44	Dorset	67	4.14
Hampshire	45	2.74	Hampshire	53	3.27
Berkshire	41	2.50	City of London	43	2.66
City of London	40	2.44	Berkshire	34	2.10
Oxfordshire	32	1.95	Surrey	24	1.48
Surrey	32	1.95	Military	23	1.42
Cornwall	25	1.52	Ireland	20	1.24
Hertfordshire	17	1.03	Herefordshire	20	1.24
Kent	14	0.85	Monmouthshire	19	1.17
Huntingdonshire	13	0.79	Oxfordshire	17	1.05
Leicestershire	12	0.73	Warwickshire	10	0.62
Bedfordshire	11	0.67	Carmarthenshire	8	0.49
Herefordshire	10	0.61	Kent	8	0.49
Abroad	10	0.61	Buckinghamshire	8	0.49
Other	176	10.71	Other	173	10.69
Not recorded	116	7.06	Not recorded	219	13.53
Total	1 643	100.00	Total	1 619	100.00

Note: Percentages have been rounded up or down and so do not always total exactly 100.00.

Sources: Admissions Register; Casebook; *The Clergy List for 1864* (London: George Cox, 1864); Thomas Moule, *The County Maps of Old England*, introduced by Roderick Barron, first pub. 1830, repr. (London: Studio Editions Ltd, 1990); Frederic A. Youngs, *Guide to the Local Administrative Units of England*, 2 vols (London: Royal Historical Society, 1979), vol. 1: *Southern England*; Frederic A. Youngs, *Guide to the Local Administrative Units of England*, 2 vols (London: Royal Historical Society, 1991), vol. 2: *Northern England.*

during 1825 originated from the three most proximate counties.[128] Even patients from the local region could face a difficult journey, given the rudimentary nature of Georgian transport, but for those from further afield, the trip was formidable. This geographical barrier made it difficult for local élites to enforce application to a faraway institution, especially since without formal sponsorship rights they could not guarantee admission. Therefore, we can assume that most patients were not driven to Bath because they 'lacked any other choice'.[129] Their chronic ailments, in conjunction with their financial circumstances, may have left few other medical possibilities, but there was always the option of staying put. Just as poor relief was manipulated with creativity, so the lower orders resorted to the charity of the General Hospital when what was on offer matched their self-perceived needs.[130]

Since home towns and villages were locationally scattered, and patients followed a variety of paths to entry, the initial stages of the selection process are difficult to uncover, even where Poor Law authorities were involved. The incomplete caution money records contained within the House Visitors Books suggest that although parishes were more regular sponsors than private individuals at mid-century, many patients provided their own deposits (Table 10.3). This apparent self-sufficiency may conceal the extent to which raising the prerequisite funds was a collective endeavour, for the letter proposing Cornelius Gengell, a 50-year-old man from Christian Malford in Wiltshire, maintained that he was 'advised also by his friends to make trial of the Hospital who will readily make a collection for him of the three pounds caution money hoping he will find benefit by it'.[131] But whatever the source of caution money, the potential patient had to have a clean bill of moral health because admission was restricted to proper objects of charity whose cases were 'duly attested by the ministers and church wardens of their parish of residence'.[132] Not all the letters of recommendation preserved in the 1750s Casebook referred directly to moral character; indeed, some openly acknowledged shortcomings. With Thomas Miller from Ensham in Dorset who was 'Afflicted with a violent jaundice ... The cause', his sponsor believed, was 'drinking large quantities of spiritous liquors'.[133] Thomas Price of Builth in Breconshire, on the other hand, was 'pretty much injured by hard work', although he too drank 'too freely of malt liquors'.[134] More common, however, was a stress on the worthiness of applicants like John Matthews, an 'industrious' mason from Shaftesbury, who had a 'sober honest character',[135] or the 'sober industrious' husband of Mary Tuck from Hampshire.[136] The slim occupational profile of patients also intimates their rectitude. Employment details were not specifically requested, but the job of the applicant was mentioned in a small proportion of the Casebook letters (Table 10.4). The dependent status of the pauper, like the special conditions surrounding the admission of soldiers, encouraged their more frequent specification, and the undifferentiated label of labourer is

Table 10.3 Bath General Hospital: sources of caution money, 1742–43 and 1755–56

Date	*Source*	*No.*
1 January 1742/3 to 16 November 1742	Patient	33
	Parish	28
	Private sponsor	25
	Not recorded	25
	Total	111
1 May 1754 to 30 April 1755	Patient	111
	Parish	65
	Private sponsor	33
	Not recorded	14
	Total	223
1 May 1755 to 30 April 1756	Patient	71
	Parish	39
	Private sponsor	18
	Not recorded	158
	Total	286

Note: The house visitors' records on which these sources for caution money have been based are incomplete. This is demonstrated by the 'not recorded' and the 'total' figures, which are derived from the Admissions Register for 1742–43 and the *Annual Reports* for 1754–55 and 1755–56.

Sources: House Visitors Book 1; House Visitors Book 2.

difficult to evaluate in socio-economic terms. However, servants and skilled craftsmen predominate among the other occupations in which more than one patient worked. Thus, it would seem that among inmates of the mid-eighteenth century Bath Infirmary there was a hard core from the respectable lower orders.

The need for patient co-operation within an admissions process which sought proven moral credentials produced a population predisposed to accept the disciplined regime. The deference of the deserving poor also enabled any breaches of order to be managed without recourse to brutal punishment.[137] In 1756, for example, the house visitors noted that Evan Philip had been caught by one of the honorary surgeons not wearing his medallion when out in the city. He was duly contrite, begging 'pardon for appearing without a badge' and promising 'to offend in that manner no more'.[138] There is no evidence that patients were sentenced, denounced or forced to admit their guilt in public; nor

Table 10.4 Bath General Hospital: the occupational profile of patients, 1750–58

Occupation	*No.*
Pauper	49
Soldier	40
Labourer	35
Servant/coachman	15
Painter	12
Mariner/seaman	11
Chairman	8
Plumber	7
Shoemaker	7
Husbandman	6
Carpenter	5
Glazier	4
Weaver/woolcomber	4
Gardener	3
Potter	3
Barber	2
Mason	2
Lead/silver worker	2
Shepherd	2
Other	27
Not recorded	1 375
Total	1 619

Source: Casebook.

were they threatened with the publication of their names in the newspapers.[139] However, the Minute Books for the early nineteenth century show the weekly committee reinforcing the disciplinary function of the house visitors by summoning and reprimanding a patient from Nash's Ward who had already 'humbly apologized for his fault'.[140] On another occasion, it was the chairman of the committee who warned William Gilbert for 'using rude language to one of the nurses' and other 'improper conduct'. He was 'To be expelled ... in case of any further complaint against him'.[141] Where a dismissal did result from misbehaviour, previous propriety was taken into account. Thus, when Richard Green was discharged for being absent overnight, a minute was taken of the 'extenuating circumstances' so that his case could be considered if he applied for readmission; Green, it was argued, had been 'led astray' by William Street, who was ejected at the same time 'for intoxication and sleeping out ... two nights'.[142] Whereas aberrant culprits were met with leniency, consistent misbehaviour prompted the governors to inform the patient's sponsor of the reasons for dismissal.[143] Therefore, when Robert Petworth and John Kinsman were 'discharged ... for repeated acts of drunkenness and ill behaviour', their respective parishes were told of their sins.[144] Given the local support which patients had to organize in order to gain admission, any ignominious expulsion endangered their future positions, for by returning home with dishonour, they risked alienating themselves from influential figures in the community with whom their subsequent security might rest. It was force of this threat for an essentially pliant patient body that accounts for the ability of the Bath governors to implement their rational plan of moral reform in an institution where there was neither closure nor a rigid staff–inmate split.

The transaction of power

In a sermon preached during 1740s, Josiah Tucker maintained that the Bristol Infirmary was innocent of authoritarianism because, although it aimed to correct the poor, their decision to seek admission signalled consent and hence the retention of liberty.[145] The relations of confinement at the Bath Hospital suggest a more complicated transaction of power, in which collaboration took place over the pursuit of objectives that were at least partially shared. From the late eighteenth century, the surveillance of behaviour outside the institution intensified, and the distinction between inmates and servants increased. Unfortunately, we cannot recover how the internal routine evolved, but throughout the Georgian period patients continued to occupy communal wards and hence their individuality was undermined by the constant company of others. Paradoxically, this batch living also enabled a 'local solidarity' to flourish in contrast to the seclusion of the single-celled Panopticon.[146] Therefore, at no stage before 1830 was power concentrated exclusively in the hands of the governors and their senior paid officers. This argument is consistent with Foucault's thesis[147] that 'Power is not to be taken to be a phenomenon of one individual's consolidated and homogenous domination over others, or that of one group or class over others'. However, it does not imply that the political interaction engaged in at the Bath Hospital was 'local and unstable', 'never in anybody's hands, never appropriated as a commodity or piece of wealth'. On the contrary, the Infirmary was structured according to the paternalist values for which it stood. Under this moral system, patients of voluntary and deserving status enjoyed a modicum of autonomy, manifest in wearing personal clothing, expressing grievances and mixing with peers. However, these were not rights but concessions granted by the governors towards whom power was inexorably skewed. Their commitment to a rule which was firm but fair helped to safeguard patients against abuses and ensure a minimum standard of care. What it did not do was permit patients to become 'a multiplicity of points of resistance', capable of reconstituting the boundaries of influence by winning disputes where the governors were unwilling to surrender. Therefore, though the politics of the Bath Infirmary were not tyrannical, they did not embody a 'mobile and transitory' model of power.

As well as acting as a site for the negotiation of paternalism, the social relations of the General Hospital served as a political symbol which augmented its architectural statement of order. In her study of *Medicine and Society in Wakefield and Huddersfield*, Hilary Marland is sceptical of moral reform as a motive for nineteenth-century medical charities, arguing that their rules and regulations were 'just as likely' to have been imposed to achieve 'the smooth functioning of the institutions'.[148] But pragmatism was not incompatible with an ideological agenda. Since Georgian voluntary infirmaries were few in number and generally recruited from the respectable poor, their effect on the behaviour of the lower orders was minimal. Far more important was the figurative role of the regime. Selecting only worthy cases offered institutional affirmation of their differentiation from the feckless poor. Furthermore, commendation from a patron, and the public expression of gratitude for recovery,[149] encapsulated the reciprocal obligations of rich and poor. At the Bath Infirmary, there were no direct sponsorship rights, but governors were an important source for the caution money of patients admitted in the 1740s and 1750s.[150] The paternalist relationship was also played out when former inmates praised the care of the General Hospital in returning 'humble and hearty thanks to Almighty God' in their home parishes.[151] However, it was church attendance *en masse* – when patients joined with the visiting Company in Bath Abbey to offer 'thanks for the benefit received by the Bath-waters'[152] – which best relayed the image of an orderly, social hierarchy with all in their rightful place.[153] This is why the contingent at a charity service in 1766 so moved the Reverend John Penrose, who was visiting from Cornwall:

> It was a very affecting sight to see all the patients ranged in two lines, the men on one side, the women on the other, making a lane from the outer door of the Abbey to the door of the inner part, where service is performed, for the mayor and magistrates and all the congregation to pass through. Eight beadles, in an uniform

> dress, (brown great coats, with yellow capes, and sleeves turned up with yellow) with each a staff in his hand with a brass knob at the top attended them. And when they went from the church, they all walked two and two very orderly, for beadles with staves preceding, then the men patients, then two more beadles, then the women patients, then the two other beadles closing the procession.[154]

Such public displays were a drama in 'the ritual theatre of patrician power',[155] but the regularity which they paraded both educated the poor and reassured the affluent. Like the penitentiary, therefore, the Georgian voluntary infirmary 'exerted a hold on men's imaginations because it represented in microcosm the hierarchical, obedient, and godly social order, which they felt was coming apart around them'.[156]

In this part, we have used the Bath Hospital to examine the emergence of a broader social élite in Georgian Britain and to assess both its level of political integration and its command of the poor. Chapter 8 argued that as politeness replaced landownership as the entrée to gentility, the General Infirmary offered the middling men who ran its affairs a means of satisfying their desire for kudos and esteem. Chapter 9 pondered whether the social cohesion achieved through participation in an array of philanthropic, economic and cultural networks was accompanied by a truce over religion and politics. Although the Hospital was ecumenical in its attitude to non-Anglican sects and recruited governors from opposing factions and parties, the low attendance at most administrative gatherings ensured that any eirenic effect was slight. None the less, the willingness of opponents to collaborate in purveying charitable health care enabled the institution to symbolize an integrated élite. The means by which the Bath Infirmary applied itself to the moral education of the lower orders has been the subject of this chapter. Designed in an austere classical style, the building itself personified the authority of the governing classes, while its internal division of space mapped the subordination of patients and servants. Reinforcing the architecture of order were the socio-political relations of confinement. Being paternalist in outlook, the governors responded humanely to the health and welfare needs of servants, and sought to guarantee a minimum standard of care and provision for patients. Equally, however, they shaped a rational plan of control, inspired by the materialist philosophy of the Enlightenment, which embraced the supervision of external activities as well as behaviour within the Hospital. From the later eighteenth century, measures were taken to improve the calibre of staff; their interaction with patients was restricted; and greater formality in disciplinary procedures was adopted. This more bureaucratic style was part of the wider programme of managerial change in progress as a result of increased influence from the middling sort. Throughout the Georgian period, however, implementation of the moral agenda was heavily dependent upon servants who, though only infrequently dismissed for delinquency, were not removed from their charges in the way that staff and inmates were split in the total institution. Yet few patients were expelled for their misdemeanours. The reason was that they were willing entrants – drawn from the upright poor and endorsed by their local communities – who had a vested interest in conforming to the regulations. Their obedience enabled the Hospital to serve as an icon of order, representing the endurance of hierarchy in the same way that it signified the political integration of an enlarged social élite.

Notes

1. Borsay, *English Urban Renaissance*, pp. 284–6, 294–6, 300–301; Jacques Carré, 'The Lady and the Poor Man; or, the Philanthropists's Etiquette', in Jacques Carré (ed.), *The Crisis of Courtesy: Studies in the Conduct-Book in Britain 1600–1900* (Leiden: E.J. Brill, 1994), pp. 157–8, 165–6; Fissell, 'Physic of Charity', pp. 114–15; Langford, *Public Life*, pp. 449–52; Thompson, 'Patrician Society', pp. 388–93.
2. Ignatieff, *Just Measure*, pp. 11–14.
3. Roy Porter, 'Madness and its Institutions', in A. Wear (ed.), *Medicine in Society: Historical Essays* (Cambridge: Cambridge University Press, 1992), pp. 281–5.
4. Akihito Suzuki, 'Anti-Lockean Enlightenment?: Mind and Body in Early Eighteenth-Century English Medicine', in Roy Porter (ed.), *Medicine in the Enlightenment* (Amsterdam: Rodopi, 1995), p. 337.
5. Ignatieff, *Just Measure*, p. 67.
6. Suzuki, 'Anti-Lockean Enlightenment?', p. 338.
7. J. Barry, 'Piety', p. 170; Porter, 'Reforming the Patient', pp. 9–44; Porter, 'Civilization and Disease', pp. 154–83.
8. Blizard, *Suggestions*, pp. 34, 80–81.
9. *An Account of the Establishment of the County Hospital at Winchester*, quoted in Woodward, *To Do the Sick No Harm*, p. 152. See also Andrew, *Philanthropy and Police*, p. 53; 'An Address to the Nobility, Gentry, Clergy, and Others on Behalf of a Public Infirmary now Erected at Liverpool', quoted in McLoughlin, *Liverpool Infirmary*, p. 17; Hume, *Newcastle Infirmary*, p. ix; McMenemey, *Worcester Royal Infirmary*, p. 21.
10. Smith, *Bristol Royal Infirmary*, p. 26.
11. Minute Book, 16 February 1738, 'Plan and Elevation'; Olive, *Particular Excellence*, p. 22.
12. Wood, *Bath*, p. 291; Nikolaus Pevsner, *A History of Building Types* (London: Thames and Hudson, 1976), pp. 148–9; Thompson and Goldin, *Hospital*, pp. 87–96.
13. Adrian Forty, 'The Modern Hospital in England and France: The Social

and Medical Uses of Architecture', in Anthony D. King (ed.), *Buildings and Society: Essays on the Social Development of the Built Environment* (London: Routledge and Kegan Paul, 1980), p. 72; Thompson and Goldin, *Hospital*, p. 87.
14. Matthew Johnson, *An Archaeology of Capitalism* (Oxford: Blackwell, 1996), p. 143.
15. Borsay, *English Urban Renaissance*, pp. 260–61, 265, 270, 305–7.
16. Robin Evans, *The Fabrication of Virtue: English Prison Architecture 1750–1840* (Cambridge: Cambridge University Press, 1982), pp. 6, 75, 393–4. See also Michael Donnelly, *Managing the Mind: A Study of Medical Psychology in Early Nineteenth-Century Britain* (London: Tavistock, 1983), pp. 48–9, 56.
17. Wood, *Bath*, pp. 291–2.
18. Forty, 'Modern Hospital', pp. 69–70.
19. Wood, *Bath*, pp. 290–92.
20. Forty, 'Modern Hospital', pp. 69–70.
21. Erving Goffman, *Asylums: Essays on the Social Situation of Mental Patients and Other Inmates* (London: Pelican Books, 1968), pp. 24, 51–3.
22. Goffman, *Asylums*, pp. 17–18. For an excellent summary of the 'total institution', see Tom Burns, *Erving Goffman* (London: Routledge, 1992), pp. 144–54.
23. Porter and Porter, *In Sickness*, p. 197.
24. Wood, *Bath*, pp. 295, 297–9. For examples of the rules applied to patients at other Georgian voluntary infirmaries, see Brockbank, *Royal Infirmary, Manchester*, pp. 210–12; Eade, *Norfolk and Norwich Hospital*, pp. 221–2; Howie, 'Royal Salop Infirmary', pp. 52–3; Jacob, *General Hospital*, pp. 342–3; McLoughlin, *Liverpool Infirmary*, pp. 83–4.
25. Rules. Minute Book, 21 May 1760; 29 February 1764.
26. Minute Book, 6 April 1774.
27. Howie, 'Salop Royal Infirmary', pp. 45–8. For job descriptions of the apothecary and matron at other infirmaries, see Anning, *General Infirmary at Leeds*, pp. 44–5, 61–2; Brockbank, *Royal Infirmary, Manchester*, pp. 208–10; Clark-Kennedy, *The London*, p. 45; Eade, *Norfolk and Norwich Hospital*, pp. 339–40, 342; McLoughlin, *Liverpool Infirmary*, pp. 77–81. For a comparison of the duties of patients and servants elsewhere, see note 24.
28. Wood, *Bath*, pp. 298–9; Minute Book, 6 April 1774.
29. Minute Book, 24 June 1742. See also Wood, *Bath*, p. 294; Minute Book, 27 August 1828.
30. Minute Book, 8 June 1803; 12 October 1825.
31. Minute Book, 27 August 1828
32. Wood, *Bath*, p. 294.
33. Minute Book, 28 July 1756; 5 September 1775; 15 December 1819.
34. Minute Book, 22 April 1812; 10 June 1812; 26 January 1820.
35. Minute Book, 3 June 1742; 27 December 1749.
36. Minute Book, 8 December 1819.
37. Kersley and Cosh, *Royal National Hospital*, p. 15.
38. Wood, *Bath*, p. 297. Rules. Minute Book, 9 January 1751.
39. *Gentleman's Magazine*, 30 (1760), pp. 525–6.
40. Minute Book, 6 April 1774; 1 May 1775; 18 May 1775.

41. Minute Book, 30 September 1830.
42. Wood, *Bath*, p. 299.
43. See, for example, Brockbank, *Royal Infirmary, Manchester*, p. 211; Frizelle and Martin, *Leicester Royal Infirmary*, pp. 58–9; Jacob, *General Hospital*, p. 343; McLoughlin, *Liverpool Infirmary*, p. 83; Turner, *Hampshire County Hospital*, p. 41.
44. Wood, *Bath*, p. 297.
45. See, for example, E.H. Phelps Brown and Sheila V. Hopkins, 'Seven Centuries of Building Wages', in E.M. Carus-Wilson (ed.), *Essays in Economic History*, 2 vols (London: Edward Arnold, 1962), vol. 2, p. 177–8.
46. Minute Book, 6 May 1742.
47. *London Evening Post*, 8 July 1738.
48. Minute Book, 15 March 1786; 5 November 1800; 18 February 1807; 26 January 1816.
49. Minute Book, 2 May 1763; 1 May 1793; 14 May 1817; 28 January 1824.
50. Minute Book, 29 May 1771; 1 May 1826.
51. Minute Book, 10 October 1792; 2 May 1796; 13 February 1805.
52. Minute Book, 13 February 1828.
53. Minute Book, 9 November 1738.
54. Minute Book, 17 August 1743.
55. Minute Book, 1 April 1747.
56. Minute Book, 21 May 1828. See also Minute Book, 24 June 1807.
57. Minute Book, 1 April 1747. See also Minute Book, 17 August 1808.
58. Minute Book, 29 October 1817.
59. Minute Book, 13 June 1744.
60. Minute Book, 29 October 1828; 18 February 1829; 8 April 1829; 22 April 1829; 1 July 1829.
61. Wood, *Bath*, p. 298. Rules.
62. House Visitors Book 2, 27 August 1756.
63. House Visitors Book 1, 17 July 1742; 26 July 1742.
64. For a review of complaints against nursing staff at the Salop and Exeter Infirmaries, see Howie, 'Complaints', pp. 355–6.
65. Jordanova, 'Representation of the Family', p. 130.
66. Minute Book, 23 May 1775. See also Minute Book, 13 December 1826; 19 December 1827.
67. See, for example, Minute Book, 23 December 1801; 15 September 1813; 24 August 1816; 28 March 1821; 1 July 1829.
68. Minute Book, 27 August 1828. When the porter's yearly wage was fixed at £12, for example, he was allowed up to three annual increases of £1 for good behaviour. See Minute Book, 2 June 1830.
69. Minute Book, 29 October 1828; 10 June 1829.
70. Minute Book, 29 October 1828; 18 February 1829; 8 April 1829; 22 April 1829; 1 July 1829.
71. Minute Book, 29 October 1828.
72. Wood, *Bath*, p. 298. Rules. See also Brockbank, *Royal Infirmary, Manchester*, p. 211; Clark-Kennedy, *The London*, p. 35; Eade, *Norfolk and Norwich Hopital*, p. 342; Langford, 'Hereford General Hospital', p. 154; McLoughlin, *Liverpool Infirmary*, p. 82.
73. Robert Dingwall, Anne Marie Rafferty and Charles Webster, *An Intro-*

duction to the Social History of Nursing (London: Routledge, 1988), p. 11.
74. Wood, *Bath*, p. 298. Rules. See also Woodward, *To Do the Sick No Harm*, pp. 30–31
75. Minute Book, 10 June 1829.
76. Dingwall, Rafferty and Webster, *Social History of Nursing*, pp. 22–3.
77. See Table 10.1. For examples of complaints apparently relating to patient care and/or domestic duties, see House Visitors Book 1, 15 April 1743; House Visitors Book 2, 4 August 1758.
78. Dingwall, Rafferty and Webster, *Social History of Nursing*, p. 19. See also Perry Williams, 'Religion, Respectability and the Origins of the Modern Nurse', in R. French and A. Wear (eds), *British Medicine in an Age of Reform* (London: Routledge, 1991), pp. 231–50.
79. Minute Book, 1 July 1829.
80. Minute Book, 27 August 1828.
81. Dingwall, Rafferty and Webster, *Social History of Nursing*, p. 19; Williams, 'Religion', p. 234.
82. Minute Book, 19 December 1827; 10 June 1829.
83. See, for instance, Minute Book, 10 March 1830.
84. See, for example, Minute Book, 17 January 1753; 4 December 1799.
85. Minute Book, 20 October 1802.
86. House Visitors Book 2, 9 June 1754; Minute Book, 17 February 1830.
87. Minute Book, 3 March 1830.
88. Minute Book, 21 January 1778; 28 January 1778; 14 April 1831.
89. House Visitors Book 2, 9 June 1754.
90. House Visitors Book 1, 6 July 1747.
91. Minute Book, 10 February 1830.
92. Wood, *Bath*, p. 297; Rules.
93. *Annual Reports*, 1756/57–1765/66. See also *Bath and Bristol Guide*, p. 19.
94. Minute Book, 3 June 1742; 11 January 1763. Rules. See also Risse, *Hospital Life*, p. 220.
95. Minute Book, 5 November 1800. See also Strange, *Royal Sea Bathing Hospital*, p. 53.
96. Minute Book, 18 July 1827; 8 July 1829; 15 July 1829.
97. *Appeal*, pp. 11–13; *Short Vindication*, p. 10.
98. Wood, *Bath*, p. 295; Minute Book, 26 January 1826. See also Howie, 'Complaints', pp. 347–51.
99. See, for example, House Visitors Book 2, 27 July 1754; 23 October 1755; 10 May 1756; 15 January 1757; 1 December 1758; 12 September 1759.
100. For a rare case of a recorded grievance, see House Visitors Book 1, 25 October 1742, when there were 'Great complaints from patients in the Duke's Ward of the ill behaviour of ... Richardson'.
101. Minute Book, 14 April 1830.
102. The Minute Book also records this procedure occurring on 15 July 1742, when John Green was 'continued in the House upon his future good behaviour' after making an acceptable submission.
103. Minute Book, 21 April 1830.
104. See also W.B. Howie, 'Consumer reaction: a patient's view of hospital

life in 1809', *British Medical Journal*, **3** (8 September 1973), p. 536; Risse, *Hospital Life*, pp. 24, 57–8.

105. House Visitors Book 1, 8 August 1742. Minute Book, 16 January 1754; 18 June 1817; 10 March 1819; 16 May 1827.
106. Minute Book, 3 February 1796; 29 March 1815.
107. Minute Book, 14 April 1830. See also Howie, 'Complaints', p. 356.
108. Minute Book, 13 September 1789.
109. Minute Book, 8 April 1795. See also Minute Book, 13 February 1754.
110. Minute Book, 16 January 1754; 11 August 1802; 19 December 1804; 16 December 1807; 25 March 1818; 9 September 1818; 24 August 1825; 7 February 1827; 18 April 1827; 16 May 1827; 19 March 1828.
111. Minute Book, 9 October 1793; 5 March 1800; 28 October 1807. For a review of the nature of complaints against patients at the Salop and Exeter Infirmaries, see Howie, 'Complaints', pp. 351–5.
112. House Visitors Book 1, 6 July 1742. House Visitors Book 2, 13 October 1756. Minute Book, 7 December 1803; 3 March 1819; 6 January 1830; 16 June 1830; 30 September 1830.
113. See, for example, McMenemey, *Worcester Royal Infirmary*, p. 65; Smith, *Bristol Royal Infirmary*, p. 34.
114. This happened at the spa hospital for the poor in Harrogate during the nineteenth century. See Bernard Jennings (ed.), *A History of Harrogate and Knaresborough* (Huddersfield: Advertiser Press, 1970), p. 298.
115. House Visitors Book 1, 5 July 1742.
116. House Visitors Book 2, 13 November 1757. See also House Visitors Book 2, 25 December 1757; 2 April 1758; 11 February 1759.
117. House Visitors Book 1, 4 July 1743. See also House Visitors Book 1, 26 June 1742.
118. Minute Book, 19 May 1779.
119. House Visitors Book 1, 7 June 1743; 30 August 1743. House Visitors Book 2, 21 June 1756.
120. Minute Book, 23 August 1786.
121. House Visitors Book 1, 6 July 1742; 8 August 1742. House Visitors Book 2, 13 October 1756.
122. Minute Book, 23 May 1775.
123. Minute Book, 25 October 1786.
124. Bath Chronicle, *Hot Water Hospital*, pp. 3, 11–12. See also Rolls, *Hospital of the Nation*, pp. 27–30.
125. Bevan, *Salop Infirmary*, 'A Comparative Average Statement of In and Out-Patients'.
126. *Annual Report*, 1742–59. The category was dropped from the patient statistics in 1760.
127. Minute Book, 25 January 1744. See also Minute Book, 13 July 1743; 27 July 1743; 19 October 1743.
128. *Bath Journal*, 10 January 1825; 14 February 1825; 14 March 1825; 11 April 1825; 16 May 1825; 13 June 1825; 11 July 1825; 8 August 1825; 12 September 1825; 14 November 1825; 12 December 1825. It seems that no figures were published for October.
129. Arthur E. Imhof, 'The Hospital in the Eighteenth Century: For Whom?', *Journal of Social History*, 10 (1970), p. 451.
130. Fissell, 'Physic of Charity', pp. 5, 202–19; Slack, *English Poor Law*, p. 56. See also Morris, 'Voluntary Societies', pp. 364–5.

131. Casebook, admitted 7 October 1753.
132. Minute Book, 16 February 1738, 'Plan and Elevation'.
133. Casebook, admitted 25 May 1756.
134. Casebook, admitted 18 June 1752.
135. Casebook, admitted 20 September 1757. See also Casebook, admitted 16 May 1753; 13 October 1753.
136. Casebook, admitted 15 September 1758.
137. In 1755, Mary Jones was sentenced to a public whipping for stealing clothes from the Worcester Infirmary where she had been an in-patient. See McMenemey, *Worcester Royal Infirmary*, pp. 64–5.
138. House Visitors Book 2, 17 May 1756; 24 May 1756.
139. Howie, 'Complaints', p. 352; Hume, *Newcastle Infirmary*, p. 25.
140. Minute Book, 27 January 1831.
141. Minute Book, 23 September 1829.
142. Minute Book, 6 January 1830.
143. See also Waddy, *Northampton General Hospital*, p. 31.
144. Minute Book, 8 February 1804. See also Minute Book, 11 January 1826.
145. Josiah Tucker, *A Sermon Preached in the Parish Church in Bristol* (Bristol: William Crossley, 1746), p. 15.
146. Thomas A. Markus, *Buildings and Power: Freedom and Control in the Origin of Modern Building Types* (London: Routledge, 1993), p. 18.
147. Michel Foucault, 'Two Lectures', in Colin Gordon (ed.), *Michel Foucault Power/Knowledge: Selected Interviews and Other Writings 1972–1977* (Brighton: Harvester Press, 1980), p. 98; Michel Foucault, *The History of Sexuality*, trans. R. Hurley, 3 vols (Harmondsworth: Penguin Books, 1981), vol. 1: *An Introduction* p. 94.
148. Marland, *Medicine and Society*, p. 150.
149. See, for example, Brockbank, *Royal Infirmary, Manchester*, p. 208; Davies, *Deeds Not Words*, p. 28; Fissell, *Patients*, p. 87; Jacob, *General Hospital*, pp. 340–41; McLoughlin, *Liverpool Infirmary*, p. 74; John Whyman, *Aspects of Holidaymaking and Resort Development Within the Isle of Thanet, With Particular Reference to Margate, c. 1736–1840* (New York: Arno Press, 1981), p. 712.
150. Some identifications are uncertain because Christian names were not always stated. However, almost half of the private sponsors who supplied caution money between June 1742 and November 1743 were governors, and approximately 30 per cent between March 1754 and April 1756. See House Visitors Books 1 and 2.
151. A standard form was printed for this purpose. See Minute Book, 25 October 1786.
152. John Penrose, *Letters from Bath 1766–1767*, ed. by Brigitte Mitchell and Hubert Penrose (Gloucester: Alan Sutton, 1983), p. 125.
153. Borsay, *English Urban Renaissance*, p. 297.
154. Penrose, *Letters*, p. 59.
155. Roy Porter, 'Medical Enlightenment?', p. 55. See also Thompson, 'Patrician Society', pp. 389–90
156. Ignatieff, *Just Measure*, p. 84. See also Michael Ignatieff, 'Total Institutions and Working Classes: A Review Essay', *History Workshop Journal*, 15 (1983), p. 169.

PART SIX

Conclusion

CHAPTER ELEVEN

Medical Charity and the Middling Sort

The overarching objective of this book has been to understand the General Infirmary as a manifestation of Georgian society and Georgian Bath. Unlike the absolutist states of continental Europe, Britain during the long eighteenth century was not an *ancien régime* still under the thumb of a patrician élite and a clerical intelligensia. Rather, a series of fundamental changes were afoot which signalled the onset of modernity. Formative to this process were commercial prosperity and the Enlightenment. The Financial Revolution of the post-Restoration period combined with a pre-existing growth in trade to set the economy on an upward path which generated new wealth. This then provided the means to implement the progressive optimism of the Enlightenment which in England had been evident since the later seventeenth century in the Scientific Revolution, religious pluralism and the constitutional monarchy. But from the 1760s, confidence began to wane. Challenged by political radicalism at home and abroad, by the Romantic and Evangelical Movements and by industrialization, the beliefs of the Enlightenment were gradually overtaken by *laissez-faire* and utilitarian thinking. The Georgian Bath Hospital not only inhabited this shifting economic and intellectual environment; it also occupied a place in local society at a time when Bath was developing from an exclusive but lively resort into a populous and respectable residential town. The Infirmary's history has been interpreted as the product of both these contexts interlocking to shape a particular variation on the voluntary hospital theme.

The commercial economy

The principle of associated philanthropy which underpinned the voluntary infirmary was an effective way of tapping the resources of the commercial economy. In return for their gifts, donors and subscribers – like joint-stock investors – were normally permitted to attend meetings and elect officers. Such opportunities for participation made these charities increasingly popular at a time when the traditional bequest was being undermined by concerns about the abuse of inheritance rights and the misappropriation of posthumous benevolence. No less important was the suitability of collective schemes to the modest surplus incomes of the middling sort. Yet despite this appeal, voluntary hospitals had difficulty in absorbing the volatilities of the market economy. At Bath, annual deficits broadly coincided with points of national crisis, and after 1750 the impact of inflation was relentless. The practice of spa therapy seemingly reduced expenditure on the apothecary's shop relative to other institutions, and although the general problem of spiralling household costs was experienced during the Napoleonic Wars, they remained below the price index for consumer goods. What undercut these advantages was the structure of income. For many voluntary hospitals, stable annual subscriptions were the major revenue. However, the lack of patient sponsorship and the ban on local residents reduced the incentive to support the Bath Infirmary on a regular basis and annual subscriptions typically accounted for no more than 15 per cent of incomings. Therefore, highly variable casual benefactions, primarily from personal donors and charity sermons, were the mainstay. Only the trend for church collections followed the line of inflation, leaving the governors with little option after 1793 but to dispose of stocks and shares in response to economic pressures. Not until the late 1820s did such accumulated assets yield a substantial income which delivered financial security.

The vagaries in the supply of wealth from the commercial economy did not prevent its money from being perceived as a threat to public morality. This disquiet was most intense before 1750 due to fall-out from the South Sea Bubble, embezzlement at the Charitable Corporation and a series of political misdemeanours. Critics blamed commerce and resorted to a classical, paternalist notion of civic virtue to attack the new 'monied interest'; without landed property, it was argued, these men lacked the independence to pursue the public good with impunity. The campaign for political reform kept the ethic of civic virtue alive after 1760. However, commercial prosperity also allowed the emergence of an alternative moral code which in philanthropy harnessed 'shareholder' association to non-profit-making ventures. The application of this economic concept to the propagation of good works helped to defuse fears of corruption. But in order so to arbitrate the charities had to be free of clientage. At the Bath Infirmary, the high financial threshold for automatic admission to governorships and the exclusion of annual subscribers contravened the ideal of an open administration by requiring smaller contributors to seek the patronage of existing members if they wished to join the governing body. Once appointed or elected, however, all governors entered a management structure comprising a general court, a weekly committee, rotating house visitors and, increasingly, subcommittees to handle specific briefs. Although courts and committees were often poorly attended after the first flush of enthusiasm, both the visiting system and the subcommittee network achieved better staffing levels. But more important than participation for civic virtue were the strategies adopted by governors who were active. The Bath Infirmary was able to maintain accurate financial accounts and records of its proceedings, and expenditure was carefully supervised. These good practices were evident from *Annual Reports*, and they were made public in the press and in charity sermons and the reports attached to them. Furthermore, steps were taken early to counter corruption by proscribing the acceptance of gratuities by staff, and at later stages bonds were demanded of the steward and the register. Indeed, by the close of the Georgian period, even the activities of governors were being subjected to more formal scrutiny and to the advice of experts – procedures no doubt imported from the business practices of the middling sort. These efforts were not entirely successful, but the dishonesties to which the Hospital occasionally fell victim were relatively minor. Consequently, it was able to promote reconciliation between the commercial economy and civic virtue.

The medical profession

The application of associated philanthropy to medicine channelled the wealth of the eighteenth century towards a project that was central to the Enlightenment agenda. Georgian doctors acquired money plus social and cultural status from their alliance with voluntary infirmaries, but medical knowledge and clinical autonomy were also at issue in relation to patients, governors and fellow practitioners. Although medicine responded sluggishly to the theoretical challenges of the Scientific Revolution, the empirical methodology was embraced more willingly and the Bath Hospital followed the example of other infirmaries in claiming to extend medical knowledge by exposing physicians and surgeons to a rich variety of patients. Founded with the aim of testing the spa waters, the Hospital was drawn into the sulphur controversy during the 1750s when it faced accusations of publishing inaccurate case histories, and of entering into a conspiracy with the Corporation and the local medical establishment to frustrate the scientific analysis of the springs. The sulphur dispute was a complex confrontation which revolved around radical politics, professional hierarchies and market competition as much as medical knowledge. None the less, until Rice Charleton and William Falconer prepared their sophisticated statistical evaluations towards the end of the century, the routine data collected by the General Hospital was only sporadically deployed by its medical practitioners.

That the research of Charleton and Falconer was not continued is indicative of the conservative nature of balneology. At the Bristol Infirmary after 1750, a rigid anti-phlogistic regime of bleeding, purging, blisters and a bland diet was evolved in which the patient's voice became redundant. At the Bath Infirmary, too, there were moves in this direction with standardized treatment programmes, a clinical language alien to patients, more regular visits by the physicians and surgeons, and the appointment of an assistant to the apothecary in 1830 on the grounds that the auxiliary remedies which had always accompanied drinking and bathing were being prescribed more extensively. At the same time, however, Bath patients were not reduced to their diseases, but kept possession of individual identities in case histories which detailed occupation, complexion and the personal reaction to symptoms. It is important not to overplay this comparison because Bristol may have been atypical of not just provincial infirmaries but even the London teaching hospitals. None the less, the anti-phlogistic regimen accorded with the localized pathology that was gaining ground in late Georgian medicine, whereas the resilient patient narrative matched the holism of humoral theory that informed spa therapy. The implication is that the Bath Hospital was becoming isolated from modern medical practice.

If the clinical knowledge to be acquired was increasingly outmoded, the General Infirmary remained an effective site for the negotiation of clinical autonomy, supplying a compliant patient body and an arena in which conflicts between practitioners and relationships with lay governors were acted out. The sulphur controversy saw the Hospital governors augmenting the authority of prestigious local physicians and colluding with them to exclude Charles Lucas and William Baylies from working in the city when they threatened the resort by questioning the uniqueness of its springs and criticizing its amenities. Whereas Lucas and Baylies were 'outsiders' who never won an honorary post, Archibald Cleland was a surgeon at the Infirmary when in 1743 he was subjected to the machinations of its doctors. The case against Cleland rested on his conduct of vaginal examinations which were construed by colleagues as considerable operations which required prior notification. Although the ensuing trial by the governors raised a series of issues relative to medical theory and practice, and the role of women in Georgian society, Cleland insisted that he was being dismissed because he had previously attacked the spa. His arguments are convincing. But for the lay governors – caught up in a breach of medical respectability cleverly manipulated by Cleland's enemies – the risk of harbouring sexual impropriety was too great to bear.

The relationship between doctors and governors that was so vital in the Cleland affair altered over the course of the Georgian period. Financial patrons enjoyed no sponsorship rights at Bath, but physicians and surgeons were not autonomous in admitting patients. First, they were dependent upon the written recommendations which accompanied applications, the quality of which led to repeated complaints. Secondly, both the processing of admissions, and decisions about discharge, were undertaken in conjunction with non-medical governors. By the turn of the century, physicians and surgeons were no longer exercising regularly the right to attend the weekly committee. However, their ability in the 1790s to stall plans for new premises based on a radical environmental pathology, and the whittling down of the clinical conditions that the Hospital was willing to treat during the 1820s, reveals power gravitating towards the medical staff. This increased autonomy – together with the ongoing opportunities for patient control, medical knowledge, economic gain, and the accumulation of social and cultural capital – meant that the General Infirmary enhanced the occupational standing of medical practitioners in Bath. Medicine's gains triggered a multiplier effect, boosting the confidence of the professional classes and also their commercial peers with whom values and experiences were shared. Therefore, if servicing the Bath Infirmary delivered specific occupational rewards to the honorary physicians and surgeons, they were also drawn by economic and moral, social and political returns which were common to the middling sort as a whole.

The moral economy

The moral economy of Georgian medical philanthropy – and its mediation of social status, political conflict and power – oiled the emergence of a wider élite in which doctors and fellow members of the affluent professional and commercial classes gradually fused with aristocrats and landed gentry. This process was visible in the changing attitudes to giving and receiving that were refracted through the Bath Infirmary. Two moral discourses shaped the ethics of the patron. The first discourse, associated with the civic humanism also used by the landed interest to critique corrupt commercial exchanges, advocated a tributary relationship in which poverty was construed as providential and charity as a duty of stewardship incumbent upon property owners. The second discourse arose from the adaptation of this civic virtue to plenty by acknowledging not only that the increased consumption of non-essential goods created wealth but also that benevolence spurred by private conscience rather than public obligation was no less genteel.

The resulting social virtue was codified in a proprietary relationship where property was seen as divinely ordained and charity as an optional mark of politeness. The early eighteenth-century Bath Infirmary was dominated by the tributary relationship. Clerics preaching on its behalf advised their congregations that the intercessionary prayers of the poor which followed from good stewardship were a useful antidote to the spiritual dangers of wealth. Illness also retained its didactic function and whilst science and religion were no longer opposed, recovery was still in the hands of a God who was less sympathetically inclined towards the uncharitable. Finally, the embarrassment of riches, derived from commerce and compounded by the Evangelical restatement of frugality, was exploited to fuel guilt about luxury and comfort, and anxiety about man's temporal and eternal fate.

Yet although charity sermons were in the tributary mode, the Bath Infirmary, being based on the joint-stock principle, was an institution of commercial society. Moreover, it inspired from the beginning a less austere moral sensibility that was to grow into the proprietary relationship. Early publicity stressed the common predicament of humanity and the pleasure of compassionate giving. A cultural event dedicated to fund raising also praised the audience for its sensibility. Even charity sermons carried a complementary message which urged pity for the poor and argued that good works brought more lasting enjoyment than trivial amusements or vices. These ideas found a mature expression in 1810 with Joseph Hunter's *The Ameliorated Condition of the Poor*, in which he emphasized that Christian love had liberated the lower orders from slavery and induced the rich voluntarily to be charitable. Later Georgian Bath, however, remained ambivalent about its frivolous past; and local histories and guidebooks, together with the appointment of Evangelical ministers during the 1820s, indicate a residual worry which survived in the respectable residential town. This local scenario – with charity hanging on to its redemptive qualities – challenges Donna Andrew's contention that the tributary relationship had died out by 1740. Rather, the moral discourses surrounding the Bath Infirmary point to a hybrid of civic and social virtue in which the proprietary relationship became dominant but not all-encompassing.

If the ethics of giving were in transition, so too were attitudes to the recipient. Since mercantilism was the prevailing economic theory up to 1750, population was equated with prosperity. Although voluntary hospitals claimed to reduce the mortality and morbidity which depleted national wealth, the number of beds and the influence of other health-related factors ensured that their practical impact was minimal. At the Bath Infirmary, even the espousal of this therapeutic rationale was undercut by the chronic disease profile, but the preponderance of young male patients with employment potential enabled the institution to exemplify mercantilist ends. After 1750, demographic increase led to doubts that population growth was necessarily beneficial. Furthermore, whilst the ascendant *laissez-faire* philosophy assumed that the lower orders were responsible moral agents, its economic individualism was easily hijacked by the Malthusian view that they were naturally lazy and degenerate. From this harsher moral economy a new model of charity was born. Whereas the rational benevolence of the early Georgian period aimed only to distinguish between the impostor and the genuinely needy, the scientific philanthropy of the 1790s followed utilitarianism in seeking to identify the poor who were capable of independence through the closely supervised dispensation of aid. Though medicine furnished voluntary hospitals with a scientific legitimacy, they responded nevertheless to the new charitable habitat by developing their out-patient facilities and by encouraging corporate subscribers. Neither of these strategies were open to the Bath Infirmary due to the exclusion of local townspeople and the denial of sponsorship rights to patrons. In addition, the reliance on recommendatory letters from distant medical practitioners prevented the admissions procedure from implementing scientific discrimination. It was this variance from the up-and-coming philanthropic ethos which over time slowly denuded the position of the General Infirmary as Bath's leading charity.

Status, politics and power

The reconstitution of donor and recipient embodied within the moral economy of the long eighteenth century was connected to critical social and political changes. The divorce of gentility from lineage and inheritance, which permitted charity to be rooted in social rather than civic virtue, also enabled the middling sort to acquire status which had previously been genetically ascribed and confined to the aristocracy and gentry. The voluntary hospital offered an ideal setting for this transfer, its associated philanthropy bringing together benefactors from different social backgrounds. Taking snapshots of donors and subscribers at fifteen-year intervals between 1741 and 1830 demonstrates that the financial viability of the Bath Infirmary was not primarily dependent upon the aristocracy. Quinquennial analysis of engagement in hospital management also indicates a minor role. Although grandees, baronets and knights were more prominent as governors than contributors and often chosen to fill the honorific post of president, they participated rarely in the general court and when infrequently chosen to staff the weekly committee, their attendance was typically poor. Consequently, gentlemen or esquires essentially ran the Infirmary, with stalwart support first from physicians and surgeons and later from clergymen.

During the course of the Georgian period, men entitled Mr – initially uppermost on the weekly committee – virtually disappeared from hospital government, to be replaced by esquires. The fluidity of status labels compels a cautious interpretation, but biographical research intimates that occupational continuity underpinned this loss of gentlemen. The governors active in administration were heavily recruited from Bath's élite tradesmen who catered for the visiting Company. Like all other patrons, they desired the public esteem that came from doing good; and like the professional middling sort, they also wished to satisfy their social aspirations. The General Infirmary met this status requirement mainly through its printed publicity which linked the middle orders to their patrician superiors. However, the seasonal appearance of aristocrats and gentry presented gentlemen with the opportunity for face-to-face interaction, and meeting regularly with their peers fostered a feeling of collective consciousness which was reinforced through membership of other local networks – economic, social and philanthropic. Therefore, the Bath Hospital helped the prospering commercial classes to consolidate their position at the top of the urban hierarchy and negotiate the status of esquire.

Although absorbing urban gentlemen into a wider élite assisted in fusing the old and new gentry, sociability alone was not enough to heal the religious and political wounds which had afflicted Britain since the Restoration. Medical charities were among the philanthropic bodies which pursued assimilation by providing an enterprise around which the warring groups could unite. The Bath Infirmary was in this peace-making mould. An early circulation of leaflets thus included Dissenting congregations in London. The appointment of an Anglican chaplain from the 1770s was accompanied by clear statements that he was voluntarily supported. And the patrons and governors drawn from the religious minorities included several Presbyterian ministers whose active governorships in the later Georgian period may have compensated for their political disabilities. Competing factions and parties were also represented on the governing body: Tories as well as Whigs during the Jacobite era, different coalitions during the long Whig oligarchy, radicals as well as conservatives during the campaigns for electoral reform. In a spa town dedicated to maximizing its custom, religious toleration and political neutrality had an economic logic independent of the General Hospital. Furthermore, the infrequent attendance of the governors whose political affiliations were identified from national biographical tools seriously constrained any eirenic effect. None the less, the selection of politicians from rival factions and parties did let the Bath Infirmary convey an integrated image of the governing élite.

Local government and the voluntary sector, as much a part of Georgian Britain's political culture as its parliamentary contests, were no more consensual. At Bath, the Corporation objected to the General Hospital on the grounds that it would attract vagrants, and the strict arrangements for the admission and discharge of patients were put in place to address this complaint. Resistance to the spa water Infirmary was bound up with conflict between visitors and residents. By the later eighteenth century, tensions were subsiding as the financial advantages of the resort to the tradesmen who controlled the Corporation became ever more apparent. The rapprochement was evident in the growing number of doctors and governors who were elected as councilmen, but the General Hospital rarely featured in Corporation business and received none of the grants awarded to other charities; accused of distracting attention from the indigenous sick poor, it served as a focus for residual resentment towards the peripatetic Company. Similarly, there was little scope for the appeasement of local party divisions. Although the voting behaviour of governors on the Bath Corporation shows the Infirmary accommodating a range of political opinion during parliamentary contests, its oligarchic constitution restricted automatic membership of the governing body to high-paying benefactors. The low turnout for administrative events, including those at which hospital posts were filled, also contrasted sharply with the democratic ethos. Therefore, instead of deflecting the reform prospectus of the middling sort, the Bath Infirmary reiterated existing structures of power.

The consolidation of traditional authority was extended to the education of patients in the ways of healthy, sober and godly living: a policy underwritten by the materialist psychology of the Enlightenment which deduced from the oneness of mind and body that morality was learnt and hence susceptible to improvement. Built in the orderly classical style, the Bath Infirmary projected the mastery of the governing classes, while its ground plan configured the subservience of servants and patients. Both groups were protected by a paternalist concern for their welfare and a mechanism for the redress of grievances, but the relations of confinement were also defined by a set of rules which were systematically transmitted and later endowed with religious approval. Since supervision by the governors was episodic, the enforcement of this moral code relied heavily upon lowly servants. Yet despite the lack of a rigid staff–inmate split before the end of the Georgian period, few patients were expelled for misbehaviour. This was not because delinquency went unchecked. Rather, admission depended upon sound moral credentials and an ignominious discharge risked alienating the source of that assurance. Therefore, the Bath Infirmary treated the respectable lower orders who were predisposed to accept the disciplined regime and sufficiently subordinate to stand as a reassuring symbol of the obedient poor.

Towards a middle class

A recurring theme in this study has been the influence of the middling sort in managing the General Hospital and shaping the values which it represented. It is, therefore, apposite to conclude by asking whether a middle class was made during the long eighteenth century. The seminal influence of Marxist theory on historical conceptions of class has led to a preoccupation with political struggle[1] from which not even post-modernist writing has escaped. Dror Wahrman's recent work on the language of electoral reform thus insists that before 1830, 'middle class' was 'an *imagined* constituency' without 'distinctive interests' or 'a concrete socio-political programme'; only as a consequence of the 1832 Reform Bill did the 'category of "middle class" ... play a central role in organizing and understanding social and political experience'.[2] The social history of the Bath Infirmary muddies this chronology which, though aligned with the high politics of the later Georgian era, ignores both the complementary sources of political power and the range of political issues of significance to the middling sort. Not only did the paternalist ethos sensitize the governing élite to interests besides those of the narrow electorate, but central government was also responsive to local government, pressure groups, petitioning, the press and voluntary societies – of which infirmaries were but one example. Above all, the hospital movement pursued rationales in economics, social status and ethics which were no less important than political confrontation in the maturation of a middle class.

The economic underpinnings for a flourishing middling sort were supplied by the commercial prosperity of post-Restoration Britain, and the later Agrarian and Industrial Revolutions. Arising from the intersection of this wealth with the Enlightenment, voluntary infirmaries seized upon the paternalist idea of civic virtue, translating it into a polite social virtue that was accessible to a wider élite. The Bath Hospital facilitated the dispersal of gentility both by enhancing the occupational prestige of physicians and surgeons, and by hosting a trade in social status for the more successful members of Bath's professional and commercial classes. Reinforcing this quest for social status, and the resulting sense of identity among urban gentlemen, was a set of moral values over which the landed and middling orders were in broad agreement.

Applying the joint-stock company to charity and managing it with propriety was an effective means of cleansing the commercial economy in the eyes of the landed interest. Conversely, the General Infirmary's administrative procedures underwent adaptation during the Georgian period as the paternalist reliance on the integrity of governors was supplemented with a bourgeois emphasis on formality and expert advice. The General Infirmary also responded to the mind set of middling men in addressing personal morality. Although the paternalist, tributary relationship was durable in Bath, an alternative proprietary relationship unfolded from the 1760s, replacing compulsory stewardship with optional giving. Attitudes to the lower orders were changing in tandem as, from the late eighteenth century, the poor were increasingly regarded as degenerates in need of detailed supervision if charity was to deliver moral rehabilitation. The origins of this new medicine for poverty were in *laissez-faire* economics, Evangelical religion and utilitarianism, with all of which the middling sort were closely identified. Therefore, despite the lack of direct political power, an accommodation was reached in which the moral system of the landowning élite gradually assimilated values bearing the imprint of the middle orders.

The practice of medical charity in Georgian Bath offers counter-indications to the view that no middle class emerged in Britain before 1830. By the final decade of the eighteenth century, middling men had grown in number and in affluence; they had won social status through genteel pursuits; and, critically, they had aquired a distinctive ideological position in relation to the poor which was infiltrating the political consciousness of the landed élite. Far from being disinterested Good Samaritans, therefore, Georgian patrons of the Bath Infirmary were able to follow a series of economic, social, political and ethical goals which, for the middling sort, contributed to their development as a class.

Notes

1. Karl Marx, 'Communist Manifesto', in T.B. Bottomore and Maximilien Rubel (eds), *Karl Marx: Selected Writings in Sociology and Social Philosophy* (Harmondsworth: Penguin Books, 1961), p. 207.
2. Dror Wahrman, *Imagining the Middle Class: The Political Representation of Class in Britain c.1780–1840* (Cambridge: Cambridge University Press, 1995), pp. 18, 263.

Appendices

Appendix A Bath General Hospital: the condition of patients at discharge, 1742–55 and 1760–1830

(a) 1742–55

Condition at discharge	*Patients discharged*	
	No.	*%*
1742/43		
Cured	23	30.67
Great benefit	18	24.00
Better	—	—
No better	—	—
Incurable	29	38.67
Dead	3	4.00
Improper	—	—
Hectical	—	—
At own request	—	—
Misbehaviour	2	2.67
Eloped	—	—
Total	75	100.00
1745/46		
Cured	33	30.00
Great benefit	36	32.73
Better	—	—
No better	—	—
Incurable	9	8.18
Dead	6	5.45
Improper	10	9.09
Hectical	—	—
At own request	14	12.73
Misbehaviour	2	1.82
Eloped	—	—
Total	110	100.00
1750/51		
Cured	48	20.60
Great benefit	113	48.50

Appendix A continued

(a) 1742–55 continued

Condition at discharge	*Patients discharged*	
	No.	*%*
Better	—	—
No better	—	—
Incurable	12	5.15
Dead	14	6.01
Improper	5	2.15
Hectical	—	—
At own request	40	17.17
Misbehaviour	—	—
Eloped	1	0.43
Total	233	100.00
1755/56		
Cured	87	32.10
Great benefit	76	28.04
Better	37	13.65
No better	17	6.27
Incurable	2	0.74
Dead	8	2.95
Improper	18	6.64
Hectical	3	1.11
At own request	17	6.27
Misbehaviour	5	1.85
Eloped	1	0.37
Total	271	100.00

(b) 1760–1830

Condition at discharge	*Patients discharged*	
	No.	*%*
1760/61		
Cured	62	31.16
Much better	88	44.22
Incurable	—	—

Appendix A continued

(b) 1760–1830 continued

Condition at discharge	*Patients discharged*	
	No.	%
Improper	42	21.11
Irregular	2	1.01
Dead	5	2.51
Total	199	100.00
1765/66		
Cured	107	31.94
Much better	160	47.76
Incurable	—	—
Improper	55	16.42
Irregular	1	0.30
Dead	12	3.58
Total	335	100.00
1770/71		
Cured	72	26.18
Much better	137	49.82
Incurable	—	—
Improper	57	20.73
Irregular	3	1.09
Dead	6	2.18
Total	275	100.00
1775/76		
Cured	80	26.23
Much better	182	59.67
Incurable	—	—
Improper	38	12.46
Irregular	1	0.33
Dead	4	1.31
Total	305	100.00
1780/81		
Cured	120	35.82
Much better	146	43.58
Incurable	—	—
Improper	60	17.91

Appendix A continued

(b) 1760–1830 continued

Condition at discharge	*Patients discharged*	
	No.	%
Irregular	5	1.49
Dead	4	1.19
Total	335	100.00
1785/86		
Cured	82	28.87
Much better	149	52.47
Incurable	29	10.21
Improper	15	5.28
Irregular	4	1.41
Dead	5	1.76
Total	284	100.00
1790/91		
Cured	109	34.82
Much better	144	46.01
Incurable	23	7.35
Improper	30	9.59
Irregular	—	—
Dead	7	2.24
Total	313	100.00
1795/96		
Cured	96	28.40
Much better	154	45.56
Incurable	18	5.33
Improper	55	16.27
Irregular	7	2.07
Dead	8	2.37
Total	338	100.00
1800/01		
Cured	68	24.46
Much better	139	50.00
Incurable	13	4.68
Improper	49	17.63
Irregular	3	1.08

Appendix A continued

(b) 1760–1830 continued

Condition at discharge	*Patients discharged*	
	No.	%
Dead	6	2.16
Total	278	100.00
1805/06		
Cured	70	25.27
Much better	132	47.65
Incurable	10	3.61
Improper	44	15.89
Irregular	5	1.81
Dead	16	5.78
Total	277	100.00
1810/11		
Cured	68	25.37
Much better	142	52.99
Incurable	12	4.48
Improper	34	12.69
Irregular	5	1.87
Dead	7	2.61
Total	268	100.00
1815/16		
Cured	71	23.67
Much better	160	53.33
Incurable	20	6.67
Improper	33	11.00
Irregular	5	1.67
Dead	11	3.67
Total	300	100.00

Appendix A concluded

(b) 1760–1830 concluded

Condition at discharge	*Patients discharged*	
	No.	%
1820/21		
Cured	81	23.55
Much better	198	57.56
Incurable	25	7.27
Improper	32	9.30
Irregular	2	0.58
Dead	6	1.74
Total	344	100.00
1825/26		
Cured	128	33.51
Much better	179	46.86
Incurable	39	10.21
Improper	28	7.33
Irregular	3	0.79
Dead	5	1.31
Total	382	100.00
1830/31		
Cured	120	31.50
Much better	181	47.51
Incurable	69	18.11
Improper	4	1.05
Irregular	3	0.79
Dead	4	1.05
Total	381	100.00

Note: Percentages have been rounded up or down and so do not always total exactly 100.00.

Source: *Annual Reports*.

Appendix B Bath General Hospital: presidents, 1739–1830

Year	*President*	*Year*	*President*
1739	Thomas Carew Esq. MP	1785	Hon. John Jefferys Pratt MP
1740	Thomas Carew Esq. MP	1786	Lord Vernon
1741	Hon. Marshall Wade MP	1787	Earl of Mansfield
1742	Ralph Allen Esq.	1788	Earl Nugent
1743	Lord Bishop of Bath and Wells	1789	Lord Primate of Ireland
1744	Earl of Chesterfield	1790	Marquis of Bath
1745	Francis Colston Esq.	1791	Earl of Harewood
	HRH Prince of Wales	1792	Earl of Chesterfield
1746	HRH Prince of Wales	1793	Lord Bishop of Durham
1747	HRH Prince of Wales	1794	Lord Viscount Weymouth MP
1748	Duke of Beaufort	1795	Sir R.P. Arden MP
1749	Duke of Bedford	1796	Duke of Northumberland
1750	Lord Viscount Palmerston	1797	HRH Prince of Wales
1751	Lord Viscount Dupplin MP	1798	HRH Duke of York
1752	Duke of Devonshire	1799	Lord Gwydir
1753	Nathaniel Curzon Esq. MP	1800	Marquis of Stafford
1754	Marquis of Rockingham	1801	William Gore Langdon Esq. MP
1755	Sir John Ligonier MP	1802	William Dickinson Esq. MP
1756	Lord Ilchester	1803	Lord Bishop of Bath and Wells
1757	Duke of Kingston	1804	Lord John Thynne MP
1758	Rt Hon. William Pitt MP	1805	John Palmer Esq. MP
1759	Marquis of Carnarvon MP	1806	Earl Manvers
1760	Lord Archbishop of Canterbury	1807	Earl of Pembroke

1761	Lord Henley	1808	Thomas Buckler Lethbridge Esq. MP
1762	Duke of Marlborough	1809	William Dickinson Esq. MP
1763	Sir John Sebright Bart MP	1810	Earl of Bridgwater
1764	Walter Long Esq.	1811	Duke of Leeds
1765	Earl of Lincoln	1812	Earl of Guildford
1766	Duke of Beaufort	1813	Sir Benjamin Hobhouse MP
1767	HRH Duke of York	1814	Sir James Mansfield Bart
1768	Duke of Montagu	1815	Lieut-Col Charles Palmer MP
1769	Sir Lawrence Dundas MP	1816	Lord Bishop of Gloucester
1770	Earl of Kerry	1817	John Parish Esq.
1771	John Smith Esq. MP	1818	Sir T. Shelley Bart MP
1772	Revd. Mr. Hethrington	1819	Lieutenant-General Popham
1773	Revd. Dr. Domville	1820	Charles Knatchbull Esq.
1774	Duke of Devonshire	1821	Sir Walter James Bart
1775	Duke of Leeds	1822	Charles Phillott Esq.
1776	Henry Hoare Esq.	1823	Earl of Brecknock
1777	Lord Clifford	1824	Earl of Liverpool
1778	Lord Bishop of Bath and Wells	1825	Lord Bishop of Bath and Wells
1779	Earl of Guildford	1826	Edward Berkeley Portman Esq.
1780	Earl Spencer	1827	Sir William Draper Best MP
1781	Earl of Ailesbury	1828	John H. Smyth Pigott Esq.
1782	Earl Camden	1829	Marquis of Landsdowne
1783	Lord Rodney	1830	Lord Bexley
1784	Abel Moysey Esq. MP		

Principal sources: 12 Geo. II, p. 579; Minute Books, 1 May 1740, 1 May 1741, 1 May 1742, 2 May 1743, 1 May 1744, 1 May 1745, 1 May 1746, 1 May 1747, 25 May 1748; *Annual Reports*, 1748/49–1830/31.

Appendix C Bath General Hospital: treasurers, 1739–1830

Name	*Year of appointment*
Francis Fauquier Esq.	1739
Richard Nash Esq.	1739
Dr William Oliver	1739
Hon. Benjamin Bathurst	1745
Daniel Danvers Esq.	1760
James Roffey Esq.	1762
Giles Jones Esq.	1764
Henry Cornwall Legh Esq.	1766
Ralph Allen Esq.	1767
Benjamin Colbourne Esq.	1770
Samuel Campbell Esq.	1778
Mr Charles Phillott	1780
William Watson Esq.	1792
Thomas Lowfield Esq.	1794
Dr Henry Harington	1798
Wyndham Goodden Esq.	1816
Edmund Anderdon Esq.	1822
Johnson Phillott Esq.	1825

Notes:

1. Giles Jones Esq. was probably the surgeon who served the General Hospital in a voluntary capacity between 1744 and 1755.
2. Charles Phillott later acquired the status of esquire in the early 1790s.
3. It is likely that William Watson Esq. was the physician who received a knighthood in 1796. See *DNB*, vol. 6, p. 45.

Sources: 12 Geo. II, p. 579; *Annual Reports*.

Appendix D Bath General Hospital: the social status of governors attending at least one general court, 1742–1830

	Social status									
Year	*Aristocrats* No.	*Baronets or knights* No.	*'Honourables'* No.	*Esquires* No.	*Gentlemen* No.	*Doctors* No.	*Clergymen* No.	*Military officers* No.	*Political appointments* No.	*Total* No.
1742/43				3	10	1	2			16
1745/46			1	6	12	4	3			26
1750/51	1		1	2	17	7	1			29
1755/56			1	5	14	8	3		1	32
1760/61			1	6	12	4	2			25
1765/66				6	10	4	3			23
1770/71	1			12	13	2	3		1	32
1775/76				25	8	5	4		1	43
1780/81		1		13	11	2	4			31
1785/86				14	9	2	6			31
1790/91	1			13	8	4	8	1		35
1795/96				8	7	3	5			23
1800/01				14		3	4			21
1805/06				13	1	1	4			19
1810/11				13		1	6		1	21
1815/16				17	1		3			21
1820/21				19		4	7			30
1825/26		1		27	2	2	8	2		42
1830/31	1	1		19		4	10	1	1	37

Notes:
1. The administrative year, 1742/43, has been chosen as the starting point for the analysis of attendance at both general courts and weekly committees because the General Hospital opened to patients in May 1742 and meetings then settled into a regular pattern. Only one general court was held during this first year of operation.
2. The aristocrat attending the general court in 1770/71 was Lord Londonderry, who was not a governor.

Source: Minute Books.

Appendix E Bath General Hospital: the social status of governors appointed to the weekly committee, 1742–1830

	Social status									
Year	*Aristocrats* No.	*Baronets or knights* No.	*'Honourables'* No.	*Esquires* No.	*Gentlemen* No.	*Doctors* No.	*Clergymen* No.	*Military officers* No.	*Political appointments* No.	*Total* No.
1742/43				7	12	6	6		1	32
1750/51			1	4	17	7	3		1	33
1755/56			1	3	19	8	3		1	35
1760/61			1	7	16	4	3		1	32
1765/66				11	13	6	3		1	34
1770/71				11	14	5	3		1	34
1775/76				14	10	5	3		1	33
1780/81		1		11	9	6	4		1	32
1785/86		1		14	7	5	4		1	32
1790/91		1		15	7	4	7	1	1	36
1795/96				12	7	4	8		1	32
1800/01				22		5	4		1	32
1805/06				19	1	6	4		1	31
1810/11		1		20		5	5		1	32

1815/16	1		20	1	5	4		1	32
1820/21	1		22		3	5		1	32
1825/26			20		4	7		1	32
1830/31	1		19		4	6	1	1	32

Notes:

1. Since no annual list was published until 1749/50, the governors appointed to the weekly committee for 1742/43 have been compiled from the Minute Books.
2. Whereas the Hospital's year began on 1 May, the Bath Corporation's year began on a variable date in the Autumn. This led to problems with classifying the political appointment only in 1742/43 when both mayors attended the weekly committee during their terms of office. Since Ralph Allen Esq. was present at more meetings (12) than Mr Henry Atwood (4), he was designated the political appointee.
3. The 'Total' column excludes governors appointed to the weekly committee for whom no social status is available: one in 1760/61 and one in 1790/91.

Sources: *Annual Reports*; Minute Books.

Appendix F Bath General Hospital: the social status of governors attending the weekly committee, 1742–1830

Social status	*No. of governors appointed*	*No. of governors present at one or more meetings*	*No. of governors present at 10 or more meetings*
1742/43			
Aristocrats	—	1	—
Baronets and knights	—	—	—
'Honourables'	—	—	—
Esquires	7	5	2
Gentlemen	12	15	10
Doctors	6	5	5
Clergy	6	4	3
Military officers	—	—	—
Political appointments	1	1	1
Unattributed	—	—	—
Total	32	31	21
1755/56			
Aristocrats	—	—	—
Baronets and knights	—	—	—
'Honourables'	1	1	1
Esquires	3	2	—
Gentlemen	19	14	8
Doctors	8	6	3
Clergy	3	2	1
Military officers	—	—	—
Political appointments	1	1	—
Unattributed	—	—	—
Total	35	26	13
1770/71			
Aristocrats	—	—	—
Baronets and knights	—	—	—
'Honourables'	—	—	—
Esquires	11	7	2
Gentlemen	14	11	8
Doctors	5	3	—
Clergy	3	3	1
Military officers	—	—	—

Appendix F continued

Social status	*No. of governors appointed*	*No. of governors present at one or more meetings*	*No. of governors present at 10 or more meetings*
Political appointments	1	—	—
Unattributed	—	—	—
Total	34	24	11
1785/86			
Aristocrats	—	—	—
Baronets and knights	1	—	—
'Honourables'	—	—	—
Esquires	14	9	2
Gentlemen	7	7	5
Doctors	5	4	2
Clergy	4	3	2
Military officers	—	1	—
Political appointments	1	1	1
Unattributed	—	—	—
Total	32	25	12
1800/01			
Aristocrats	—	—	—
Baronets and knights	—	—	—
'Honourables'	—	—	—
Esquires	22	17	4
Gentlemen	—	—	—
Doctors	5	3	—
Clergy	4	3	1
Military officers	—	—	—
Political appointments	1	1	—
Unattributed	—	—	—
Total	32	24	5
1815/16			
Aristocrats	—	—	—
Baronets and knights	1	—	—
'Honourables'	—	—	—
Esquires	20	11	5
Gentlemen	1	1	—

Appendix F concluded

Social status	*No. of governors appointed*	*No. of governors present at one or more meetings*	*No. of governors present at 10 or more meetings*
Doctors	5	1	—
Clergy	4	1	—
Military officers	—	—	—
Political appointments	1	1	1
Unattributed	—	—	—
Total	32	15	6
1830/31			
Aristocrats	—	—	—
Baronets and knights	1	1	1
'Honourables'	—	—	—
Esquires	19	11	6
Gentlemen	—	—	—
Doctors	4	1	—
Clergy	6	4	4
Military officers	1	1	1
Political appointments	1	1	—
Unattributed	—	—	—
Total	32	19	12

Notes:

1. Since no annual list was published until 1749/50, the governors appointed to the weekly committees for 1742/43 have been compiled from the Minute Books.
2. Whereas the Hospital's year began on 1 May, the Bath Corporation's year began on a variable date in the autumn. This led to problems with classifying the political appointment only in 1742/43 when both mayors attended the weekly committee during their terms of office. Since Ralph Allen Esq. was present at more meetings (12) than Mr Henry Atwood (4), he was designated the political appointee.
3. In 1742/43, the Earl of Chesterfield, two esquires and two gentlemen who had not been appointed to the weekly committee attended meetings. Ralph Allen, president of the Hospital in this year, was present at 12 meetings, but the others only at one each.
4. For five-yearly samples of governors attending at least one meeting of the weekly committee, see Appendix G.

Sources: *Annual Reports*; Minute Books.

Appendix G Bath General Hospital: the occupations of governors attending one or more weekly committees per annum, 1742–1830

No mention of William but there are gaps in years

	No. of attendances	*Occupation*
1742/43		
Dr William Oliver	49	Physician [honorary] [treasurer]
Mr John Morris	46	Apothecary [paid employee]
Mr Philip Allen	34	Brother of Ralph Allen Esq., local businessman
Mr Paul Bertrand	33	Jeweller and toy-maker
Mr James Leake	31	Bookseller
Dr Edward Harington	30	Physician [honorary]
Francis Fauquier Esq.	29	Financial writer [treasurer]
Revd Mr James Sparrow	29	Rector of Walcot, Bath
Dr David Hartley	28	Physician; philosopher
Revd Dr Benet Stevenson	27	Presbyterian minister
Mr John Harford	25	Apothecary
Mr William Hoare	25	Portrait painter
Mr John Stagg	25	Boarding/dancing school master
Mr James Grist	24	Apothecary
Dr Thomas Brewster	21	Physician; translator
Mr Jeremiah Peirce	18	Surgeon [honorary]
Dr Alexander Rayner	17	Physician [honorary]
Revd John Chapman	16	Chaplain to Ralph Allen Esq.

	No. of attendances	*Occupation*
Ralph Allen Esq.	12	Postal contractor and quarry owner; Mayor of Bath from autumn 1742
Mr Samuel Bush	10	Apothecary
Richard Nash Esq.	10	Master of Ceremonies [treasurer]
Mr Evans Thomas	8	Wine merchant
Mr John Wood	7	Architect
Richard Roberts Esq.	6	Not known
Edward Andrews Esq.	5	Of Mangotsfield, Gloucestershire
Mr Henry Atwood	4	Glazier; Mayor of Bath to autumn 1742
Revd Mr Walter Chapman	3	Master of St John's Hospital, Bath
Earl of Chesterfield	1	Politician, wit and letter-writer
Mr Philip Bennet	1	Of Widcombe, near Bath; MP for Bath, 1741–47
Mr Richard Matravers	1	Apothecary; Justice of Bath to autumn 1742
John Roberts Esq.	1	Secretary to Henry Pelham; political associate of Lord Dupplin; MP for Harwich, 1761–72
1745/46		
Mr John Morris	43	Apothecary [paid employee]
Mr Paul Bertrand	36	Jeweller and toy-maker
Dr David Hartley	35	Physician [honorary]; philosopher
Mr William Hoare	32	Portrait painter

Dr William Oliver	32	Physician [honorary] [treasurer]
Mr Philip Allen	28	Brother of Ralph Allen Esq., local businessman
Mr John Stagg	20	Boarding/dancing school master
Revd Mr James Sparrow	18	Rector of Walcott, Bath
Richard Luther Esq.	17	Of Myless, near Ongar, Essex
Mr John Harford	15	Apothecary
Dr Thomas Brewster	14	Physician [honorary]; translator
Revd John Chapman	12	Chaplain to Ralph Allen Esq.
Hon. Benjamin Bathurst	9	Of Siddington, Gloucestershire [treasurer]
Dr Alexander Rayner	9	Physician [honorary]
Mr Jeremiah Peirce	8	Surgeon [honorary]
Revd Mr Freind	7	Rector of Witney, Oxfordshire
Samuel Strode Esq.	7	*Either* London barber-surgeon and South Sea broker of Ponsbourne, Hertfordshire and Mapledurham, Oxfordshire; *or* of Southill, near Shepton Mallet and/or Barrington Court, near Ilminster, both in Somerset
John Carew Esq.	6	Of Camerton, Somerset
Mr Evans Thomas	6	Wine merchant
Mr James Grist	4	Apothecary
Dr Richard Bostock	3	Physician [honorary]
Dr Edward Harington	3	Physican [honorary]
Thomas Perrot Esq.	3	Of Northleigh, Oxfordshire
John Roberts Esq.	3	Secretary to Henry Pelham; political associate of Lord Dupplin; MP for Harwich, 1761–72
Ralph Allen Esq.	2	Postal contractor and quarry owner
Richard Nash Esq.	2	Master of Ceremonies [treasurer]

Appendix G continued

	No. of attendances	*Occupation*
Mr John Wood	2	Architect
Mr Samuel Bush	1	Apothecary
Thomas Carew Esq.	1	Of Crowcombe, Somerset; MP for Minehead, 1739–47
Francis Colston Esq.	1	Of Bristol [?]
Francis Fauquier Esq.	1	Financial writer
Mr Samuel Purlewent	1	Attorney
1750/51		
Mr Thomas Palmer	41	Surgeon [honorary]
Mr John Morris	40	Apothecary [paid employee]
Mr Paul Bertrand	39	Jeweller and toy-maker
Dr David Hartley	38	Physician; philosopher
Mr Philip Allen	25	Brother of Ralph Allen Esq., local businessman
Mr William Hoare	24	Portrait painter
Mr James Leake	23	Bookseller
Mr Henry Wright	22	Surgeon [honorary]
Dr Richard Davies	21	Physician; medical and scientific writer
Dr William Oliver	20	Physician [honorary] [treasurer]
Dr Thomas Brewster	19	Physician [honorary]; translator
Revd Mr James Sparrow	18	Rector of Walcot, Bath
Hon. Benjamin Bathurst	14	Of Siddington, Gloucestershire [treasurer]

Mr John Harford	13	Apothecary
Mr Robert Dingley	12	London merchant
Dr William Woodford	12	Physician [honorary]
Dr John Summers	11	Physician [honorary]
Dr Abel Moysey	9	Physician [honorary]
Revd Mr Knipe	8	Clergyman
Mr Jeremiah Peirce	8	Surgeon [honorary]
Mr James Grist	7	Apothecary
Mr John Stagg	7	Boarding/dancing school master
Revd Mr Freind	5	Rector of Witney, Oxfordshire
Richard Nash Esq.	5	Master of Ceremonies [treasurer]
Mr John Donne	3	Surgeon [honorary]
Mr Samuel Purlewent	3	Attorney
Mr Samuel Bush	2	Apothecary
Mr Philip Ditcher	1	Surgeon [honorary]
Rt Hon. Lord Dupplin	1	MP for Cambridge, 1741–58; member of the Board of Trade
Mr Evans Thomas	1	Wine merchant
1755/56		
Dr Abel Moysey	32	Physician [honorary]
Mr Thomas Palmer	30	Surgeon [honorary]
Dr William Oliver	27	Physician [honorary] [treasurer]
Mr Philip Ditcher	26	Surgeon [honorary]
Mr John Morris	26	Apothecary [paid employee]
Revd Mr James Sparrow	24	Rector of Walcot, Bath
Hon. Benjamin Bathurst	22	Of Siddington, Gloucestershire; MP for Cirencester, 1754–61 [treasurer]

Appendix G continued

	No. of attendances	*Occupation*
Mr Jonathan Henshaw	20	Apothecary
Mr William Hoare	19	Portrait painter
Dr David Hartley	17	Physician; philosopher
Mr James Leake	16	Bookseller
Mr John Harford	11	Apothecary
Mr Henry Wright	11	Surgeon [honorary]
Mr John Donne	9	Surgeon [honorary]
Mr Philip Allen	8	Brother of Ralph Allen Esq., local businessman
James Roffey Esq.	6	Of York and Bath
Dr Thomas Brewster	4	Physician [honorary]; translator
Revd Mr Duel Taylor	3	Rector of Bath
Mr William Gallaway	3	Apothecary
Mr Giles Jones	2	Surgeon [honorary]
Mr Paul Bertrand	1	Jeweller and toy-maker
Mr Samuel Bush	1	Apothecary; Mayor of Bath from autumn 1755
Dr Rice Charleton	1	Physician
Dr Richard Davies	1	Physician; medical and scientific writer
Anthony Keck Esq.	1	Serjeant at Law
Mr Jeremiah Peirce	1	Surgeon [honorary]

1760/61		
Dr William Oliver	30	Physician [honorary]
Mr Samuel Howse	27	Draper
Dr Abel Moysey	25	Physician [honorary]
Mr Henry Wright	23	Surgeon [honorary]
Mr Philip Ditcher	22	Surgeon [honorary]
Mr Thomas Palmer	22	Surgeon [honorary]
Mr John Stagg	21	Boarding/dancing school master
Mr James Leake	20	Bookseller
Daniel Danvers Esq.	15	Banker [treasurer]
Dr Rice Charleton	14	Physician [honorary]
Revd Mr James Sparrow	12	Rector of Walcot, Bath
Thomas Deeke Esq.	10	Coal works owner of Timsbury, Somerset [?]
Mr Jonathan Henshaw	9	Apothecary
Mr William Hoare	9	Portrait painter
Mr Prince Hoare	8	Statuary
Mr Philip Allen	6	Brother of Ralph Allen Esq., local businessman
Revd Mr Duel Taylor	5	Rector of Bath
Mr John Donne	5	Surgeon [honorary]
Dr Robert Gusthart	2	Physician
Mr Robert Dingley	1	London merchant
Mr Giles Jones	1	Surgeon
James Roffey Esq.	1	Of York and Bath
1765/66		
Mr Edward Parker	46	Wine merchant

	No. of attendances	*Occupation*
Revd Mr Frank	26	Presbyterian minister
Mr Henry Wright	24	Surgeon [honorary]
Mr Philip Ditcher	23	Surgeon [honorary]
Revd Mr James Sparrow	23	Rector of Walcot, Bath
Henry Cornwall Legh Esq.	18	Of High Legh, Cheshire
Mr William Hoare	17	Portrait painter
Benjamin Colbourne Esq.	16	London apothecary who moved to Bath
John Lloyd Esq.	16	Of Ford, near Winscombe, Somerset
Mr John Stagg	16	Boarding/dancing school master
Mr Thomas West	15	Apothecary
Mr Prince Hoare	14	Statuary
Mr Giles Jones	12	Surgeon [treasurer]
Mr Samuel Howse	8	Draper
Dr Abel Moysey	8	Physician [honorary]
Mr Philip Allen	5	Brother of the late Ralph Allen Esq., local businessman
James Roffey Esq.	5	Of York and Bath
John Braithwaite Esq.	4	Of Dyrham Park, near Bath, Gloucestershire
Revd Mr Duel Taylor	3	Rector of Bath
Dr Rice Charleton	3	Physician [honorary]
Daniel Danvers Esq.	2	Banker [treasurer]
Mr John Donne	2	Surgeon [honorary]

Dr Robert Gusthart	2	Physician [honorary]
John D. Birkhead Esq.	1	Not known
Dr John Brent	1	Physician
Mr Lewis Clutterbuck	1	Town Clerk of Bath
William Gregory Esq.	1	Bookseller [?]
Dr Henry Harington	1	Physician
Dr Ralph Schomberg	1	Physician; miscellaneous writer
1770/71		
Mr Edward Parker	38	Wine merchant
Mr Joseph Phillott	33	Surgeon [honorary]
Mr Henry Wright	26	Surgeon [honorary]; Justice of Bath from autumn 1770
Daniel Danvers Esq.	24	Banker [treasurer]
Revd Mr Frank	21	Presbyterian minister
Mr William Hoare	20	Portrait painter
Mr Thomas West	19	Apothecary
Mr William Anderdon	18	Apothecary
John Lloyd Esq.	14	Of Ford, near Winscombe, Somerset
Mr Richard Roberts	12	Not known
Mr Philip Ditcher	11	Surgeon [honorary]
Mr Simon Crook	8	Apothecary
Samuel Campbell Esq.	7	Not known
Ralph Allen Esq.	5	Postal contractor; relative of the late Ralph Allen Esq., local businessman
Revd Mr James Sparrow	4	Rector of Walcot, Bath
Benjamin Colbourne Esq.	3	London apothecary who moved to Bath [treasurer]

	No. of attendances	*Occupation*
Mr Thomas Creaser	3	Surgeon
Revd Mr Hele	3	Master of the Grammar School, Bath
Dr Henry Harington	2	Physician
Dr Rice Charleton	1	Physician [honorary]
John Roberts Esq.	1	Secretary to Henry Pelham; political associate of Lord Dupplin; MP for Harwich, 1761–72
Dr Ralph Schomberg	1	Physician; miscellaneous writer
Mr William Street	1	Apothecary and banker
William Wade Esq.	1	Master of Ceremonies
1775/76		
Mr Edward Parker	42	Wine merchant
Mr Joseph Phillott	38	Surgeon [honorary]
Mr Charles Phillott	31	Apothecary and banker
Mr Leonard Coward	29	Lacemaker
Mr Henry Wright	29	Surgeon [honorary]; Justice of Bath from autumn 1775
Dr Daniel Lysons	25	Physician
Revd Mr Frank	22	Presbyterian minister
Mr William Hoare	20	Portrait painter
Richard Wilsonn Esq.	18	Not known
Mr Thomas West	17	Apothecary

Daniel Danvers Esq.	16	Banker [treasurer]
Philip Ditcher Esq.	10	Surgeon [honorary]; Mayor of Bath to autumn 1775; Justice of Bath from autumn 1775
Samuel Campbell Esq.	7	Not known
John Lloyd Esq.	7	Of Ford, near Winscombe, Somerset
Ralph Allen Esq.	6	Postal contractor; relative of the late Ralph Allen Esq., local businessman
Mr William Anderdon	5	Apothecary
Ven. Archdeacon Chapman	4	Rector of Bath
Samuel Eyre Esq.	4	Of New House, near Salisbury, Wiltshire
Dr Ralph Schomberg	2	Physician; miscellaneous writer
Walter Wiltshire Esq.	2	Carrier
James Clutterbuck Esq.	1	Lawyer
Mr Simon Crook	1	Apothecary
John Donne Esq.	1	Surgeon
Dr Robert Gusthart	1	Physician [honorary]
Revd Mr John Sibley	1	Rector of Walcot, Bath
William Wade Esq.	1	Master of Ceremonies
1780/81		
Mr Edward Parker	47	Wine merchant
Mr Charles Phillott	43	Apothecary and banker [treasurer]
Mr Leonard Coward	37	Lacemaker
Mr Joseph Phillott	37	Surgeon [honorary]
Dr Daniel Lysons	32	Physician [honorary from 10 January 1781]
Mr Thomas West	28	Apothecary

Appendix G continued

	No. of attendances	*Occupation*
Henry Wright Esq.	23	Surgeon [honorary]
Thomas Curtis Esq.	22	Not known
Mr Harry Atwood	21	Surgeon [honorary from 31 January 1781]
William Hoare Esq.	19	Portrait painter
Revd Mr Edward Armstrong	11	Clergyman
Ven. Archdeacon Chapman	9	Rector of Bath
Revd Mr Nathaniel Morgan	5	Incumbent of Charlecombe, near Bath; master of the Grammar School, Bath
Mr William Anderdon	4	Apothecary
Samuel Campbell Esq.	4	[treasurer]
Benjamin Colbourne Esq.	3	London apothecary who moved to Bath [treasurer]
Simon Crook Esq.	2	Apothecary; Justice of Bath to autumn 1780
John Donne Esq.	2	Surgeon
Revd Mr John Sibley	2	Rector of Walcot, Bath
Francis Bennett Esq.	1	Draper; Justice of Bath 1779/81
Revd Dean Clarke	1	Clergyman
Mr S. Howse	1	Wine merchant
John Jefferys Esq.	1	Lawyer; Town Clerk of Bath
Sir John Miller Bart	1	Of Bath Easton, Somerset
Mr Thomas Rundell	1	Surgeon

1785/86

Mr Charles Phillott	39	Apothecary and banker [treasurer]
Mr Henry Howse jun.	37	Draper
Dr William Falconer	26	Physician [honorary]
Dr Daniel Lysons	25	Physician [honorary]
Mr George Chapman	23	Linen draper
John Toke Esq.	23	Not known
Mr Joseph Phillott	22	Surgeon [honorary]
Henry Wright Esq.	22	Surgeon [honorary]; Justice of Bath to autumn 1785
Mr Thomas West	15	Apothecary
Leonard Coward Esq.	12	Lacemaker; Mayor of Bath to autumn 1785
Revd Mr Edward Armstrong	10	Clergyman
Revd Mr John Sibley	10	Rector of Walcot, Bath
Mr William Anderdon	6	Apothecary
Mr Harry Atwood	4	Surgeon [honorary]
Dr Henry Harington	3	Physician [honorary]
William Hoare Esq.	3	Portrait painter
Dr Caleb Hillier Parry	3	Physician
Edward Rudge Esq.	3	Merchant and alderman of Salisbury; owner of much of the Abbey Estate at Evesham, Worcestershire
Christopher Anstey Esq.	2	Poet
Samuel Campbell Esq.	2	[treasurer]
Simon Crook Esq.	2	Apothecary
Benjamin Colbourne Esq.	1	London apothecary who moved to Bath [treasurer]
Captain King	1	Master of Ceremonies

	No. of attendances	*Occupation*
Revd Mr Nathaniel Morgan	1	Incumbent of Charlecombe, near Bath; master of the Grammar School, Bath
Walter Wiltshire Esq.	1	Carrier
1790/91		
Dr Daniel Lysons	36	Physician [honorary]
Major William Brooke	35	Not known
Mr Charles Phillott	34	Apothecary and banker [treasurer]
Mr Charles Brett	26	Not known
Henry Wright Esq.	26	Surgeon [honorary]
Mr Henry Edward Howse	25	Draper, grocer and Stamp Office agent
John Toke Esq.	23	Not known
Mr George Chapman	22	Linen draper
Ven. Dr James Phillott	15	Rector and Archdeacon of Bath; vicar of Widcombe and Lyncombe
Mr Joseph Phillott	11	Surgeon [honorary]
Revd Samuel Griffith	8	Minister of the Margaret Chapel, Bath
Mr Thomas West	7	Apothecary
Revd Robert B. Gabriel	6	Minister of the Octagon Chapel, Bath
George Ramsey Esq.	6	Not known
Thomas Bowdler Esq.	5	Philanthropist; author; editor of *The Family Shakespeare*

Revd Mr John Sibley	5	Rector of Walcot, Bath
Dr William Falconer	4	Physician [honorary]
Revd William Leigh	4	Absentee rector of Little Plumstead, Norfolk
Benjamin Colbourne Esq.	3	London apothecary who moved to Bath [treasurer]
Dr Henry Harington	3	Physician [honorary]
Revd Edward Armstrong	2	Clergyman
Leonard Coward Esq.	2	Lacemaker; Mayor of Bath to autumn 1790
Revd Mr Nathaniel Morgan	2	Incumbent of Charlecombe, near Bath; master of the Grammar School, Bath
Mr William Anderdon	1	Apothecary
Christopher Anstey Esq.	1	Poet
Thomas Hicks Esq.	1	Surgeon [?]
Walter Wiltshire Esq.	1	Carrier; Justice of Bath from autumn 1790
1795/96		
Mr Morgan Nichols	35	Surgeon [honorary]
Dr Daniel Lysons	33	Physician [honorary]
Charles Phillott Esq.	32	Apothecary and banker [treasurer]
Mr Thomas West	18	Apothecary
Revd Thomas Fothergill	17	Clergyman
Gill Baddeley Esq.	12	Of Oxford Row, Bath
Mr George Chapman	12	Linen draper
Ven. Dr James Phillott	12	Rector and Archdeacon of Bath; vicar of Widcombe and Lyncombe
Mr Joseph Phillott	10	Surgeon [honorary]
John Horton Esq.	9	Apothecary; Justice of Bath 1794/96
Richard Atwood Esq.	5	Not known

Appendix G continued

	No. of attendances	*Occupation*
Mr Charles Crook	5	Apothecary
Revd Mr John Sibley	5	Rector of Walcot, Bath
Dr Henry Harington	4	Physician [honorary]; Justice of Bath 1794/96
Mr Henry Edward Howse	4	Draper, grocer and Stamp Office agent
George Ramsey Esq.	4	Not known
Winthrop Baldwin Esq.	3	Of the Royal Crescent, Bath
Dr William Falconer	3	Physician [honorary]
Revd Edward Armstrong	2	Clergyman
J.L. Boissier Esq.	2	Of Marlborough Buildings, Bath
Simon Crook Esq.	2	Apothecary
Revd Humphrey Sumner	2	Clergyman
Thomas Bowdler Esq.	1	Philanthropist; author; editor of *The Family Shakespeare*
Revd Samuel Griffith	1	Minister of the Margaret Chapel, Bath
Grenado Pigott Esq.	1	Of Marlborough Buildings, Bath
Revd Dr Francis Randolph	1	Minister of the Laura Chapel, Bath
John Symons	1	Surgeon; Mayor of Bath from autumn 1795
1800/01		
Charles Phillott Esq.	33	Apothecary and banker; Justice of Bath 1799/1801 [treasurer]
Ven. Dr James Phillott	19	Rector and Archdeacon of Bath; vicar of Widcombe and Lyncombe
Thomas West Esq.	19	Apothecary

William Dawson Esq.	11	Master of Ceremonies
Samuel Howse Esq.	11	Wine merchant
George Chapman Esq.	9	Linen draper; Justice of Bath to autumn 1800
Henry Edward Howse Esq.	9	Draper, grocer and Stamp Office agent
John Morris Esq.	8	Attorney
Morgan Nichols Esq.	7	Surgeon [honorary]
Joseph Phillott Esq.	7	Surgeon [honorary]
Dr William Falconer	6	Physician [honorary]
John Horton Esq.	5	Apothecary; Mayor of Bath to autumn 1800; Justice of Bath from autumn 1800
William Abraham Esq.	4	Grain merchant and/or banker
Richard Atwood Esq.	4	Not known
J.L. Boissier Esq.	4	Of Marlborough Buildings, Bath
Dr James Holman	4	Physician [honorary]
Gill Baddeley Esq.	3	Of Oxford Row, Bath
Thomas Barrow Esq.	2	Of Laura Place, Bath
Thomas Bowdler Esq.	1	Philanthropist; author; editor of *The Family Shakespeare*
Charles Crook Esq.	1	Apothecary
Simon Crook Esq.	1	Apothecary
Revd Dr John Gardiner	1	Minister of the Octagon Chapel, Bath
Dr Henry Harington	1	Physician; Justice of Bath 1799/1801 [treasurer]
Revd Mr John Sibley	1	Rector of Walcot, Bath
1805/06		
Charles Phillott Esq.	35	Apothecary and banker; Justice of Bath to autumn 1805; Mayor of Bath from autumn 1805 [treasurer]

	No. of attendances	*Occupation*
Samuel Howse Esq.	18	Wine merchant
Dr William Perry	10	Physician
Ven. Dr James Phillott	9	Rector and Archdeacon of Bath; vicar of Widcombe and Lyncombe
J.L. Boissier Esq.	6	Of Marlborough Buildings, Bath
Mr Henry Knight	6	Tea dealer
Charles Crook Esq.	4	Apothecary
John Morris Esq.	4	Attorney
Revd Mr John Sibley	3	Rector of Walcot, Bath
Dr William Falconer	2	Physician [honorary]
Revd Dr John Gardiner	2	Minister of the Octagon Chapel, Bath
Joseph Phillott Esq.	2	Surgeon [honorary]
George Simon Crook Esq.	2	Apothecary
George Chapman Esq.	1	Linen draper
Philip George Esq.	1	Attorney; Town Clerk of Bath
Henry Edward Howse Esq.	1	Draper, grocer and Stamp Office agent
Revd Dr Francis Randolph	1	Minister of the Laura Chapel, Bath
Thomas West Esq.	1	Apothecary
1810/11		
Edmund Anderdon Esq.	37	Apothecary
Charles Phillott Esq.	32	Apothecary and banker; Justice of Bath 1809/11 [treasurer]

Revd Joseph Hunter	25	Presbyterian minister
John Kitson Esq.	25	Apothecary
Johnson Phillott Esq.	23	Banker
Robert Moody Esq.	16	Truss-maker and surgical mechanist
Revd Robert Jacomb	12	Clergyman
George Kitson Esq.	8	Surgeon
Samuel Howse Esq.	7	Wine merchant
Philip George Esq.	6	Attorney; Town Clerk of Bath
Ven. Dr James Phillott	4	Rector and Archdeacon of Bath; vicar of Widcombe and Lyncombe
Eleazer Pickwick Esq.	3	Coach proprietor
Dr John Ford Davis	2	Physician
Henry Knight Esq.	2	Tea dealer
Revd Mr John Sibley	2	Rector of Walcot, Bath
Wyndham Goodden Esq.	1	Barrister
Dr Henry Harington	1	Physician; Justice of Bath 1809/11 [treasurer]
Morgan Nichols Esq.	1	Surgeon [honorary]
Joseph Phillott Esq.	1	Surgeon [honorary]
1815/16		
Edmund Anderdon Esq.	41	Apothecary; Justice of Bath from autumn 1815
John Kitson Esq.	36	Apothecary
Charles Phillott Esq.	36	Apothecary and banker; Mayor of Bath to autumn 1815; Justice of Bath from autumn 1815 [treasurer]
Johnson Phillott Esq.	20	Banker
Noah Chivers Esq.	14	Of Axford Buildings, Bath
Henry Edward Howse Esq.	11	Draper, grocer and Stamp Office agent

Appendix G continued

	No. of attendances	*Occupation*
Mr John Knight	8	Chemist and druggist
Philip George Esq.	6	Attorney; Town Clerk of Bath
Charles Crook Esq.	5	Apothecary; Justice of Bath 1814/16
Revd Josiah Thomas	4	Minister of Christ Church, Bath
Dr John Ford Davis	3	Physician
Philip George Esq. jun.	1	Attorney
Wyndham Goodden Esq.	1	Barrister
Henry Knight Esq.	1	Tea dealer
Robert Moody Esq.	1	Truss-maker and surgical mechanist
1820/21		
Edmund Anderdon Esq.	35	Apothecary; Justice of Bath 1819/21
Mr Henry Howse jun.	33	Not known
Charles Phillott Esq.	25	Apothecary and banker; Justice of Bath to autumn 1820 [treasurer]
Henry Edward Howse Esq.	18	Draper, grocer and Stamp Office agent
Revd William Marshall	18	Curate of Bath Abbey
James Sloper Esq.	14	Apothecary
John Kitson Esq.	11	Apothecary; Justice of Bath 1819/21
George Lye Esq.	11	Of North Parade, Bath
Revd Thomas Falconer	8	Clergyman
Noah Chivers Esq.	5	Of Axford Buildings, Bath

Joseph Phillott Esq.	3	Surgeon; Justice of Bath 1819/21
Dr John Ford Davis	2	Physician [honorary]
Revd Thomas Wilkins	2	Rector of Charlecombe; vicar of Weston; master of the Grammar School, Bath
Dr Edward Barlow	1	Physician [honorary]
Charles Crook Esq.	1	Apothecary; Justice of Bath 1819/21
1825/26		
Edmund Anderdon Esq.	41	Apothecary; Mayor of Bath to autumn 1825; Justice of Bath from Autumn 1825 [treasurer]
Revd Thomas Falconer	34	Clergyman
Revd Joseph Hunter	28	Presbyterian minister
Mr Henry Howse jun.	24	Not known
Revd William Marshall	19	Curate of Bath Abbey
Revd Thomas Broadhurst	15	Minister of the Unitarian Chapel, Bath; boarding school master
James Sloper Esq.	9	Apothecary
Henry Edward Howse Esq.	6	Draper, grocer and Stamp Office agent
Joseph Phillott Esq.	5	Surgeon; Justice of Bath 1824/26
Charles Phillott Esq.	3	Apothecary and banker; Justice of Bath 1824/26
John Knight Esq.	2	Chemist and druggist
Dr James Muttlebury	2	Physician [honorary]
Dr Edward Barlow	1	Physician [honorary]
Dr John Ford Davis	1	Physician [honorary]
Revd Dr John Gardiner	1	Minister of the Octagon Chapel, Bath
Johnson Phillott Esq.	1	Banker [treasurer]
Thomas Thackeray Esq.	1	Of Burlington Street, Bath

	No. of attendances	*Occupation*
1830/31		
William Basnet Esq.	36	Of Cran Hill Villa, Weston Road, Bath
M.T. Langton Esq.	33	Of South Parade, Bath
Captain W.J. Lye RN	32	Of North Parade, Bath
Johnson Phillott Esq.	29	Banker [treasurer]
Revd William Marshall	27	Curate of Bath Abbey
Revd Joseph Hunter	22	Presbyterian minister
Joseph Barrat Esq.	18	Ran a circulating library, and religious and moral tract warehouse; also sold proprietary medicines
B.L. Lye Esq.	17	Of Seymour Street, Bath
Revd Thomas Broadhurst	16	Minister of the Unitarian Chapel, Bath; boarding school master
Sir Orford Gordon Bart	14	Of Pulteney Street, Bath
Walter Capper Esq.	11	Of Green Park Buildings, Bath [?]; *Charles* Capper was a consulting engineer in Birmingham, who advised on the refurbishment of the Hospital
Revd E.J. Crawley	11	Clergyman
F.H. Falkner Esq.	9	Surgeon [?]
Dr John Ford Davis	5	Physician [honorary]; Mayor of Bath from autumn 1830
John Davis Esq.	4	Not known
Dr Charles Henry Parry	3	Physician
Richard Francis George Esq.	2	Surgeon [honorary]

Richard Shuttleworth Crutwell Esq.	1	Printer, bookseller and publisher
Peter Marriott Esq.	1	Surgeon [?]

Notes:

1. Where no occupational details are available, residential information is given.
2. Identities which are uncertain are followed by a question mark.
3. Mayors and justices of Bath are only indicated where they attended the weekly committee during their periods of office. Whereas the Hospital's year began on the 1 May, the Corporation's year began on a variable date in the Autumn.
4. Paid staff, honorary physicians and surgeons, and office holders are indicated in brackets.
5. I am grateful to Trevor Fawcett for his help in tracing these identities.

Principal sources: 12 Geo. II, pp. 572–3; *Annual Reports*; Minute Books; Bath Corporation Minute Book; *Bath Journal*; *Improved Bath Guide*; Collinson, *Somerset*; *DNB*; Sedgwick, *The House of Commons 1715–1754*, vol. 1: *Introductory Survey, Constituencies, Members A–D*; Sedgwick, *The House of Commons 1715–1754*, vol. 2: *Members E–Y*; Namier and Brooke, *The House of Commons 1754–1790*, vol. 2: *Members A–J*; Namier and Brooke, *The House of Commons 1754–1790*, vol. 3: *Members K–Y*; *The Clerical Guide or Ecclesiastical Directory*, 2nd edn (London: F.C. and J. Rivington, 1822); *Fasti Ecclesiae Anglicanae 1541–1857: Bath and Wells Diocese*, compiled by Joyce M. Horn and Derrick Sherwin Bailey (London: Institute of Historical Research, 1979); *Robbins' Bath Directory*; *The New Bath Directory* [1805]; *The New Bath Directory for the Year 1809* (Bath: J. Browne, 1809); *The New Bath Directory* (Bath: Wood and Cunningham, 1812); *Gye's Bath Directory*; *Keene's Improved Bath Directory* (Bath: John and James Keene, 1824); *Bath Directory* (Bath: John and James Keene, 1826); *Keene's Bath Directory* [1829]; P.S. Brown, 'The Vendors of Medicines Advertised in Eighteenth-Century Bath Newspapers', *Medical History*, **19** (1975); Trevor Fawcett, 'Eighteenth-Century Shops and the Luxury Trade', *Bath History*, **3** (1990); Fletcher and Harris, 'Pharmacy in Bath'; Hembry, *English Spa*; Jenkins, 'A History of the Proprietary Chapels of Bath'; J.F. Meehan, *Famous Houses of Bath and District* (Bath: B. and J.F. Meehan, 1901); Meehan, *More Famous Houses of Bath and District*; Peach, *Historic Houses in Bath*; Thomas, 'The Phillotts of Bath'.

Appendix H Bath General Hospital: the seasonal attendance of governors at weekly committees, 1742–1830

Year	*Month*	*Total attendances*	*Esquires attendances*	*Gentlemen attendances*
1742/43	May	81	12	36
	June	52	9	21
	July	45	4	20
	August	35	2	12
	September	46	5	17
	October	42	3	19
	November	38	2	13
	December	55	8	25
	January	51	4	22
	February	36	—	17
	March	50	6	16
	April	45	8	24
	Total	576	63	242
1745/46	May	60	12	20
	June	32	4	16
	July	36	3	16
	August	25	2	8
	September	28	1	13
	October	33	3	12
	November	38	4	19
	December	30	4	7
	January	28	2	13
	February	16	3	7
	March	19	2	8
	April	35	3	14
	Total	380	43	153
1750/51	May	49	—	23
	June	35	—	15
	July	24	—	15
	August	27	—	13
	September	35	1	15
	October	51	2	28
	November	35	—	18
	December	45	—	22
	January	46	—	25
	February	31	—	14

Appendix H continued

Year	*Month*	*Total attendances*	*Esquires attendances*	*Gentlemen attendances*
	March	37	1	20
	April	41	1	23
	Total	456	5	231
1755/56	May	32	—	19
	June	24	—	9
	July	16	—	6
	August	15	—	7
	September	20	—	10
	October	35	—	20
	November	28	—	16
	December	44	1	21
	January	22	1	10
	February	19	—	11
	March	36	2	17
	April	31	3	12
	Total	322	7	158
1760/61	May	18	3	11
	June	28	4	18
	July	21	3	12
	August	19	3	9
	September	19	3	11
	October	33	6	17
	November	29	—	19
	December	23	—	14
	January	17	—	13
	February	18	—	11
	March	24	1	14
	April	38	3	24
	Total	287	26	173
1765/66	May	33	4	17
	June	25	2	16
	July	25	7	14
	August	25	7	15
	September	23	7	13
	October	32	10	18
	November	30	6	18

Appendix H continued

Year	*Month*	*Total attendances*	*Esquires attendances*	*Gentlemen attendances*
	December	17	2	12
	January	23	5	13
	February	27	4	18
	March	25	3	13
	April	29	6	16
	Total	314	63	183
1770/71	May	33	9	20
	June	28	5	18
	July	12	1	9
	August	18	3	13
	September	21	3	14
	October	30	5	21
	November	23	8	14
	December	17	4	12
	January	18	1	14
	February	21	2	18
	March	20	5	13
	April	35	9	23
	Total	276	55	189
1775/76	May	58	27	22
	June	26	3	17
	July	16	5	8
	August	27	7	17
	September	21	2	17
	October	28	8	17
	November	26	3	17
	December	34	5	19
	January	24	1	18
	February	24	1	21
	March	20	4	14
	April	30	7	19
	Total	334	73	206
1780/81	May	39	7	24
	June	27	5	19
	July	17	2	14
	August	28	4	19

Appendix H continued

Year	*Month*	*Total attendances*	*Esquires attendances*	*Gentlemen attendances*
	September	35	7	22
	October	27	3	20
	November	30	8	17
	December	34	9	19
	January	21	4	12
	February	28	6	17
	March	38	11	21
	April	33	11	15
	Total	357	77	219
1785/86	May	31	15	11
	June	36	6	20
	July	16	4	11
	August	19	4	11
	September	18	2	11
	October	18	2	11
	November	34	8	11
	December	29	11	11
	January	13	2	8
	February	23	4	14
	March	34	7	13
	April	25	6	14
	Total	296	71	146
1790/91	May	27	5	11
	June	29	7	16
	July	14	3	7
	August	17	2	9
	September	25	3	13
	October	21	3	11
	November	23	4	10
	December	39	12	10
	January	11	5	3
	February	34	6	10
	March	42	11	15
	April	32	7	11
	Total	314	68	126

Appendix H continued

Year	*Month*	*Total attendances*	*Esquires attendances*	*Gentlemen attendances*
1795/96	May	13	1	7
	June	14	2	6
	July	22	3	11
	August	10	1	6
	September	13	2	8
	October	8	2	4
	November	27	5	14
	December	24	1	11
	January	25	7	12
	February	30	6	14
	March	26	4	13
	April	24	5	10
	Total	236	39	116
1800/01	May	15	13	—
	June	25	22	—
	July	9	7	—
	August	5	5	—
	September	8	8	—
	October	12	11	—
	November	13	9	—
	December	18	14	—
	January	13	10	—
	February	10	8	—
	March	27	21	—
	April	16	11	—
	Total	171	139	—
1805/06	May	10	7	—
	June	10	6	—
	July	9	6	—
	August	7	6	—
	September	6	5	—
	October	8	5	1
	November	12	9	—
	December	7	4	—
	January	11	9	1
	February	10	7	2
	March	9	5	1

Appendix H continued

Year	*Month*	*Total attendances*	*Esquires attendances*	*Gentlemen attendances*
	April	9	6	1
	Total	108	75	6
1810/11	May	32	24	—
	June	26	19	—
	July	13	10	—
	August	23	18	—
	September	26	21	—
	October	19	14	—
	November	11	9	—
	December	8	6	—
	January	15	13	—
	February	7	6	—
	March	12	9	—
	April	16	13	—
	Total	208	162	—
1815/16	May	25	21	1
	June	16	15	—
	July	10	9	1
	August	13	13	—
	September	14	14	—
	October	9	8	1
	November	26	23	2
	December	18	17	1
	January	11	11	—
	February	13	12	1
	March	15	15	—
	April	18	15	1
	Total	188	173	8
1820/21	May	21	14	3
	June	21	17	3
	July	11	7	2
	August	11	7	2
	September	16	10	2
	October	11	7	2
	November	23	16	3
	December	17	12	4

Appendix H concluded

Year	*Month*	*Total attendances*	*Esquires attendances*	*Gentlemen attendances*
	January	13	10	2
	February	11	6	2
	March	12	7	4
	April	20	10	4
	Total	187	123	33
1825/26	May	15	6	2
	June	17	6	2
	July	8	3	2
	August	15	3	4
	September	16	4	2
	October	14	4	2
	November	17	8	1
	December	15	7	1
	January	9	3	—
	February	17	4	2
	March	36	15	4
	April	14	5	2
	Total	193	68	24
1830/31	May	22	14	—
	June	29	15	—
	July	11	9	—
	August	27	15	—
	September	31	14	—
	October	21	12	—
	November	32	14	—
	December	30	15	—
	January	22	14	—
	February	19	11	—
	March	21	12	—
	April	26	16	—
	Total	291	161	—

Source: Minute Books.

Appendix I Bath General Hospital: the geographical origins of governors not permanently resident in the immediate vicinity of the city, 1760/61 and 1765/66

Governor	*Origin*
Jacob Bosanquet Esq.	Merchant in London
Thomas Carew Esq.	Of Croakham
Awnsham Churchill Esq.	Of Dorsetshire
William Colbourne Esq.	Of Highgate
Thomas Deeke Esq.	Of Timsbury
Peter Delme Esq.	Of Wiltshire
Mr Robert Dingley	Merchant in London
Francis Fauquier Esq.	Governor of the Island of Virginia
Revd Dr Freind	Canon of Christ-Church, Oxford
Richard Frewin MD	Of Oxford
William Gardiner Esq.	Of Richmond
George Heathcote Esq.	Of Hereford
Henry Hoare Esq.	Of London
Frazer Honeywood Esq.	Of London
Richard Luther Esq.	Of Essex
Smart Lethieullier	Of Essex
Thomas Master Esq.	Of Cirencester
Hon. Robert Needham	Of Stoke in Hampshire
William Oliver MD jun.	Of London
Thomas Prowse Esq.	Of Somersetshire
Joseph Percival Esq.	Of Bristol
George Randolf MD	Of Bristol
Robert Smith Esq.	Of Bristol
George Scott Esq. MA FRS	Of Essex
Sir Robert Thockmorton Bart	Of Berkshire
Sir William Wentworth Bart	Of Yorkshire

Source: *Annual Reports*, 1760/61 and 1765/66.

Appendix J Bath General Hospital: the political affiliations of governors, 1739/42–1830

(a) 1739/42: Robert Walpole (1721–42)

Name	*Constituency*	*Affiliations*
Ralph Allen Esq.		Whig
Duke of Beaufort		Tory
Thomas Carew Esq.	Minehead, 1739–47	Tory
Earl of Chesterfield		Walpole opposition
John Codrington Esq.	Bath, 1734–41	Tory
Thomas Coster Esq.	Bristol, 1734–39	Tory
Henry Hoare Esq.	Salisbury, 1734–41	Tory
Samuel Holden Esq.	East Looe, 1735–40	Walpole administration; Chairman of the Dissenting Deputies Committee
Thomas Strangeways Horner Esq.	Somerset, 1727–41	Tory
Sir John Jennings		Whig
Dr Richard Mead		Whig
Robert Needham Esq.	Old Sarum, 1734–41	Walpole administration
Dr William Oliver		Whig
Hon. Arthur Onslow	Surrey, 1727–61	Speaker of the House of Commons
Sir Philip Parker Long		Whig
Viscount Palmerston	Bossiney, 1734–41 Weobley, 1741–47	Walpole administration
Thomas Prowse Esq.	Somerset, 1740–67	Moderate Tory
Hon. William Pulteney	Middlesex, 1734–42	Walpole opposition

Sir Thomas Lumley Saunderson	Lincolnshire, 1727–40	Walpole opposition
Hon. Edward Southwell	Bristol, 1739–54	Walpole opposition
Lord Sundon	Westminster, 1727–41 Plympton, 1742–47	Walpole administration
Sir William Thompson		Whig
Lt Gen. George Wade	Bath, 1722–48	Walpole administration
Sir William Wentworth	Malton, 1731–41	Walpole administration
William Woolaston Esq.	Ipswich, 1733–41	Walpole administration
Sir William Wyndham	Somerset, 1710–40	Tory

(b) 1755/56: Duke of Newcastle (1754–56)

Ralph Allen Esq.		Whig
Lord George Anson		Newcastle administration
Hon. William Bateman		Commissioner of the Navy, 1756–61
Earl of Bath [formerly William Pulteney]		Whig
Duke of Beaufort		Tory
Duke of Bedford		Whig
Sir Walter Blackett	Newcastle-upon-Tyne, 1734–77	Tory
Thomas Carew Esq.		Tory
Earl of Chesterfield		Whig
Duke of Devonshire		Whig
Lord Viscount Dupplin	Cambridge, 1741–58	Newcastle administration
George Heathcote Esq.		Whig
Henry Hoare Esq.		Tory
Frazier Honeywood Esq.		Whig

Appendix J continued

(b) 1755/56: Duke of Newcastle (1754–56) continued

Name	*Constituency*	*Affiliations*
Field-Marshall Ligonier	Bath, 1748–63	
Duke of Marlborough		Whig
Thomas Master Esq.		Tory
Hon. Arthur Onslow	Surrey, 1727–61	Speaker of the House of Commons
Hon. William Pitt	Aldborough, 1754–56; Okehampton, 1756–57	Whig; Newcastle administration > opposition
Thomas Prowse Esq.	Somerset, 1740–67	Moderate Tory
Marquis of Rockingham		Whig
Humphry Sydenham Esq.		Tory
Sir William Wentworth		Whig
William Woolaston Esq.		Whig
(c) 1770/71: Lord North (1770–82)		
Hon. William Bateman		Commissioner of the Navy, 1756–61
Duke of Bedford		Whig
Sir Walter Blackett	Newcastle upon Tyne, 1734–77	Tory
Lord Camden		North opposition
Marquis of Carnarvon		North administration
Earl of Chatham [formerly William Pitt]		North opposition
Earl of Chesterfield		Whig

Lord Clive	Shrewsbury, 1761–74	North opposition
Richard Hippisley Coxe Esq.	Somerset, 1768–84	North opposition
Sir Peter Denis		Whig
Samuel Eyre Esq.		Independent
Henry Hoare Esq.		Tory
Anthony James Keck Esq.	Newton, 1768–80	North opposition
Sir Charles Kemys Tynte	Somerset, 1747–74	Tory
Earl Kinnoul [formerly Lord Viscount Dupplin]		Whig
Peter Legh Esq.	Newton, 1743–74	North opposition
Duke of Newcastle		Whig
Duke of Northington [formerly Robert Henley]		Whig
Marquis of Rockingham		Whig
Sir John Sebright	Bath, 1763–74	North administration
John Smith Esq.	Bath, 1766–75	North administration

(d) 1785/86: William Pitt the Younger, first period (1783–1801)

Sir Charles Barrow	Gloucester, 1751–89	Pitt opposition
Lord Camden		Whig
Henry Hoare Esq.		Tory
John Hunter Esq.	Leominster, 1784–97	Pitt administration
Earl Kinnoul [formerly Lord Viscount Dupplin]		Whig
Sir James Tylney Long	Devizes, 1780–88	Pitt administration
Paul Methuen Esq.	Great Bedwyn, 1774–81	North opposition [up to 1781]

(d) 1785/86: William Pitt the Younger, first period (1783–1801) continued

Name	*Constituency*	*Affiliations*
Paul Cobb Methuen Esq.	Great Bedwyn, 1781–84	Independent [up to 1784]
Sir John Miller	Newport, 1784–90	Independent
Abel Moysey Esq.	Bath, 1774–90	Pitt opposition
Lord Constantine Mulgrave	Newark, 1784–90	Pitt administration
Duke of Newcastle		Whig [?]
Earl Nugent	St. Mawes, 1774–84	Pitt administration [up to 1784]
Edward Phelips Esq.	Somerset, 1784–92	Pitt administration
Rt Hon. John Jeffreys Pratt	Bath, 1780–94	Pitt administration
Sir John Trevelyan	Somerset, 1780–96	Pitt administration
Sir Charles Kemys Tynte		Tory
Lord Vernon	Glamorgan, 1768–80	North opposition [up to 1780]
(e) 1800/01: William Pitt the Younger, second period – after Whig realignment (1783–1801)		
Sir Richard Pepper Arden	Bath, 1794–1801	Pitt administration [Master of the Rolls]
Marquis of Bath [formerly Hon. Thomas Thynne]	Bath, 1790–96	Pitt administration [up to 1796]
Francis John Brown Esq.	Dorset, 1784–1806	Independent

Earl Camden [formerly Rt Hon. John Jeffreys Pratt]		Pitt administration
Earl Eardley	Wallingford, 1796–1802	Pitt administration
Sir Benjamin Hobhouse	Bletchingey, 1797–1802	Pitt administration
William Gore Langton Esq.	Somerset, 1795–1807	Whig
Duke of Northumberland		Pitt opposition
Sir Matthew White Ridley	Newcastle upon Tyne, 1774–1812	Independent
Marquis of Stafford		Whig
Lord John Thynne	Bath, 1796–1832	Tory

Notes:
1. Both the constituency and the affiliation relate to the sample year.
2. A question mark indicates that the political affiliation of the governor is uncertain.
3. Governors who were MPs for Bath or Somerset have been included irrespective of whether their political affiliation has been ascertained.

Principal sources: 12 Geo. II, pp. 572–3; *Annual Reports*; *DNB*; Sedgwick, *The House of Commons 1715–1754*, vol. 1: *Introductory Survey, Constituencies and Members A–D*; Sedgwick, *The House of Commons 1715–1754*, vol. 2: *Members E–Y*; Namier and Brooke, *The House of Commons 1754–1790*, vol. 2: *Members A–J*; Namier and Brooke, *The House of Commons 1754–1790*, vol. 3: *Members K–Y*; Stenton, *Who's Who of British Members of Parliament*, vol. 1: *1832–1885*; Cannon, 'Bath Politics'; David Harley, 'Religious and Professional Interests in Northern Spa Literature, 1625–1775', *Bulletin of the Society for the Social History of Medicine*, 35 (1984); Hembry, *English Spa*; McIntyre, 'Towns'; Meehan, *More Famous Houses of Bath and District*; Peach, *Ralph Allen*.

Appendix K Bath General Hospital: the dismissal of officers and servants, 1742–1831

Post	*Name*	*Date*	*Reason*
Steward	Noah Elliot	6 Jan. 1773	Corruption
Matron	Margaret Morris	3 Mar. 1773	‘improper conduct’
	—	10 June 1778	—
Cook	Ann Jordan	25 Apr. 1744	—
	Elizabeth Goodnaugh	1 July 1829	‘incapable’
	—	14 Apr. 1830	‘misconduct’
Laundry maid/house maid	Mary Londy	20 May 1778	—
	Alice Gray	8 Mar. 1786	—
Baker/brewer	Benjamin Silcox	10 Oct. 1775	‘misbehaviour’
	James Pullen	26 May 1779	—
	Thomas Biggs	13 Dec. 1826	‘neglect of duty’
Porter	—	13 Jan. 1790	—
	—	22 Feb. 1826	‘misconduct’
	Samuel Spear	18 May 1830	Asked patient’s friends for alcohol
Laboratory man/boy	Richard Turner	15 Jan. 1783	‘ill behaviour’
	Henry Lamb	6 Jan. 1830	‘extremely improper conduct’
Nurse	Macklinton	14 Oct. 1742	‘misbehaviour’
	Eccles	31 Dec. 1742	—
	Dagger	28 Jan. 1746/7	—
	Russell	9 Mar. 1747/8	‘misbehaviour’
	Grey	13 Mar. 1748/9	‘taking money of the patients’
	Haward	13 Mar. 1748/9	‘taking money of the patients’
	Ann Wiltshire	24 Jan. 1753	—
	Hester Walters	6 Oct. 1756	‘disguised in liquor’
	Vezey	14 Feb. 1781	‘insolent behaviour to the matron’
	Reeves	3 Dec. 1783	‘disguised in liquor’

	Hitcock	29 Sept. 1784	'permitting spiritous liquors to be drank in her ward'
	Morris	30 July 1794	'having taken money of the patients'
	Gay	2 Mar. 1796	—
	Porter	4 June 1800	'pawned ten blankets'
	Jane Whittern	30 Nov. 1803	'having taken money from the patients'
	Wakefield	27 Dec. 1826	'neglect of duty'
	Davey	19 Dec. 1827	'misconduct'
	Pitman	19 Dec. 1827	'misconduct'
	Edwards	17 Feb. 1830	Allowing provisions to be brought into the Hospital without the permission of the physicians and surgeons
	White	16 June 1830	Staying out late
	Morris	14 Apr. 1831	'improper language'
Chairman	Rudman	29 July 1742	'misbehaviour in the House'
	Benjamin Burges	30 May 1744	—
	Thomas Peirce	15 June 1750	—
	Joseph Bull	13 Apr. 1768	—
	Henry Stevens	4 June 1777	—
	Richard Glanfield	15 Sept. 1779	—
	Samuel Stockwell	12 Nov. 1783	—
	Henry Vincent	26 Jan. 1803	'misbehaviour'
	William Holbrook	22 June 1803	'misconduct'
	Samuel Lewis	17 July 1816	'misbehaviour'
	Samuel Bowman	30 Dec. 1818	'drunkenness and other misconduct'
	James Pike	5 Sept. 1827	'abusive language and drunkenness'
	James Holman	19 Dec. 1827	'neglect of duty'
	Daniel Martin	21 May 1828	'very improper conduct in neglecting his duty'
	William Russell	21 May 1828	'neglect of duty'

Source: Minute Books.

Bibliography

Manuscript sources

Spelling, punctuation and dates have been modernized.

Bath City Record Office

Royal National Hospital for Rheumatic Diseases (formerly Bath General Hospital)

1/1–1/17	Committee Minute Books, 16 February 1737–26 December 1833.
1/38	Copies of Letters, 1737–57 [Letter Book].
1/39	Folder of Letters and Other Items 1737 Onwards [Letter Folder]
1/40	House Visitors Book, 25 June 1742–16 November 1743 [House Visitors Book 1]
1/41	House Visitors Book, 28 March 1754–27 September 1759 [House Visitors Book 2]
1/42	Subcommittee Book, 5 November 1778–27 January 1823.
1/43	Rules and Duties of Staff 18th Century Onwards.
2/1	Ledger, 1737–60.
2/3	Journal, 1737–61.
2/4	House Incidents Book, 1742–57.
2/11	Benefactions of £50 and Upwards to 1883.
3/1	Admissions, 1742–52 [Admissions Register].
4/1	Casebook, 1750–58.
7/6	*Annual Reports*, 1738–1842.

Royal United Hospital (formerly Bath United Hospital)

RUH/1 Minute Book, June 1827–October 1832.

Bath Corporation

Minute Books, 1738–1830.

Somerset County Record Office

Bath Abbey

D/P/ba.ab Overseers Accounts, 1729–1831.
D/Pba.ab Vestry Minutes, 1819–84.

Acts of Parliament

12 Geo. II, *An Act for Establishing and Well Governing an Hospital or Infirmary in the City of Bath* (London: 1739).

19 Geo. III, *An Act More Effectually to Enable the President and Governors of the Hospital or Infirmary at Bath, Established by an Act, Passed in the Twelfth Year of the Reign of ... King George the Second ... to Take or Acquire, and Hold, Any Lands, Tenements, or Hereditaments, or Any Interest in Lands, Tenements, or Hereditaments, and Any Money or Personal Property, to be Laid Out in Lands, Tenements, or Hereditaments, Pursuant to Any Will, or Otherwise, to the Amount Limited in the Said Act* (London: 1779).

11 Geo. IV, *An Act for Altering and Amending an Act Passed in the Twelfth Year of the Reign of His Majesty King George the Second ... ; and for Constructing Baths Therein, and Supplying the Same with Water from the Hot Baths in the Said City* (London: 1830).

Newspapers and periodicals

Bath Chronicle.
Bath Journal.
Gentleman's Magazine.
London Evening Post.
London Magazine.
Public Ledger.
Spectator.

Printed sources and unpublished theses

Abbott, M. *Family Ties: English Families 1540–1920* (London: Routledge, 1993).

Abel-Smith, B., *The Hospitals 1800–1948: A Study in Social Administration in England and Wales* (London: Heinemann, 1964).

Addison, W., *English Spas* (London: Batsford, 1951).

An Address to the Governors of the Bath Hospital on the Propriety of Extending the Benefits of that Humane and Laudable Institution (Bath: R. Cruttwell, 1792).

Aikin, J., *Thoughts on Hospitals with a Letter to the Author by Thomas Percival* (London: Joseph Johnson, 1771).

Alumni Cantabrigienses: Part I to 1751, 4 vols (Cambridge: Cambridge University Press, 1922–27).

Alumni Cantabrigienses: Part II 1752–1900, 6 vols (Cambridge: Cambridge University Press, 1940–54).

Alumni Oxoniensis: The Members of the University of Oxford 1715–1886, 4 vols (London: Joseph Foster, 1888).

Andrew, D., *Philanthropy and Police: London Charity in the Eighteenth Century* (Princeton: Princeton University Press, 1989).

Andrew, D., 'On Reading Charity Sermons: Eighteenth-Century Anglican Solicitation and Exhortation', *Journal of Ecclesiastical History*, 43 (1992).

Anning, S.T., *The General Infirmary at Leeds*, 2 vols (Edinburgh: Livingstone, 1963–66), vol. 1: *The First Hundred Years 1767–1869* (1963).

Anstey, C., *The New Bath Guide*, ed. Gavin Turner, first pub. 1766, repr. (Bristol: Broadcast Books, 1994).

An Appeal to the Public ... Relating to the Proceedings of a Party of the Governors of the New General Hospital at Bath Against Mr Archibald Cleland (London and Bath: A. Dodd and W. Frederick, 1743).

Baly, M., 'The Care of the Sick Poor in Bath from the Late Eighteenth Century to the First Half of the Nineteenth Century' (unpublished and undated typescript, supplied by the author).

Barbeau, A., *Life and Letters at Bath in the Eighteenth Century* (London: William Heinemann, 1904).

Barber, W.J., *A History of Economic Thought* (Harmondsworth: Penguin Books, 1967).

Barlow, E., *An Essay on the Medicinal Efficacy and Employment of the Bath Waters* (Bath: Longman, Hurst, Rees, Orme and Brown, 1822).

Barnard, E.A.B., 'An Eighteenth-Century Worcestershire Doctor: William Baylies of Evesham, 1724–1787', *Transactions of the Worcestershire Archaeological Society*, 4 (1945).

Barrell, J., *The Political Theory of Painting from Reynolds to Hazlitt* (New Haven: Yale University Press, 1986).

Barrett, J., 'Spas and Seaside Resorts, 1660–1780', in *The Rise of the New Urban Society*, Open University Third Level Course, English Urban History 1500–1780, Units 13, 14, 15 and 16 (Milton Keynes: Open University Press, 1977).

Barry, J., 'Piety and the Patient: Medicine and Religion in Eighteenth-Century Bristol', in R. Porter (ed.), *Patients and Practioners: Lay Perceptions of Medicine in Pre-Industrial Society* (Cambridge: Cambridge University Press, 1985).

Barry, J., 'Bourgeois Collectivism? Urban Association and the Middling Sort', in J. Barry and C. Brooks (eds), *The Middling Sort of People: Culture, Society and Politics in England 1550–1800* (London: Macmillan, 1994).

Barry, J., 'Introduction', in J. Barry and C. Brooks (eds), *The Middling Sort of People: Culture, Society and Politics in England 1550–1800* (London: Macmillan, 1994).

The Bath and Bristol Guide; Or, The Tradesman's and Traveller's Pocket-Companion, 3rd edn (Bath: T. Boddely, 1755).

Bath Chronicle, *The Bath General or Hot Water Hospital* (Bath: H.E. Carrington, 1857).

Bath Directory (Bath: John and James Keene, 1826).

The Bath Eye Infirmary 1811 to 1948 (no place of publication, publisher or date).

[Bath General Infirmary], *Narrative of the Efficacy of the Bath Waters, in Various Kinds of Paralytic Disorders Admitted into the Bath Hospital* (Bath: R. Cruttwell, 1787).

[Bath General Infirmary], 'A Short Account of the Nature, Rise and Progress of the General Infirmary at Bath', in E. Bayly, *A Sermon Preached at the Abbey-Church at Bath* (Bath: Thomas Boddely, 1749).

[Bath General Infirmary], 'A Short Account of the Nature, Rise and Progress of the General Infirmary at Bath', in J. Dalton, *The Religious Use of the Visitation of Sickness* (Bath: Thomas Boddely, 1746).

[Bath General Infirmary], 'A Short Account of the Nature, Rise and Progress of the General Infirmary at Bath', in R. Leyborne, *Charity Conducive to God's Glory: A Sermon for the Benefit of the General Hospital, in Bath* (Bath: Thomas Bodely, 1754).

[Bath General Infirmary], 'A Short Account of the Nature, Rise and Progress of the General Infirmary at Bath', in R. Olive, *The Particular Excellence and True State of the Bath Infirmary* (Bristol: E. Farley, 1759).

[Bath General Infirmary], 'A Short Account of the Nature, Rise and Progress of the General Infirmary at Bath', in W. Warburton, *A Sermon Preached at the Abbey-Church at Bath* (London: J. Leake, 1742).

The Bath Infirmary for the Cure of Diseases of the Eye, Instituted November 1811: Fourth Annual Report, from January 1st, 1815, to January 1st, 1816 (Bath: Richard Cruttwell, 1816).

Bath: Official Guide Book 1986 (Bath: Bath City Council 1986).

Batty Shaw, A., *Norfolk and Norwich Medicine: A Retrospect* (Norwich: Norwich Medico-Chirurgical Society, 1992).

Baugh, D.A., 'Poverty, Protestantism and Political Economy: English Attitudes toward the Poor, 1660–1800', in S. Baxter (ed.), *England's Rise to Greatness 1660–1763* (Berkeley: University of California, 1983).

Baylies, W., *A Narrative of Facts Demonstrating the Actual Existence and True Cause of that Physical Confederacy in Bath made Known to the Public in the Printed Letters of Dr. Lucas and Dr. Oliver* (London: A. Millar, 1757).

Baylies, W., *Practical Reflections on the Uses and Abuses of Bath Waters* (London: A. Millar, 1757).

Baylies, W., *An Historical Account of the Rise, Progress and Management of the General Hospital or Infirmary in the City of Bath* (Bath: James Leake, 1758).

Bayly, E., *A Sermon Preached at the Abbey-Church at Bath* (Bath: Thomas Boddely, 1749).

Bebbington, D.W., *Evangelicalism in Modern Britain: A History from the 1730s to the 1980s* (London: Unwin Hyman, 1989).

Beckett, J.V., *The Aristocracy in England 1660–1914* (Oxford: Basil Blackwell, 1986).

Beier, A.L., *The Problem of the Poor in Tudor and Early Stuart England* (London: Methuen, 1983).

Bellers, J., 'An Essay Towards the Improvement of Physick', in G. Clarke (ed.), *John Bellers: His Life, Times and Writings* (London: Routledge and Kegan Paul, 1987).

Berg, M., *The Age of Manufactures: Industry, Innovation and Work in Britain 1700–1820* (London: Fontana Press, 1985).

Berry, A., 'Patterns of Patronage: English Voluntary Hospitals in the Eighteenth Century', (unpublished paper to the Annual Conference of the Society for the Social History of Medicine, University of Southampton, July 1993).

Berry, A., 'Patronage, Funding and the Hospital Patient, c.1750–1815' (unpublished doctoral thesis, University of Oxford, 1995).

Berry, C.J., *The Idea of Luxury: A Conceptual and Historical Investigation* (Cambridge: Cambridge University Press, 1994).

Bevan, H., *Records of the Salop Infirmary from the Commencement of the Charity to the Present Time* (Shrewsbury: Sandford and Howell, 1847).

Bindman, D., *Hogarth* (London: Thames and Hudson, 1981).

Birken, W., 'The Dissenting Tradition in English Medicine of the Seventeenth and Eighteenth Centuries', *Medical History*, 39 (1995).

Black, J., *The English Press in the Eighteenth Century* (London: Croom Helm, 1987).

Blackstone, W., *Commentaries on the Laws of England*, 4 vols (Oxford: Clarendon Press, 1765–69).

Blaug, M., *Economic Theory in Retrospect*, 3rd edn (Cambridge: Cambridge University Press, 1978).

Blizard, W., *Suggestions for the Improvement of Hospitals and Other Charitable Institutions* (London: C. Dilly: 1796).

Blomfield, J., *St George's 1733–1933* (London: Medici Society, 1933).

Borsay, P., *The English Urban Renaissance: Culture and Society in the Provincial Town 1660–1760* (Oxford: Clarendon Press, 1989).

Borsay, P., 'Image and Counter Image in Georgian Bath', *British Journal for Eighteenth-Century Studies*, **17** (1994).

Borsay, P., 'Health and leisure resorts, 1700–1840', in P. Clark (ed.), *The Cambridge Urban History of Britain*, 3 vols (Cambridge: Cambridge University Press, forthcoming), vol. 2.

Boyce, B., *The Benevolent Man: A Life of Ralph Allen of Bath* (Cambridge, MA: Harvard University Press, 1967).

Brewer, J., *The Sinews of Power: War, Money and the English State 1688–1783* (London: Unwin Hyman, 1989).

Brewer, J., *The Pleasures of the Imagination: English Culture in the Eighteenth Century* (London: HarperCollins, 1997).

A Brief Memoir of the Late Joseph Hunter FSA (Lincoln's Inn Fields, London: printed for private distribution only by John Edward Taylor, 1861).

Briggs, A., *The Age of Improvement 1783–1867* (London: Longmans, 1959).

'Britannicus', *Remarks on an Appeal to the Public by Mr Cleland* (London: J. Woon, W. Owen, E. Amey and W. Frederick, 1748).

British Medical Association, *The Book of Bath: Written for the Ninety Third Annual Meeting of the BMA held at Bath in July 1925* (Bath: BMA, 1925).

Brockbank, W., *Portrait of a Hospital 1752–1948 to Commemorate the Bi-Centenary of the Royal Infirmary, Manchester* (London: William Heinemann, 1952).

Brown, J., *On the Pursuit of False Pleasure, and the Mischiefs of Immoderate Gaming* (Bath: James Leake, 1750).

Brown, M. and Samuel, J., 'The Jews of Bath', *Bath History*, **1** (1986).

Brown, P.S., 'The Vendors of Medicines Advertised in Eighteenth-Century Bath Newspapers', *Medical History*, **19** (1975).

Buer, M.C., *Health, Wealth and Population in the Early Days of the Industrial Revolution* (London: George Routledge, 1926).

Bunce, J.T., *A History of the Birmingham General Hospital and Music Festivals* (Birmingham: Cornish Brothers, 1873).

Burke, P. 'Overture: The New History, its Past and its Future', in P. Burke (ed.), *New Perspectives on Historical Writing* (Cambridge: Polity Press, 1991).

Burnby, J.G.L., *A Study of the English Apothecary From 1660 to 1760*, *Medical History* Supplement No. 3 (London: Wellcome Institute for the History of Medicine, 1983).

Burns, T., *Erving Goffman* (London: Routledge, 1992).

Bynum, W.F., 'Health, Disease and Medical Care', in G.S. Rousseau and R. Porter (eds), *The Ferment of Knowledge: Studies in the Historiography of Eighteenth-Century Science* (Cambridge: Cambridge University Press, 1980).

Bynum, W.F., *Science and the Practice of Medicine in the Nineteenth Century* (Cambridge: Cambridge University Press, 1994).

Cameron, H.C., *Mr Guy's Hospital 1726–1948* (London: Longmans, Green and Co., 1954).

Cannadine, D., 'Conspicuous Consumption by the Landed Classes, 1790–1830', in M. Turner (ed.), *Malthus and his Time* (London: Macmillan, 1986).

Cannon, J., 'Bath Politics in the Eighteenth Century', *Somerset Archaeological and Natural History Society Proceedings*, 105 (1960–61).

Cannon, J., *Aristocratic Century: The Peerage of Eighteenth-Century England* (Cambridge: Cambridge University Press, 1984).

Cannon, J., *Samuel Johnson and the Politics of Hanoverian England* (Oxford: Clarendon Press, 1994).

Cantor, D., 'Contracting Cancer?: The Politics of Commissioned Histories', *Social History of Medicine*, 5 (1992).

Carlyle, T. 'The Signs of the Times', in *Thomas Carlyle: Selected Writings*, ed. Alan Shelston, repr. (Harmondsworth: Penguin Books, 1986).

Carré, J., 'The Lady and the Poor Man; or, the Philanthropist's Etiquette', in J. Carré (ed.), *The Crisis of Courtesy: Studies in the Conduct-Book in Britain 1600–1900* (Leiden: E.J. Brill, 1994).

Cartwright, F.F., *A Social History of Medicine* (London: Longman, 1977).

Cavallo, S., *Charity and Power in Early Modern Italy: Benefactors and their Motives in Turin 1541–1789* (Cambridge: Cambridge University Press, 1995).

Chandler, M., *The Description of Bath: A Poem Humbly Inscribed to Her Royal Highness the Princess Amelia, with Several Other Poems*, 6th edn (London and Bath: James Leake, 1744).

Charleton, R., *Three Tracts on the Bath Waters*, 2nd edn (Bath: R. Cruttwell, 1774).

Checkland, S., *British Public Policy 1776–1939: An Economic, Social and Political Perspective* (Cambridge: Cambridge University Press, 1983).

Cherry, S., 'The Role of a Provincial Hospital: The Norfolk and Norwich Hospital, 1771–1880', *Population Studies*, **26** (1972).

Cherry, S., 'The Role of English Provincial Voluntary General Hospitals in the Eighteenth and Nineteenth Centuries', 2 vols (unpublished doctoral thesis, University of East Anglia, 1976).

Cherry, S., *Medical Services and the Hospitals in Britain 1860–1939* (Cambridge: Cambridge University Press, 1996).

Christie, I.R., *British 'Non-Elite' MPs 1715–1820* (Oxford: Clarendon Press, 1995).

Clark, J.C.D., *English Society 1688–1932* (Cambridge: Cambridge University Press, 1985).

Clark, J.C.D., *Revolution and Rebellion: State and Society in England in the Seventeenth and Eighteenth Centuries* (Cambridge: Cambridge University Press, 1986).

Clark, J.C.D., 'On Hitting the Buffers: The Historiography of England's *ancien régime* – a Response', *Past and Present*, **117** (1987).

Clark, P., 'Migration in England during the Late Seventeenth and Early Eighteenth Centuries', *Past and Present*, 83 (1979).

Clark, P., *Sociability and Urbanity: Clubs and Societies in the Eighteenth-Century City*, Eighth H.J. Dyos Memorial Lecture (Leicester: University of Leicester Victorian Studies Centre, 1986).

Clark-Kennedy, A.E., *The London: A Study in the Voluntary Hospital System*, 2 vols (London: Pitman Medical, 1962), vol. 1: *1740–1840*.

Cleland, A., *A Full Vindication of Mr Cleland's Appeal to the Public* (Bath and London: W. Frederick and A. Dodd, 1744).

The Clergy List for 1864 (London: George Cox, 1864).

The Clerical Guide or Ecclesiastical Directory, 2nd edn (London: F.C. and J. Rivington, 1822).

Coley, N.G., 'Physicians and the Chemical Analysis of Mineral Waters in Eighteenth-Century England', *Medical History*, **26** (1982).

The Collective Reports of the Bath Penitentiary and Lock Hospital, from 1816 to 1824 (Bath: Wood, Cunningham and Smith, 1824).

Colley, L., *In Defiance of Oligarchy: The Tory Party 1714–1760* (Cambridge: Cambridge University Press, 1982).

Collinson, J., *The History and Antiquities of the County of Somerset*, introduced by Robert Dunning, 3 vols, first pub. 1791, repr. (Gloucester: Alan Sutton, 1983).

Cooter, R., *Surgery and Society in Peace and War: Orthopaedics and the Organization of Modern Medicine 1880–1948* (London: Macmillan, 1993).

Copeman, E., *Brief History of the Norfolk and Norwich Hospital* (Norwich: Charles Muskett, 1856).

Corfield, P.J., 'Class by Name and Number in Eighteenth-Century Britain', *History*, **72** (1987).

Corfield, P.J., *Power and the Professions in Britain 1700–1850* (London: Routledge, 1995).

Crafts, N.F.R., 'British Economic Growth, 1700–1831: A Review of the Evidence', *Economic History Review*, **36** (1983).

Cragg, G.R., *The Church and the Age of Reason 1648–1789*, repr. (Harmondsworth: Penguin Books, 1990).

Crawford, P., 'Sexual Knowledge in England, 1500–1750', in R. Porter and M. Teich (eds), *Sexual Knowledge, Sexual Science: The History of Attitudes to Sexuality* (Cambridge: Cambridge University Press, 1994).

Crofts, B. (ed.), *At Satan's Throne: The Story of Methodism in Bath over 250 Years* (Bristol: White Tree Books, 1990).

Croxson, B., 'An Economic Analysis of a Voluntary Hospital: The Foundation and Institutional Structure of the Middlesex Hospital, 1745–1900 (unpublished doctoral thesis, University of Cambridge, 1994).

Croxson, B., 'The Public and the Private Faces of Eighteenth-Century London Dispensary Charity', *Medical History*, **41** (1997).

Dabydeen, D., *Hogarth, Walpole and Commercial Britain* (London: Hansib Publications, 1987).

Dakers, W.S., *John Wood and His Times* (Bath: Mendip Press, 1954).

Dalton, J., *The Religious Use of the Visitation of Sickness* (Bath: Thomas Boddely, 1746).

Dalton, J., *A Sermon Preached ... Before the Governors of the Middlesex Hospital* (London: John Whiston, Benjamin White and S. Baker, 1751).

Dandeker, C., *Surveillance, Power and Modernity: Bureaucracy and Discipline from 1700 to the Present Day* (Cambridge: Polity Press, 1990).

Daunton, C., *The London Hospital Illustrated: 250 Years* (London: B.T. Batsford, 1990).

Daunton, M., *Progress and Poverty: An Economic and Social History of Britain 1700–1850* (Oxford: Oxford University Press, 1995).

Davidoff, L. and Hall, C., *Family Fortunes: Men and Women of the English Middle Class 1780–1850* (Chicago: University of Chicago Press, 1987).

Davies, T.G., *Deeds Not Words: A History of the Swansea General and Eye Hospital 1817–1948* (Cardiff: University of Wales Press, 1988).

Davis, G., 'Entertainments in Georgian Bath: Gambling and Vice', *Bath History*, **1** (1986).

Davis, G. and Bonsall, P., *Bath: A New History* (Keele: Keele University Press, 1996).

Davison, L., 'Experiments in the Social Regulation of Industry: Gin Legislation, 1729–1751', in L. Davison, T. Hitchcock, T. Keirn and R.B. Shoemaker (eds), *Stilling the Grumbling Hive: The Response to Social and Economic Problems in England 1689–1750* (Stroud: Alan Sutton, 1992).

D'Cruze, S., 'The Middling Sort in Eighteenth-Century Colchester: Independence, Social Relations and the Community Broker', in J. Barry and C. Brooks (eds), *The Middling Sort of People: Culture, Society and Politics in England 1550–1800* (London: Macmillan, 1994).

Dean, W., *Handel* (London: Macmillan, 1982).

Defoe, D., *A Tour Thro' the Whole Island of Great Britain*, 2 vols, 4th edn (London: 1748).

Defoe, D., *A Tour through the Whole Island of Great Britain*, eds G.D.H. Cole and D.C. Browning, 2 vols, first pub. 1724–26, repr. (London: Dent, 1962).

Dickinson, H.T., *Liberty and Property: Political Ideology in Eighteenth-Century Britain* (London: Methuen, 1977).

Dickinson, H.T., 'Radicals and Reformers in the Age Wilkes and Wyvill', in J. Black (ed.), *British Politics and Society from Walpole to Pitt 1742–1789* (London: Macmillan, 1990).

Dickinson, H.T., *The Politics of the People in Eighteenth-Century Britain* (London: Macmillan, 1995).

Dictionary of National Biography [DNB], 63 vols (London: Smith, Elder and Co., 1885–1900).

Dingwall, R., Rafferty, A.M. and Webster, C., *An Introduction to the Social History of Nursing* (London: Routledge, 1988).

The Diseases of Bath: A Satire (London, 1737).

Dobson, M.J., *Contours of Death and Disease in Early Modern England*, (Cambridge: Cambridge University Press, 1997).

Donnelly, M., *Managing the Mind: A Study of Medical Psychology in Early Nineteenth-Century Britain* (London: Tavistock, 1983).

Dunkeley, P., 'Paternalism, the Magistracy and Poor Relief in England, 1795–1834', *International Review of Social History*, **24** (1979).

Dunthorne, H., *The Enlightenment* (London: Historical Association, 1991).

Dupree, M.W., 'Family Care and Hospital Care: the "Sick Poor" in Nineteenth-Century Glasgow', *Social History of Medicine*, **6** (1993).

Eade, P., *The Norfolk and Norwich Hospital 1770–1900* (London: Jarrold and Sons, 1900).

Earle, P., 'The Middling Sort in London', in J. Barry and C. Brooks (eds), *The Middling Sort of People: Culture, Society and Politics in England 1550–1800* (London: Macmillan, 1994).

Eccles, A., *Obstetrics and Gynaecology in Tudor and Stuart England* (London: Croom Helm, 1982).

Elliott, P., *The Sociology of the Professions* (London: Macmillan, 1972).

Ellis, J., *The History of the Eastern Dispensary of Bath* (Bath: W. and F. Dawson, 1855).

An Essay or a Modest Proposal of a Way to Encrease the Number of People and Consequently the Strength of the Kingdom (1693).

Evans, E.J., *The Forging of the Modern State: Early Industrial Britain 1783–1870* (London: Longman, 1983).

Evans, R., *The Fabrication of Virtue: English Prison Architecture 1750–1840* (Cambridge: Cambridge University Press, 1982).

Falconer, R.W., *History of the Royal Mineral Water Hospital, Bath*, rev. A.B. Brabazon, first pub. 1860 (Bath: Charles Hallett, 1888).

Falconer, W., *An Essay on the Bath Waters* (London: T. Lowndes, 1770).

Falconer, W., *A Practical Dissertation on the Medicinal Effects of the Bath Waters* (Bath: R. Cruttwell, 1790).

Falconer, W., *An Account of the Use, Application and Success of the Bath Waters in Rheumatic Cases* (Bath: W. Myler, 1795).

Falconer, W., *A Dissertation on Ischias; or the Disease of the Hip-Joint* (London: T. Cadell and W. Davies, 1805).

Fasti Ecclesiae Anglicanae 1541–1857: Bath and Wells Diocese, compiled by J.M. Horn and D.S. Bailey (London: Institute of Historical Research, 1979).

Fawcett, T., 'Eighteenth-Century Shops and the Luxury Trade', *Bath History*, 3 (1990).

Fawcett, T., 'Selling the Bath Waters: Medical Propaganda at an Eighteenth-Century Spa', *Somerset Archaeology and Natural History*, 134 (1990).

Fawcett, T. (ed.), *Voices of Eighteenth-Century Bath: An Anthology* (Bath: Ruton, 1995).

Fawcett, T. and Bird, S., *Bath: History and Guide* (Stroud: Alan Sutton, 1994).

Fielding, H., *The History of Tom Jones*, ed. by R.P.C. Mutter (Harmondsworth: Penguin Books, 1966).

First Report of the Society for Bettering the Conditions and Increasing the Comforts of the Poor (London: 1797).

Fisher, R., *Edward Jenner 1749–1823* (London: André Deutsch, 1991).

Fissell, M.E, 'The Physic of Charity: Health and Welfare in the West

Country 1690–1834' (unpublished doctoral dissertation, University of Pennsylvania, 1988).

Fissell, M.E., 'The "Sick and Drooping Poor" in Eighteenth-Century Bristol and its Region', *Social History of Medicine*, 2 (1989).

Fissell, M.E., 'The Disappearance of the Patient's Narrative and the Invention of Hospital Medicine', in R. French and A. Wear (eds), *British Medicine in an Age of Reform* (London: Routledge, 1991).

Fissell, M.E., *Patients, Power and the Poor in Eighteenth-Century Bristol* (Cambridge: Cambridge University Press, 1991).

Fissell, M.E., 'Innocent and Honourable Bribes: Medical Manners in Eighteenth-Century Britain', in R. Baker, D. Porter and R. Porter (eds), *The Codification of Medical Morality: Historical and Philosophical Studies of the Formalization of Western Medical Morality in the Eighteenth and Nineteenth Centuries*, 2 vols (Dordrecht, Netherlands: Kluwer Academic, 1993), vol. 1: *Medical Ethics and Etiquette in the Eighteenth Century.*

Fletcher, G. and Harris, G.I., 'Pharmacy in Bath during the Regency Period', *Pharmaceutical Historian*, 1 (1970).

Ford, W.G., (ed.), *Some Notes for Visitors* (Bath: Abbey Church of St Peter and St Paul, November 1982).

Forty, A., 'The Modern Hospital in England and France: The Social and Medical Uses of Architecture', in A. King (ed.), *Buildings and Society: Essays on the Social Development of the Built Environment* (London: Routledge and Kegan Paul, 1980).

Fosbrooke, T., *An Original History of the City of Gloucester*, introduced by Peter Ripley, first pub. 1819 (Dursley: Alan Sutton, 1976).

Foucault, *The Birth of the Clinic: An Archaeology of Medical Perception*, trans. A.M. Sheridan (London: Routledge, 1973).

Foucault, M., 'Two Lectures', in C. Gordon (ed.), *Michel Foucault Power/Knowledge: Selected Interviews and Other Writings 1972–1977* (Brighton: Harvester Press, 1980).

Foucault, M., *The History of Sexuality*, trans. R. Hurley, 3 vols (Harmondsworth: Penguin Books, 1981).

Freeman, H.W., *The Thermal Baths of Bath: Their History, Literature, Medical and Surgical Uses and Effects* (London: Hamilton, Adams and Co., and Bath: Charles Hallett, 1888).

Frith, B., *The Story of Gloucester's Infirmary* (Gloucester: Gloucester, Stroud and the Forest Hospital Management Committee, 1961).

Frizelle, E.R. and Martin, J.D., *The Leicester Royal Infirmary 1771–1971* (Leicester: Leicester No. 1 Hospital Management Committee, 1971).

Gascoigne, J., 'Anglican Latitudinarianism and Political Radicalism in the Late Eighteenth Century', *History*, 71 (1986).

Gay, P., *The Enlightenment: An Interpretation – the Rise of Modern Paganism* (London: Weidenfeld and Nicolson, 1967).

Gibbes, G.S., *A Second Treatise on the Bath Waters* (Bath: W. Meyler, 1803).

Gibson, A.G., *The Radcliffe Infirmary* (Oxford: Oxford University Press, 1926).

Gilbert, A.D., *Religion and Society in Industrial England: Church, Chapel and Social Change 1740–1914* (London: Longman, 1976).

Glaser, S., *The Spirit of Enquiry: Caleb Hillier Parry, MD. FRS* (Stroud: Alan Sutton, 1995).

Goffman, E., *Asylums: Essays on the Social Situation of Mental Patients and Other Inmates* (London: Pelican Books, 1968).

Gorsky, M., 'Charity, Mutuality and Philanthropy: Voluntary Provision in Bristol 1800–1870', (unpublished doctoral thesis, University of Bristol, 1995).

Gorsky, M., 'Medicine and Charity: Some Evidence from Bristol Infirmary, 1780–1870' (unpublished paper, Hospital Finances Seminar, Wellcome Institute for the History of Medicine, London, January 1995).

Granshaw, L., 'The Rise of the Modern Hospital in Britain', in A. Wear (ed.), *Medicine in Society: Historical Essays* (Cambridge: Cambridge University Press, 1992).

Granville, A.B., *Spas of England and Principal Sea-Bathing Places*, 2 vols, first pub. 1841, repr. (Bath: Adams and Dart, 1971), vol. 2: *The Midlands and South*.

Gray, O., 'The Rise of the Middling Sort and their Influence on Local Politics and the Economy of Seventeenth- and Eighteenth-Century Bath' (unpublished bachelor of science dissertation, University of Bath, 1985).

Gray, R., *The Aristocracy of Labour in Nineteenth-Century Britain c.1850–1914* (London: Macmillan, 1981).

Green, M.A., *The Eighteenth Century Architecture of Bath* (Bath: George Gregory, 1904).

Guerrini, A., '"A Club of Little Villains": Rhetoric, Professional Identity and Medical Pamphlet Wars', in M.M. Roberts and R. Porter (eds), *Literature and Medicine during the Eighteenth Century* (London: Routledge, 1993).

Gye's Bath Directory (Bath: H. Gye, 1819).

Hall, F.M., Stevens, R.S. and Whyman, J., *The Kent and Canterbury Hospital 1790–1987* (Canterbury: Kent Postgraduate Medical Centre, 1987).

Hamlin, C., 'Chemistry, Medicine, and the Legitimization of English Spas, 1740–1840', in R. Porter (ed.), *The Medical History of Waters and Spas, Medical History* Supplement No. 10 (London: Wellcome Institute for the History of Medicine, 1990).

Hampson, N., *The Enlightenment: An Evaluation of its Assumptions, Attitudes and Values* (Harmondsworth: Penguin Books, 1968).

Hankins, T.L., *Science and the Enlightenment* (Cambridge: Cambridge University Press, 1985).

Harley, D., 'Religious and Professional Interests in Northern Spa Literature, 1625–1775', *Bulletin of the Society for the Social History of Medicine*, 35 (1984).

Harley, D., 'Honour and Property: The Structure of Professional Disputes in Eighteenth-Century English Medicine', in A. Cunningham and R. French (eds), *The Medical Enlightenment of the Eighteenth Century* (Cambridge: Cambridge University Press, 1990).

Harley, D., 'Provincial Midwives in England: Lancashire and Cheshire, 1660–1760', in H. Marland (ed.), *The Art of Midwifery: Early Modern Midwives in Europe* (London: Routledge, 1993).

Harley, D., '"Bred up in the study of that faculty": Licensed Physicians in North-West England, 1660–1760', *Medical History*, 38 (1994).

Harley, D., 'Political Post-Mortems and Morbid Anatomy in Seventeenth-Century England', *Social History of Medicine*, 7 (1994).

Hart, H.W., 'Some Notes on the Sponsoring of Patients for Hospital Treatment under the Voluntary System', *Medical History*, 24 (1980).

Harvey, A.D., *Sex in Georgian England: Attitudes and Prejudices from the 1720s to the 1820s* (London: Duckworth, 1994).

Haskins, C., *The History of Salisbury Infirmary* (Salisbury: Salisbury and District Infirmary and Hospital League, 1922).

Hausman, W.J., 'The British Economy in Transition, 1742–1789', in J. Black (ed.) *British Politics and Society from Walpole to Pitt 1742–1789* (London: Macmillan, 1990).

Hawthorn, G., *Enlightenment and Despair: A History of Social Theory*, 2nd edn (Cambridge: Cambridge University Press, 1987).

Heal, F., *Hospitality in Early Modern England* (Oxford: Clarendon Press, 1990).

Heal, F. and Holmes, C., *The Gentry in England and Wales 1500–1700* (London: Macmillan, 1994).

Heater, D., *Citizenship: The Civic Ideal in World History, Politics and Education* (London: Longman, 1990).

Helleiner, K.F., 'The Vital Revolution Reconsidered', *Canadian Journal of Economics and Political Science*, 23 (1957).

Hembry, P., *The English Spa 1560–1815: A Social History* (London: Athlone Press, 1990).

Hembry, P., *British Spas from 1815 to the Present: A Social History*, ed. L.W. Cowie and E.E. Cowie (London: Athlone, 1997).

Hemingway, V. and Haworth, J., *Coughton Court and the Throckmortons* (Norwich: Jarrold, 1993).

Hempton, D., *Methodism and Politics in British Society 1750–1850* (London: Hutchinson, 1984).

Hempton, D., 'Religion in British Society, 1740–1790', in J. Black (ed.), *British Politics and Society from Walpole to Pitt 1742–1789* (London: Macmillan, 1990).

Hill, B., *Women, Work, and Sexual Politics in Eighteenth-Century England* (Oxford: Blackwell, 1989).

Hilton, B., *The Age of Atonement: The Influence of Evangelicalism on Social and Economic Thought 1795–1865* (Oxford: Clarendon Press, 1988).

Himmelfarb, G., *The Idea of Poverty: England in the Early Industrial Age* (London: Faber and Faber, 1984).

'Hints to Young Practitioners, and Observations for the Benefit of Those Whom They May Concern', *Edinburgh Medical and Surgical Journal*, 5 (1809).

Hitchcock, T.V., 'The English Workhouse: A Study in Institutional Poor Relief in Selected Counties 1696–1750', (unpublished doctoral thesis, University of Oxford, 1985).

Hole, R., *Pulpits, Politics and Public Order in England 1760–1832* (Cambridge: Cambridge University Press, 1989).

Holmes, G., *Augustan England: Professions, State and Society 1680–1730* (London: Macmillan, 1982).

Holmes, G., *The Making of a Great Power: Late Stuart and Early Georgian Britain 1660–1722* (London: Longman, 1993).

Holmes, G. and Szechi, D., *The Age of Oligarchy: Pre-Industrial Britain 1722–1783* (London: Longman, 1993).

Hopkins, A.E. (ed.), *Ralph Allen's Own Narrative 1720–1761*, Special Series No. 8 (no place of publication: Postal History Society, 1960).

Hoppit, J., 'Political Arithmetic in Eighteenth-Century England', *Economic History Review*, 49 (1996).

Horden, P., 'A Discipline of Relevance: The Historiography of the Later Medieval Hospital', *Social History of Medicine*, 1 (1988).

Houston, R.A., *The Population History of Britain and Ireland 1500–1750* (London: Macmillan, 1992).

Howard, J., *An Account of the Principal Lazarettos in Europe* (Warrington, 1789).

Howie, W.B., 'The Administration of an Eighteenth-Century Provincial Hospital: The Royal Salop Infirmary, 1747–1830', *Medical History*, 5 (1961).

Howie, W.B., 'Finance and Supply in an Eighteenth-Century Hospital', *Medical History*, 7, (1963).

Howie, W.B., 'Consumer Reaction: A Patient's View of Hospital Life in 1809', *British Medical Journal*, 3 (8 September 1973).

Howie, W.B., 'Complaints and Complaint Procedures in the Eighteenth- and Early Nineteenth-Century Provincial Hospitals in England' *Medical History*, 25 (1981).

Hudson, P., *The Industrial Revolution* (London: Edward Arnold, 1992).

[Hull General Infirmary], 'General Infirmary, Kingston upon Hull', in K.J. Lowson, *The Hull Royal Infirmary* (no place of publication, publisher or date).

Humble, J.G. and Hansell, P., *Westminster Hospital 1716–1974*, 2nd edn (London: Pitman Medical, 1974).

Hume, G.H., *The History of the Newcastle Infirmary* (Newcastle upon Tyne: Andrew Reid, 1906).

Hunter, J., *The Ameliorated Condition of the Poor, One Benefit Derived to the World from Christianity* (Bath: Richard Cruttwell, 1811).

Hunter, M., *Science and Society in Restoration England* (Cambridge: Cambridge University Press, 1981).

Hutchinson, T., *Before Adam Smith: The Emergence of Political Economy 1662–1776* (Oxford: Basil Blackwell, 1988).

Ignatieff, M., *A Just Measure of Pain: The Penitentiary in the Industrial Revolution* (Harmondsworth: Penguin Books, 1978).

Ignatieff, M., 'Total Institutions and Working Classes: A Review Essay', *History Workshop Journal*, 15 (1983).

Imhof, A.E., 'The Hospital in the Eighteenth Century: For Whom?', *Journal of Social History*, 10 (1970).

The Improved Bath Guide (Bath: Wood and Co., 1812).

Inkster, I., 'Marginal Men: Aspects of the Social Role of the Medical Community in Sheffield, 1790–1850', in J. Woodward and D. Richards (eds), *Health Care and Popular Medicine in Nineteenth-Century England* (London: Croom Helm, 1977).

Inkster, I., 'Variations on a Theme by Thackray: Comments upon Provincial Science Culture, c. 1780–1850', *British Society for the History of Science Newsletter*, 8 (1982).

Innes, J., 'Jonathan Clark, Social History and England's "ancien regime"', *Past and Present*, 115 (1987).

Innes, J., 'Politics and Morals: the Reformation of Manners Movement in Later Eighteenth-Century England', in E. Hellmuth (ed.), *The Transformation of Political Culture: England and Germany in the Late Eighteenth Century* (Oxford: Oxford University Press, 1990).

Innes, J., 'The Domestic Face of the Military-Fiscal State', in L. Stone (ed.), *An Imperial State at War: Britain from 1689 to 1815* (London: Routledge, 1994).

Innes, J., 'The "Mixed Economy of Welfare" in Early Modern England: Assessments of the Options from Hale to Malthus (c.1683–1803)', in M. Daunton (ed.), *Charity, Self-Interest and Welfare in the English Past* (London: UCL Press, 1996).

Ison, W., *The Georgian Buildings of Bath from 1700 to 1830*, first pub. 1948 (Bath: Kingsmead Reprints, 1969).

Jacob, F.H., *A History of the General Hospital near Nottingham* (Bristol: John Wright and Sons, and London: Simpkin Marshall, 1951).

Jenkins, K., *Re-Thinking History* (London: Routledge, 1991.

Jenkins, W.J., 'A History of the Proprietary Chapels of Bath' (unpublished typescript, Bath Central Library, 1948).

Jenkinson, J., 'The Role of Medical Societies in the Rise of the Scottish Medical Profession', *Social History of Medicine*, 4 (1991).

Jennings, B. (ed.), *A History of Harrogate and Knaresborough* (Huddersfield: Advertiser Press, 1970).

Jewson, N.D., 'Medical Knowledge and the Patronage System in Eighteenth-Century England', *Sociology*, 8 (1974).

Jewson, N.D., 'The Disappearance of the Sick-Man from Medical Cosmology, 1770–1870', *Sociology*, 10 (1976).

Johnson, M., *An Archaeology of Capitalism* (Oxford: Blackwell, 1996).

Jones, C., 'Some recent trends in the history of charity', in M. Daunton (ed.), *Charity, Self-Interest and Welfare in the English Past* (London: UCL Press, 1996).

Jones, V. (ed.), *Women in the Eighteenth Century: Constructions of Femininity* (London: Routledge, 1990).

Jordanova, L., 'Natural Facts: A Historical Perspective on Science and Sexuality', in C.P. MacCormack and M. Strathern (eds), *Nature, Culture and Gender* (Cambridge : Cambridge University Press, 1980).

Jordanova, L., *Sexual Visions: Images of Gender in Science and Medicine between the Eighteenth and Twentieth Centuries* (London: Harvester Wheatsheaf, 1989).

Jordanova, L., 'The Authoritarian Response', in P. Hulme and L. Jordanova (eds), *The Enlightenment and its Shadows* (London: Routledge, 1990).

Jordanova, L., 'The Representation of the Family in the Eighteenth Century: A Challenge for Cultural History', in J.H. Pittock and A. Wear (eds), *Interpretation and Cultural History* (London: Macmillan, 1991).

Jordanova, L., 'The Social Construction of Medical Knowledge', *Social History of Medicine*, 8 (1995).

Jorden, E., *A Discourse on Naturall Bathes, and Mineral Waters, etc.* (London, 1631).

The Journeys of Celia Fiennes, ed. C. Morris (London: Cresset Press, 1949).

Keel, O., 'The Politics of Health and the Institutionalisation of Clinical Practices in Europe in the Second Half of the Eighteenth Century', in W.F. Bynum and R. Porter (eds), *William Hunter and the Eighteenth-Century Medical World* (Cambridge: Cambridge University Press, 1985).

Keene's Bath Directory (Bath: John and James Keene, 1824).

Keene's Improved Bath Directory (Bath: John and James Keene, 1829).

Kersley, G.D., *The Three R's: Rheumatism, Rehabilitation, Research* (Bath: Ralph Allen Press, undated).

Kersley. G.D. and Cosh, J.A, 'The Royal National Hospital for Rheumatic Diseases, Bath', *The Practitioner*, **195** (1965).

Kersley, G.D. and Cosh, J.A., *The History of the Royal National Hospital for Rheumatic Diseases, Bath 1742–1965* (Bath: Royal National Hospital, 1965).

Kersley, G.D. and Cosh, J.A., *The History of the Royal National Hospital for Rheumatic Diseases, Bath 1742–1979* (Bath: Royal National Hospital, 1980).

Kilpatrick, R., '"Living in the Light": Dispensaries, Philanthropy and Medical Reform in Late-Eighteenth-Century London', in A. Cunningham and R. French (eds), *Medical Enlightenment of the Eighteenth Century* (Cambridge: Cambridge University Press, 1990).

King, A.J., 'Bath – its General History from the Norman Conquest to the Nineteenth Century', in J.W. Morris (ed.), *Handbook to Bath Prepared on the Occasion of the Visit of the British Association 1888* (Bath: Isaac Pitman and Sons, 1888).

Kingsley, N., *The Country Houses of Gloucestershire*, 2 vols (Chichester: Phillimore, 1992), vol. 1: *1660–1830*.

Kirby, T., 'Royal Mineral Water Hospital, Bath: Catalogue of the Pictures' (unpublished manuscript, Bath Central Library, undated).

Kirkup, J., 'A Pioneer Accident Service: Bath Casualty Hospital, 1788–1826', in R. Rolls, J. Guy and J.R. Guy (eds), *A Pox on the Provinces: Proceedings of the 12th Congress of the British Society for the History of Medicine* (Bath: Bath University Press, 1990).

Klein, L., 'Liberty, Manners and Politeness in Early Eighteenth-Century England', *Historical Journal*, 32 (1989).

Kramnick, I., 'Eighteenth-Century Science and Radical Social Theory: The Case of Joseph Priestley's Scientific Liberalism', *Journal of British Studies*, **25** (1986).

Lane, J., 'The Medical Practitioners of Provincial England in 1783', *Medical History*, **28** (1984).

Lane, J., '"The doctor scolds me": The Diaries and Correspondence of

Patients in Eighteenth Century England', in R. Porter (ed.), *Patients and Practitioners: Lay Perceptions of Medicine in Pre-Industrial Society* (Cambridge: Cambridge University Press, 1985).

Lane, J., 'Eighteenth-Century Medical Practice: A Case Study of Bradford Wilmer, Surgeon of Coventry, 1737–1813', *Social History of Medicine*, 3 (1990).

Lane, J., *Worcester Infirmary in the Eighteenth Century* (Worcestershire Historical Society, 1992).

Langford, A.W., 'The History of Hereford General Hospital', *Transactions of the Woolhope Naturalists' Field Club*, 37 (1959).

Langford, P., *A Polite and Commercial People: England 1727–1783* (Oxford: Clarendon Press, 1989).

Langford, P., *Public Life and the Propertied Englishman 1689–1798* (Oxford: Clarendon Press, 1991).

Laurence, A., *Women in England: A Social History 1500–1760* (London: Weidenfeld and Nicolson, 1994).

Lawrence, C., 'Ornate Physicians and Learned Artisans: Edinburgh Medical Men, 1726–1776', in W.F. Bynum and R. Porter (eds), *William Hunter and the Eighteenth-Century Medical World* (Cambridge: Cambridge University Press, 1985).

Lawrence, C., 'Priestley in Tahiti: The Medical Interests of a Dissenting Chemist', in R.G.W. Anderson and C. Lawrence (eds), *Science, Medicine and Dissent: Joseph Priestley (1733–1804)* (London: Wellcome Trust/Science Museum, 1987).

Lawrence, C., 'Democratic, Divine and Heroic: The History and Historiography of Surgery', in C. Lawrence (ed.), *Medical Theory, Surgical Practice: Studies in the History of Surgery* (London: Routledge, 1992).

Lawrence, C., *Medicine in the Making of Modern Britain 1700–1920* (London: Routledge, 1994).

Lawrence, S., *Charitable Knowledge: Hospital Pupils and Practitioners in Eighteenth-Century London* (Cambridge: Cambridge University Press, 1996).

Leader, J.D., *Sheffield General Infirmary: A Brief Sketch of a Century's Work* (Sheffield: Published on behalf of the Infirmary Board by Mr G.H. Day, Secretary, 1897).

Leake, C.D., *Percival's Medical Ethics*, first pub. 1803 (New York: Robert E. Krieger, 1975).

Lee, R.D. and Schofield, R.S., 'British Population in the Eighteenth Century', in R. Floud and D. McCloskey (eds), *The Economic History of Britain since 1700*, 2 vols (Cambridge: Cambridge University Press, 1981), vol. 1: 1700–1860.

A Letter to Mr Archibald Cleland Occasioned by his Full Vindication of his Appeal to the Public against the Proceedings of the Bath Hospital (London: J. Roberts, 1744).

Letter to the President and Governors of the Bath General Hospital from J. Parish, Esq. (Bath: Wood, 1819).

Letters of Doctor Lucas and Doctor Oliver Occasioned by a Physical Confederacy Discovered in Bath (Bath: James Leake, 1757).

The Letters of Hannah More, ed. R. Brimley Johnson (London: John Lane, 1925).

Letters from a Late Eminent Prelate to One of His Friends, 2nd edn (London: T. Cadell and W. Davies, 1809).

Levine, D., 'Industrialization and the Proletarian Family in England', *Past and Present*, 107 (1985).

Lewis, W.S. and Williams, R.M., *Private Charity in England 1747–1757* (New Haven: Yale University Press, 1938).

Leyborne, R., *Charity Conducive to God's Glory: A Sermon for the Benefit of the General Hospital, in Bath* (Bath: Thomas Boddely, 1754).

Liesenfeld, V.J., *The Licensing Act of 1737* (Madison: University of Wisconsin Press, 1987).

Linebaugh, P., *The London Hanged: Crime and Civil Society in the Eighteenth Century* (Harmondsworth: Penguin Books, 1991).

Little, B., *Selina: Countess of Huntingdon* (Bath: Huntingdon Centre, 1989).

Lloyd, J., *The Royal United Hospital, Bath: A Short History* (Bristol: Redcliffe, 1982).

Lobo, F.M., 'John Haygarth, Smallpox and Religious Dissent in Eighteenth-Century England', in A. Cunningham and R. French (eds), *The Medical Enlightenment of the Eighteenth Century* (Cambridge: Cambridge University Press, 1990).

Loudon, I., 'The Nature of Provincial Medical Practice in Eighteenth-Century England', *Medical History*, 29 (1985).

Loudon, I., *Medical Care and the General Practitioner 1750–1850* (Oxford: Clarendon Press, 1986).

Lowson, K.J., *The Hull Royal Infirmary* (no place of publication, publisher or date).

Lucas, C., *An Essay on Waters in Three Parts* (London: A. Millar, 1756).

Lucas, C., *Cursory Remarks on the Methods of Investigating the Principles and Properties of Bath and Bristol Waters* (Bath: C. Pope, 1764).

Lysons, D., *Practical Essays upon Continual and Intermitting Fevers, Dropsies, Diseases of the Liver, and the Use of Bath Waters*, 2nd edn (Bath: S. Hazard, 1783).

MacCormack, C.P., 'Nature, Culture and Gender: A Critique', in

C.P. MacCormack and M. Strathern (eds), *Nature, Culture and Gender* (Cambridge: Cambridge University Press, 1980).

Mainwaring, R., *Annals of Bath from the Year 1800 to the Passing of the New Municipal Act* (Bath: Meyler, 1838).

Malthus, T.R., *An Essay on the Principle of Population*, ed. Anthony Flew (Harmondsworth: Penguin Books, 1970).

Malthus, T.R., *A Summary View of the Principle of Population*, in T.R. Malthus, *An Essay on the Principle of Population*, ed. A. Flew (Harmondsworth: Penguin Books, 1970).

Mandeville, B., 'An Essay on Charity and Charity-Schools', in *The Fable of the Bees*, ed. Philip Harth (Harmondsworth: Penguin Books, 1970).

Manners and Morals, Hogarth and British Painting 1700–1760, introduced by Elizabeth Einberg (London: Tate Gallery, 1987).

Markus, T.A., *Buildings and Power: Freedom and Control in the Origin of Modern Building Types* (London: Routledge, 1993).

Marland, H., *Medicine and Society in Wakefield and Huddersfield 1780–1880* (Cambridge: Cambridge University Press, 1987).

Marland, H. (ed.), *The Art of Midwifery: Early Modern Midwives in Europe* (London: Routledge, 1993).

Marland, H. and Pelling, M. (eds), *The Task of Healing: Medicine, Religion and Gender in England and the Netherlands 1450–1800* (Rotterdam: Erasmus Publishing, 1996).

Martensen, R., 'The Transformation of Eve: Women's Bodies, Medicine and Culture in Early Modern England', in R. Porter and M. Teich (eds), *Sexual Knowledge, Sexual Science: The History of Attitudes to Sexuality* (Cambridge: Cambridge University Press, 1994).

Marx, K. 'Communist Manifesto', in T.B. Bottomore and M. Rubel (eds), *Karl Marx: Selected Writings in Sociology and Social Philosophy* (Harmondsworth: Penguin Books, 1961).

McClure, R., *Coram's Children: The London Foundling Hospital in the Eighteenth Century* (New Haven: Yale University Press, 1981).

McIntyre, S., 'Towns as Health and Pleasure Resorts' (unpublished doctoral thesis, University of Oxford, 1973).

McIntyre, S., 'Bath: The Rise of a Resort Town, 1660–1800', in P. Clark (ed.), *Country Towns in Pre-Industrial England* (Leicester: Leicester University Press, 1981).

McKendrick, N., 'The Consumer Revolution in Eighteenth-Century England', in N. McKendrick, J. Brewer and J.H. Plumb, *The Birth of a Consumer Society: The Commercialization of Eighteenth-Century England* (London: Hutchinson, 1982).

McKeown, T. and Brown, R.G., 'Medical Evidence Related to English

Population Changes in the Eighteenth Century', *Population Studies*, 9 (1955).
McLaren, A., 'The Pleasures of Procreation: Traditional and Biomedical Theories of Conception', in W.F. Bynum and R. Porter (eds), *William Hunter and the Eighteenth-Century Medical World* (Cambridge: Cambridge University Press, 1985).
McLoughlin, G., *A Short History of the First Liverpool Infirmary 1749–1824* (London and Chichester: Phillimore, 1978).
McLynn, F., *Crime and Punishment in Eighteenth Century England* (Oxford: Oxford University Press, 1989).
McMenemey, W.H., *A History of the Worcester Royal Infirmary* (London: Press Alliances, 1947).
McVeigh, S., *Concert Life in London from Mozart to Haydn* (Cambridge: Cambridge University Press, 1993).
Meehan, J.F., *Famous Houses of Bath and District* (Bath: B. and J.F. Meehan, 1901).
Meehan, J.F., *More Famous Houses of Bath and District* (Bath: B. and J.F. Meehan, 1906).
Melville, L., *Bath Under Beau Nash* (London: Eveleigh Nash, 1907).
Miège, G., *The Present State of Great Britain and Ireland*, 4th edn (London: A. Bell, R. Smith and J. Round, 1718).
The Miscellaneous Works of Oliver Goldsmith, introduced by David Masson, first pub. 1868, repr. (London: Macmillan, 1908).
Mitchell, B., 'English Spas', *Bath History*, 1 (1986).
Morgan, M., *Manners, Morals and Class in England 1774–1858* (London: St Martin's Press, 1994).
Morris, R.J., 'Voluntary Societies and British Urban Elites, 1780–1850: An Analysis', in P. Borsay (ed.), *The Eighteenth-Century Town: A Reader in English Urban History 1688–1820* (London: Longman, 1990).
Moscucci, O., *The Science of Woman: Gynaecology and Gender in England, 1800–1929* (Cambridge: Cambridge University Press, 1990).
Moule, T., *The County Maps of Old England*, introduced by Roderick Barron, first pub. 1830, repr. (London: Studio Editions Ltd, 1990).
Murch, J., 'Bath in its Relation to Art, Science, Literature and Education', in J.W. Morris (ed.), *Handbook to Bath Prepared on the Occasion of the Visit of the British Association, 1888* (Bath: Isaac Pitman, 1888).
Murch, J., *Biographical Sketches of Bath Celebrities, Ancient and Modern, with Some Fragments of Local History* (London: Isaac Pitman, 1893).
Namier, L. and Brooke, J., *The House of Commons*, 3 vols (London: HMSO, 1964), vol. 2: *Members A–J*.

Namier, L. and Brooke, J., *The House of Commons*, 3 vols (London: HMSO, 1964), vol. 3: *Members K–Y*.

Neale, R.S., *Bath: A Social History 1680–1850 or a Valley of Pleasure, yet a Sink of Iniquity* (London: Routledge and Kegan Paul, 1981).

Nelson, R., *An Address to Persons of Quality and Estate* (London, 1715).

Neve, M.R. 'Natural Philosophy, Medicine and the Culture of Science in Provincial England: The Cases of Bristol 1796–1850 and Bath 1750–1820' (unpublished doctoral thesis, University of London, 1984).

Neve, M., 'Orthodoxy and Fringe: Medicine in Late Georgian Bristol', in W.F. Bynum and R. Porter (eds), *Medical Fringe and Medical Orthodoxy 1750–1850* (London: Croom Helm, 1987).

The New Bath Directory (Bath: J. Browne, 1805).

The New Bath Directory (Bath: Wood and Cunningham, 1812).

The New Bath Directory for the Year 1809 (Bath: J. Browne, 1809).

Newby, E., 'The Hoares of Bath', *Bath History*, **1** (1986).

Newby, E., *William Hoare of Bath* (Stroud: Alan Sutton and Bath Museums Service, 1990).

Nicolson, M., 'The Metastatic Theory of Pathogenesis and the Professional Interests of the Eighteenth-Century Physician', *Medical History*, **32** (1988).

Nicolson, M., 'Giovanni Battista Morgagni and Eighteenth-Century Physical Examination', in C. Lawrence (ed.), *Medical Theory, Surgical Practical: Studies in the History of Surgery* (London: Routledge, 1994).

O'Brien, E., *The Charitable Infirmary, Jervis Street 1718–1987: A Farewell Tribute* (Dublin: Anniversary Press, 1987).

O'Gorman, F., *The Emergence of the British Two-Party System 1760–1832* (London: Edward Arnold, 1982).

O'Gorman, F., *Voters, Patrons and Parties: The Unreformed Electoral System of Hanoverian England 1734–1832* (Oxford: Clarendon Press, 1989).

Olive, R., *The Particular Excellence and True State of the Bath Infirmary* (Bristol: E. Farley, 1759).

Oliver, W., [the Elder], *A Practical Dissertation on Bath Waters*, 2nd edn (London: J.D. Varnam, 1716).

[Oliver, W.], *Cases of Persons Admitted into the Infirmary at Bath under the Care of Doctor Oliver* (Bath: Stephen Martin, 1760).

The Original Bath Guide (Bath: Meyler and Son, 1840).

The Original Bath Guide (Bath: Meyler and Son, 1876).

Outhwaite, R.B., *Dearth, Public Policy and Social Disturbance in England 1550–1800* (London: Macmillan, 1991).

Owen, D., *English Philanthropy 1660–1960* (Cambridge, MA: Harvard University Press, 1964).

Page, R.M., *Altruism and the British Welfare State* (Aldershot: Avebury, 1996).

Park, K., 'Healing the Poor: Hospitals and Medical Assistance in Renaissance Florence', in J. Barry and C. Jones (eds), *Medicine and Charity before the Welfare State* (London: Routledge, 1991).

Parsons, F.G., *The History of St Thomas's Hospital*, 3 vols (London: Methuen, 1932–36), vol. 2: *From 1600 to 1800*.

Parsons, F.G., *The History of St Thomas's Hospital*, 3 vols (London: Methuen, 1932–36), vol. 3: *From 1800 to 1900*.

Parsons, T., *The Social System* (London: Routledge and Kegan Paul, 1951).

Patrick, J., *A Short History of Glasgow Royal Infirmary* (Glasgow: Glasgow Royal Infirmary, 1940).

The Pauper Charity, Hereafter to be Called Bath City Infirmary and Dispensary (no place of publication, publisher or date).

Peach, R.E.M., *Historic Houses in Bath and their Associations*, 2 vols (London: Simpkin, Marshall and Co., 1883–84).

Peach, R.E.M., *Bath, Old and New: A Handy Guide and a History* (London: Simpkin, Marshall and Co., 1888).

Peach, R.E.M., *The Life and Times of Ralph Allen* (London: D. Nutt, 1895).

Pelling, M., 'Medical Practice in Early Modern England: Trade or Profession?', in W. Prest (ed.), *The Professions in Early Modern England* (Beckenham: Croom Helm, 1987).

Pemberton, A., 'Rescuing the Good Samaritan: An Exposition and Defence of the Samaritan Principle in the Welfare State', *Journal of Social Policy*, **19** (1990).

Penrose, J., *Letters from Bath 1766–67*, ed. by B. Mitchell and H. Penrose (Gloucester: Alan Sutton, 1983).

Percival, T., 'A Letter from Thomas Percival MD FRS', in J. Aikin, *Thoughts on Hospitals with a Letter to the Author by Thomas Percival* (London: Joseph Johnson, 1771).

Perry, C.B., *The Voluntary Medical Institutions of Bristol* (Bristol: Bristol Branch of the Historical Association, 1984).

Pevsner, N., *A History of Building Types* (London: Thames and Hudson, 1976).

Phelps-Brown, E.H. and Hopkins, S.V., 'Seven Centuries of Building Wages', in E.M. Carus-Wilson (ed.), *Essays in Economic History*, 2 vols (London: Edward Arnold, 1962).

Pickstone, J.V., *Medicine and Industrial Society: A History of Hospital*

Development in Manchester and its Region 1752–1946 (Manchester: Manchester University Press, 1985).

Pickstone, J.V., 'Medicine in Industrial Britain: The Uses of Local Studies', *Social History of Medicine*, 2 (1989).

Pickstone, J., 'Dearth, Dirt and Fever Epidemics: Rewriting the History of British "Public Health", 1780–1850', in T. Ranger and P. Slack (eds), *Epidemics and Ideas: Essays on the Historical Perception of Pestilence* (Cambridge: Cambridge University Press, 1992).

Pickstone, J.V. and Butler, S.V.F., 'The Politics of Medicine in Manchester, 1788–1792: Hospital Reform and Public Health Services in the Early Industrial City', *Medical History*, 28 (1984).

A Pictorial and Descriptive Guide to Bath (London: Ward Lock, 1909).

Pocock, J.G.A., *Virtue, Commerce and History: Essays on Political Thought and History, Chiefly in the Eighteenth Century* (Cambridge: Cambridge University Press, 1985).

Poems of Alexander Pope, 8 vols (London: Methuen, 1939–1967), vol. 4: *Imitations of Horace with An Epistle to Dr Arbuthnot and The Epilogue to the Satires*, ed. John Butt, 2nd edn (1953), p. 308.

Poole, S., 'Radicalism, Loyalism and the "Reign of Terror" in Bath, 1792–1804', *Bath History*, 3 (1990).

Porter, D. and Porter, R., *Patient's Progress: Doctors and Doctoring in Eighteenth-Century England* (Cambridge: Polity Press, 1989).

Porter, R., 'The Enlightenment in England', in R. Porter and M. Teich (eds), *The Enlightenment in National Context* (Cambridge: Cambridge University Press, 1981).

Porter, R., 'Mixed Feelings: The Enlightenment and Sexuality in Eighteenth-Century Britain', in P.-G. Boucé (ed.), *Sexuality in Eighteenth-Century Britain* (Manchester: Manchester University Press, 1982).

Porter, R., 'Was there a Medical Enlightenment in Eighteenth-Century England?' *British Journal for Eighteenth Century Studies*, 5 (1982).

Porter, R., 'Laymen, Doctors and Medical Knowledge in the Eighteenth Century: The Evidence of the *Gentleman's Magazine*', in R. Porter (ed.), *Patients and Practitioners: Lay Perceptions of Medicine in Pre-Industrial Society* (Cambridge: Cambridge University Press, 1985).

Porter, R., 'The Patient's View: Doing Medical History from Below', *Theory and Society*, 14 (1985).

Porter, R., *Disease, Medicine and Society in England 1550–1860* (London: Macmillan, 1987).

Porter, R., 'Medicine and Religion in Eighteenth-Century England: A Case of Conflict?' *Ideas and Production*, 7 (1987).

Porter, R., *Mind-Forg'd Manacles: A History of Madness in England from the Restoration to the Regency* (Harmondsworth: Penguin Books, 1987).

Porter, R., 'The Gift Relation', in L. Granshaw and R. Porter (eds), *The Hospital in History* (London: Routledge, 1989).

Porter, R., 'English Society in the Eighteenth Century Revisited', in J. Black (ed.), *British Politics and Society from Walpole to Pitt 1742–1789* (London: Macmillan, 1990).

Porter, R., *The Enlightenment* (London: Macmillan, 1990).

Porter, R., 'Introduction', in R. Porter (ed.), *The Medical History of Waters and Spas*, *Medical History* Supplement No. 10 (London: Wellcome Institute for the History of Medicine, 1990).

Porter, R., 'Science, Provincial Culture and Public Opinion in Enlightenment England', in P. Borsay (ed.), *The Eighteenth Century Town: A Reader in English Urban History 1688–1820* (London: Longman, 1990).

Porter, R., 'Bodies of Thought: Thoughts about the Body in Eighteenth-Century England', in J.H. Pittock and A. Wear (eds), *Interpretation and Cultural History* (London: Macmillan, 1991).

Porter, R., 'Civilization and Disease: Medical Ideology in the Enlightenment', in J. Black and J. Gregory (eds), *Culture, Politics and Society in Britain 1660–1800* (Manchester: Manchester University Press, 1991).

Porter, R., 'History of the Body', in P. Burke (ed.), *New Perspectives on Historical Writing* (Cambridge: Polity Press, 1991).

Porter, R., 'Reforming the Patient in the Age of Reform: Thomas Beddoes and Medical Practice', in R. French and A. Wear (eds), *British Medicine in an Age of Reform* (London: Routledge, 1991).

Porter, R., 'Madness and its institutions', in A. Wear (ed.), *Medicine in Society: Historical Essays* (Cambridge: Cambridge University Press, 1992).

Porter, R., 'The Rise of Physical Examination', in W.F. Bynum and R. Porter (eds) *Medicine and the Five Senses* (Cambridge: Cambridge University Press, 1993).

Porter, R., 'The Eighteenth Century', in L.I. Conrad, M. Neve, V. Nutton, R. Porter and A. Wear, *The Western Medical Tradition 800 BC to AD 1800* (Cambridge: Cambridge University Press, 1995).

Porter, R., *The Greatest Benefit to Mankind: A Medical History of Humanity from Antiquity to the Present* (London: HarperCollins, 1997).

Porter, R. and Hall, L., *The Facts of Life: The Creation of Sexual Knowledge in Britain 1650–1950* (New Haven and London: Yale University Press, 1995).

Porter, R. and Porter, D., *In Sickness and in Health: The British Experience 1650–1850* (London: Fourth Estate, 1988).

Poynton, F.J., 'An Address on the Occasion of the Unveiling of a Memorial Tablet at the Royal Literary Institution, Queen Square, to Dr. William Oliver' (unpublished typescript, Bath Central Library, 1935).

Prest, W., 'Introduction: The Professions and Society in Early Modern England', in W. Prest (ed.), *The Professions in Early Modern England* (Beckenham: Croom Helm, 1987).

Prior, M., 'Women and the Urban Economy: Oxford, 1500–1800', in M. Prior (ed.), *Women in English Society 1500–1800* (London: Routledge, 1985).

Prochaska, F.K., 'Women in English Philanthropy, 1790–1830', *International Review of Social History*, 19 (1974).

Proudfit, W.L., 'The Fleece Medical Society', *British Heart Journal*, 46 (1981).

Raphael, D.D., *Adam Smith* (Oxford: Oxford University Press, 1985).

Report of a Committee Appointed by the Governors of the Bath General Hospital, to Examine a Statement Circulated by Mr. Parish, Respecting the Finances and Administration of that Institution (Bath: Cruttwell, 1819).

Rhodes, P., *Dr John Leake's Hospital: A History of the General Lying-In Hospital, York Road, Lambeth 1765–1971* (London: Davis-Poynter, 1977).

Richardson, H., *English Hospitals 1660–1948: A Survey of their Architecture and Design* (Swindon: Royal Commission on the Historical Monuments of England, 1998).

Richardson, R., *Death, Dissection and the Destitute* (Harmondsworth: Penguin Books, 1988).

Riley, J.C., *The Eighteenth-Century Campaign to Avoid Disease* (London: Macmillan, 1987).

Risse, G.B., *Hospital Life in Enlightenment Scotland: Care and Teaching at the Royal Infirmary of Edinburgh* (Cambridge: Cambridge University Press, 1986).

Risse, G.B., 'Medicine in the Age of Enlightenment', in A. Wear (ed.), *Medicine in Society: Historical Essays* (Cambridge: Cambridge University Press, 1992).

Robbins' Bath Directory (Bath: G. Robbins, 1800).

Roberts, D., *Paternalism in Early Victorian England* (New Brunswick, NJ: Rutgers University Press, 1979).

Rodger, N.A.M., *The Wooden World: An Anatomy of the Georgian Navy* (London: Fontana, 1986).

Rogers, N., 'Paul Langford's "Age of Improvement"', *Past and Present*, 130 (1991).

Rogers, N., 'The Middling Sort in Eighteenth-Century Politics', in J. Barry and C. Brooks (eds), *The Middling Sort of People: Culture, Society and Politics in England 1550–1880* (London: Macmillan, 1994).

Rolls, R., 'Archibald Cleland: *c.* 1700–71', *British Medical Journal*, **288** (14 April 1984).

Rolls, R., *The Hospital of the Nation: The Story of Spa Medicine and the Mineral Water Hospital at Bath* (Bath: Bird, 1988).

Rolls, R., 'From Balneology to Physiotherapy: the Development of Physical Treatment at Bath', in R. Rolls, J. Guy and J.R. Guy, *A Pox on the Provinces: Proceedings of the 12th Congress of the British Society for the History of Medicine* (Bath: Bath University Press, 1990).

Rook, A., Carlton, M. and Cannon, W.G., *The History of Addenbrooke's Hospital, Cambridge* (Cambridge: Cambridge University Press, 1991).

Rosen, G., *From Medical Police to Social Medicine: Essays on the History of Medical Care* (New York: Science History Publications, 1974).

Rousseau, G.S., 'Matt Bramble and the Sulphur Controversy in the Eighteenth Century', *Journal of the History of Ideas*, **27** (1967).

Rousseau, G.S., *Perilous Enlightenment: Pre- and Post-Modern Discourses: Sexual, Historical* (Manchester: Manchester University Press, 1991).

Royal Mineral Water Hospital, 'Notes on the Pictures' (unpublished anthology of press cuttings, Bath Central Library, undated).

Rubinstein, W.D., 'The End of the "Old Corruption" in Britain, 1780–1860', *Past and Present*, **101** (1983).

Rule, J., *Albion's People: English Society 1714–1815* (London: Longman, 1992).

Rule, J., *The Vital Century: England's Developing Economy 1714–1815* (London: Longman, 1992).

Russell, P.M.G., *A History of the Exeter Hospitals 1170–1948* (Exeter: Exeter Medical Post-Graduate Institute, 1976).

Saunders, H. StG., *The Middlesex Hospital 1745–1948* (London: Max Parrish, 1949).

Schaffer, S., 'Natural Philosophy and Public Spectacle in the Eighteenth Century', *History of Science*, **21** (1983).

Schama, S., *The Embarrassment of Riches: An Interpretation of Dutch Culture in the Golden Age* (London: Fontana Press, 1987).

Schnorrenberg, B.B., 'Medical Men of Bath', *Studies in Eighteenth-Century Culture*, **13** (1984).

Secker, T., 'Sermon before the Lord Mayor,1738', in T. Secker, *Fourteen Sermons Preached on Several Occasions* (London: John Rivington, 1766).

Sedgwick, R., *The House of Commons 1715–1754*, 2 vols (London: HMSO, 1970), vol. 1: *Introductory Survey, Constituencies and Members A–D*.

Sedgwick, R., *The House of Commons 1715–1754*, 2 vols (London: HMSO, 1970), vol. 2: *Members E–Y*.

Selected Letters of Samuel Richardson, ed. John Carroll (Oxford: Clarendon Press, 1964).

Select Miscellaneous Productions of Mrs Day and Thomas Day, Esq. in Verse and Prose (London: T. Jones, 1805).

Sharpe, J.A., *Early Modern England: A Social History 1550–1760* (London: Edward Arnold, 1987).

Shemilt, P., et al., *Salisbury 200: The Bi-Centenary of Salisbury Infirmary 1766–1966* (Salisbury: Salisbury General Hospital, 1967).

Shoemaker, R.B., 'Reforming the City: The Reformation of Manners Campaign in London, 1690–1728', in L. Davison, T. Hitchcock, T. Keirn and R.B. Shoemaker (eds), *Stilling the Grumbling Hive: The Response to Social and Economic Problems in England 1689–1750* (Stroud: Alan Sutton, 1992).

A Short Vindication of the Proceedings of the Governors of the General Hospital at Bath in Relation to Mr Archibald Cleland (Bath and London: J. Leake and A. Dodd, 1744).

Sigerist, H.E., 'The History of Medicine and the History of Science', *Bulletin of the Institute of the History of Medicine*, 4 (1936).

Sigsworth, E., 'A Provincial Hospital in the Eighteenth and Early Nineteenth Centuries', *College of General Practitioners Yorkshire Faculty Journal* (June 1966).

Simond, L., *An American in Regency England: The Journal of a Tour in 1810–1811*, ed. Christopher Hibbert (London: Robert Maxwell, 1968).

The Sixth Year's State of the Casualty Hospital in the City of Bath ... for the Year 1793 (Bath: R. Cruttwell, 1794).

Slack, P., *Poverty and Policy in Tudor and Stuart England* (London: Longman, 1988).

Slack, P., *The English Poor Law 1531–1782* (London: Macmillan, 1990).

Sloman, S.L., '"The immaculate Capt. Wade": "Arbiter Elegantiae"', *Gainsborough's House Review*, (1993/94).

Smith, A., *The Theory of Moral Sentiments*, 2 vols, 9th edn (London: T. Cadell and W. Davies, 1801).

Smith, A., *An Inquiry into the Nature and Causes of the Wealth of Nations*, ed. J.R. McCulloch, 4th edn (Edinburgh: Adam and Charles Black, 1855).

Smith, F.B., *The People's Health 1830–1910* (London: Weidenfeld and Nicolson, 1979).

Smith, G., 'Prescribing the Rules of Health: Self-Help and Advice in the

Late Eighteenth Century', in R. Porter (ed.) *Patients and Practitioners: Lay Perceptions of Medicine in Pre-Industrial Society* (Cambridge: Cambridge University Press, 1985).

Smith, G.M., *A History of the Bristol Royal Infirmary* (Bristol: Arrowsmith, 1917).

Smith, R.A.L., *Bath*, 3rd edn (London: Batsford, 1948).

Smollett, T., *The Adventures of Peregrine Pickle*, ed. James L. Clifford (Oxford: Oxford University Press, 1969).

Smollett, T., *An Essay on the External Use of Water*, ed. Claude E. Jones (Baltimore: John Hopkins Press, 1935).

Souden, D., 'Migrants and the Population Structure of Later Seventeenth-Century Provincial Cities and Market Towns', in P. Clark (ed.), *The Transformation of English Provincial Towns 1600–1800* (London: Hutchinson, 1984).

Spadafora, D., *The Idea of Progress in Eighteenth-Century Britain* (New Haven: Yale University Press, 1990).

Speck, W.A., 'Conflict in Society', in G. Holmes (ed.), *Britain after the Glorious Revolution 1689–1714* (London: Macmillan, 1969).

Speck, W.A., *Stability and Strife: England 1714–1760* (London: Edward Arnold, 1977).

Spender, J.K., *The Bath Thermal Baths: Historical, Social and Medical* (London and Bath: W. Lewis, 1877).

Stafford, W., *Socialism, Radicalism and Nostalgia: Social Criticism in Britain 1775–1830* (Cambridge: Cambridge University Press, 1987).

State of the Bath City Infirmary and Dispensary ... from the 1st of October 1792 to January 1st 1794 (Bath: Cruttwell, 1794).

St Clair Strange, F.G., *The History of the Royal Sea Bathing Hospital, Margate 1791–1991* (Rainham, Kent: Meresborough Books, 1991).

Steer, F.W., *The Royal West Sussex Hospital: The First Hundred Years 1784–1884* (Chichester: Chichester City Council, 1960).

Stenton, M., *Who's Who of British Members of Parliament*, 4 vols (Brighton: Harvester Press, 1976), vol. 1: *1832–1885*.

Stone, L., 'Introduction', in L. Stone (ed.), *An Imperial State at War: Britain from 1689 to 1815* (London: Routledge, 1994).

Stone, L. and Fawtier Stone, J.C., *An Open Elite?: England 1540–1880* (Oxford: Oxford University Press, 1986).

Stourhead (London: National Trust, 1990).

Summers, J., *A Short Account of the Success of Warm Bathing in Paralytic Disorders*, 2nd edn (London: C. Hitch and L. Hawes, 1751).

Sutherland, A., *An Attempt to Ascertain and Extend the Virtues of Bath and Bristol Waters*, 2nd edn (London: W. Frederick and S. Leake, 1764).

Suzuki, A., 'Anti-Lockean Enlightenment?: Mind and Body in Early

Eighteenth-Century English Medicine', in R. Porter (ed.), *Medicine in the Enlightenment* (Amsterdam: Rodopi, 1995).

Swan, P., 'A Brief Summary of the Role and Position of Medical Societies in the Early Nineteenth-Century Medical Profession', *Journal of Local Studies*, 2 (1982).

Sympson, T., *A Short Account of the Old and of the New Lincoln County Hospitals* (Lincoln: James Williamson, 1878).

Tawney, R.H., *Religion and the Rise of Capitalism: A Historical Study* (New York: Harcourt, Brace and Co., 1926).

Taylor, J., *Hospital and Asylum Architecture in England 1840–1914: Building for Care* (London: Mansell, 1991).

Thackray, A., 'Natural Knowledge in Cultural Context: The Manchester Model', *American Historical Review*, 79 (1974).

Thicknesse, P., *The New Prose Bath Guide for the Year 1778* (printed for the author).

Thomas, J., 'The Phillotts of Bath' (unpublished typescript, Bath Central Library, 1968).

Thompson, E.P., 'Patrician Society, Plebeian Culture', *Journal of Social History*, 7 (1974).

Thompson, E.P., 'Eighteenth-Century English Society: Class Struggle without Class?' *Social History*, 3 (1978).

Thompson, J.D., and Goldin, G., *The Hospital: A Social and Architectural History* (New Haven: Yale University Press, 1975).

Titmuss, R.M., *The Gift Relationship: From Human Blood to Social Policy* (London: George Allen and Unwin, 1970).

Torrens, H., 'The Four Bath Philosophical Societies, 1779–1959', in R. Rolls, J. Guy and J.R. Guy (eds), *A Pox on the Provinces: Proceedings of the 12th Congress of the British Society for the History of Medicine* (Bath: Bath University Press, 1990).

Tregellas, W.H., *Cornish Worthies: Sketches of Some Eminent Cornish Men and Families* (London: Elliot Stock, 1884).

Trohler, U., 'Quantification in British Medicine and Surgery 1750–1830, with Special Reference to its Introduction into Therapeutics' (unpublished doctoral thesis, University of London, 1978).

Trueman, B.E.S., 'The Purchase and Management of Guy's Hospital Estates, 1726–1806', in C.W. Chalkin and J.R. Wordie (eds), *Town and Countryside: The English Landowner in the National Economy 1660–1860* (London: Unwin Hyman, 1989).

Tucker, J., *A Sermon Preached in the Parish Church in Bristol* (Bristol: William Crossley, 1746).

Tucker, R.S., 'Real Wages of Artisans in London, 1729–1935', in A.J. Taylor (ed), *The Standard of Living in Britain in the Industrial Revolution* (London: Methuen, 1975).

Turner, A.J., *Science and Music in Eighteenth-Century Bath* (Bath: University of Bath, 1977).

Turner, B.C., *A History of the Royal Hampshire County Hospital* (Chichester: Phillimore, 1986).

Turner, B.S., *Medical Power and Social Knowledge* (London: Sage, 1987).

Turner, P.V., *The Royal Mineral Water Hospital, Bath: A Brief History 1742–1921* (Bath: William Lewis and Son, 1921).

Turner, P.V., *'Charity for a Hundred Years': History of the Monmouth Street Society, Bath from 1805 to 1904* (no place of publication, publisher or date).

Tyte, W., *Bath in the Eighteenth Century: Its Progress and Life Described* (Bath: G. and F. Pickering, 1903).

Vidler, A.R., *The Church in an Age of Revolution*, repr. (Harmondsworth: Penguin Books, 1990).

Waddington, I., 'The Role of the Hospital in the Development of Modern Medicine: A Sociological Analysis', *Sociology*, 7 (1973).

Waddington, I., 'The Development of Medical Ethics: A Sociological Analysis', *Medical History*, **19** (1975).

Waddington, I., *The Medical Profession in the Industrial Revolution* (Dublin: Gill and Macmillan, 1984).

Waddy, F.F., *A History of Northampton General Hospital 1743 to 1948* (no place of publication or publisher, 1974).

Wagner, P., 'The Satire on Doctors in Hogarth's Graphic Works', in M.M. Roberts and R. Porter (eds), *Literature and Medicine during the Eighteenth Century* (London: Routledge, 1993).

Wahrman, D., *Imagining the Middle Class: The Political Representation of Class in Britain c.1780–1840* (Cambridge: Cambridge University Press, 1995).

Warburton, W., The Alliance between Church and State (London: Fletcher Gyles, 1736).

Warburton, W., *A Sermon Preached at the Abbey-Church at Bath* (London: J. Leake, 1742).

Warburton, W., *A Sermon Preached Before ... Governors of the Hospital for Smallpox* (London: H. Woodfall, 1755).

Warburton, W., 'Sermon Preached Before the Governors of the London Hospital in 1767', in W. Warburton, *Works*, ed. Richard Hurd, 12 vols (London: T. Cadell and W. Davies, 1811).

Warner, R., *The History of Bath* (Bath: R. Cruttwell, 1801).

Wear, A., 'Making Sense of Health and the Environment in Early Modern England', in A. Wear (ed.), *Medicine in Society: Historical Essays* (Cambridge: Cambridge University Press, 1992).

Wear, A., 'Religious Beliefs and Medicine in Early Modern England', in

H. Marland and M. Pelling (eds), *The Task of Healing: Medicine, Religion and Gender in England and the Netherlands 1450–1800* (Rotterdam: Erasmus, 1996).

Weber, M., 'Class, Status and Party', in R. Bendix and S.M. Lipset (eds), *Class, Status and Power: Social Stratification in Comparative Perspective* (London: Routledge and Kegan Paul, 1967).

Webster, C., 'The Crisis of Hospitals during the Industrial Revolution', in E. Forbes (ed.), *Human Implications of Scientific Advance* (Edinburgh: Edinburgh University Press, 1978).

Wesley, J., *The Journal of John Wesley*, ed. N. Curnock, 8 vols (London: Charles H. Kelly, undated).

Whyman, J., *Aspects of Holidaymaking and Resort Development Within the Isle of Thanet, With Particular Reference to Margate c. 1736–1840* (New York: Arno Press, 1981).

Wiesner, M.E., *Women and Gender in Early Modern Europe* (Cambridge: Cambridge University Press, 1993).

Wilding, P., *Professional Power and Social Welfare* (London: Routledge and Kegan Paul, 1982).

Williams, C.D., '"The Luxury of Doing Good": Benevolence, Sensibility and the Royal Humane Society', in R. Porter and M.M. Roberts (eds), *Pleasure in the Eighteenth Century* (London: Macmillan, 1996).

Williams, J.A., *Bath and Rome: The Living Link: Catholicism in Bath from 1559 to the Present Day* (Bath: Seabright's Bookshop, 1963).

Williams, J.A. (ed.), *Post-Reformation Catholicism in Bath*, 2 vols (no place of publication: Catholic Record Society, 1975).

Williams, P., 'Religion, Respectability and the Origins of the Modern Nurse', in R. French and A. Wear (eds), *British Medicine in an Age of Reform* (London: Routledge, 1991).

Williams, W.J. and Stoddart, D.M., *Bath – Some Ecounters with Science* (Bath: Kingsmead, 1978).

Wilson, A., 'William Hunter and the Varieties of Man-Midwifery', in W.F. Bynum and R. Porter (eds), *William Hunter and the Eighteenth-Century Medical World* (Cambridge: Cambridge University Press, 1985).

Wilson, A., *The Making of Man-Midwifery: Childbirth in England 1660–1770* (Cambridge, MA: Harvard University Press, 1995).

Wilson, A., 'Conflict, Consensus and Charity: Politics and the Provincial Voluntary Hospitals in the Eighteenth Century', *English Historical Review*, **111** (1996).

Wilson, A.M., 'The Enlightenment came first to England', in S. Baxter (ed.), *England's Rise to Greatness 1660–1763* (Berkeley: University of California Press, 1983).

Wilson, C., *England's Apprenticeship 1603–1763*, 2nd edn, (London: Longman, 1984).
Wilson, E., 'A Shropshire Lady in Bath, 1794–1807', *Bath History*, 4 (1992).
Wilson, K., 'Urban Culture and Political Activism in Hanoverian England: The Example of Voluntary Hospitals', in E. Hellmuth (ed.), *The Transformation of Political Culture: England and Germany in the Late Eighteenth Century* (Oxford: Oxford University Press, 1990).
Wilson, P.K., '"Sacred sanctuaries for the sick": Surgery at St Thomas's Hospital 1725–26', *London Journal*, 17 (1992).
Winch, D., *Riches and Poverty: An Intellectual History of Political Economy in Britain 1750–1865* (Cambridge: Cambridge University Press, 1996).
[Winchester County Hospital], 'An Account of the Establishment of the County Hospital at Winchester', in J. Woodward, *To Do the Sick No Harm: A Study of the British Voluntary Hospital System to 1875* (London: Routledge and Kegan Paul, 1974).
Wood, J., *A Description of Bath 1765* (Bath: Kingsmead Reprints, 1969).
Woodbridge, K., *The Stourhead Landscape* (London: National Trust, 1971).
Woodward, J., *To Do the Sick No Harm: A Study of the British Voluntary Hospital System to 1875* (London: Routledge and Kegan Paul, 1974).
The Works of Benjamin Hoadly, 3 vols (London: W. Bowyer and J. Nichols, 1773).
Wright, D.G., *Popular Radicalism: The Working Class Experience 1780–1880* (London: Longman, 1988).
Wrigley, E.A. and Schofield, R.S., *The Population History of England 1541–1871: A Reconstruction* (London: Edward Arnold, 1981).
Youngs, F.A., *Guide to the Local Administrative Units of England*, 2 vols (London: Royal Historical Society, 1979), vol. 1: *Southern England.*
Youngs, F.A., *Guide to the Local Administrative Units of England*, 2 vols (London: Royal Historical Society, 1991), vol. 2: *Northern England.*

Index